Butterworths International Medical Reviews

Neurology 4

Peripheral Nerve Disorders

Butterworths International Medical Reviews

Neurology

Editorial Board

Arthur K. Asbury, MD
Van Meter Professor of Neurology, University of Pennsylvania School of
Medicine; Hospital of the University of Pennsylvania, Philadelphia, Pennsylvania,
USA

Mark L. Dyken, MD, FACP
Professor and Chairman, Department of Neurology, University of Indiana School
of Medicine, Indianapolis, Indiana, USA

Stanley Fahn, MD
H. Houston Merritt Professor of Neurology, Columbia University College of
Physicians and Surgeons, Neurological Institute, New York, New York, USA

R. W. Gilliatt, DM, FRCP
Professor of Clinical Neurology and Chairman, Department of Clinical Neurology,
Institute of Neurology, The National Hospital, London, UK

Michael J. G. Harrison, DM, FRCP
Consultant Neurologist and Head of EEG/EMG Department, Middlesex Hospital;
Director of Research, Institute of Neurological Studies, Middlesex Hospital
Medical School, London, UK

C. David Marsden, MSc, MB, BS, MRCPsych, FRCP, FRS
Professor of Neurology, University Department of Neurology, King's College
Hospital Medical School and Institute of Psychiatry; Consultant Neurologist,
King's College Hospital and Bethlem Royal and Maudsley Hospitals, London, UK

Paolo L. Morselli
Director, Department of Clinical Research, Synthelabo LERS, Paris, France

Roger J. Porter, MD
Chief, Epilepsy Branch, Neurological Disorders Program, National Institutes of
Health, Bethesda, Maryland, USA

Erik Stålberg, MD
Associate Professor, Department of Clinical Neurophysiology,
University Hospital, Uppsala, Sweden

Robert R. Young, MD
Associate Professor, Department of Neurology, Harvard Medical School, Boston,
Massachusetts, USA

Published in this Series

Volume 1 **Clinical Neurophysiology**
Edited by Erik Stålberg and Robert R. Young

Volume 2 **Movement Disorders**
Edited by C. David Marsden and Stanley Fahn

Volume 3 **Cerebral Vascular Disease**
Edited by Michael J. G. Harrison and Mark L. Dyken

Next Volume in the Series
The Epilepsies

Butterworths
International
Medical
Reviews

Neurology 4

Peripheral Nerve Disorders

A Practical Approach

Edited by

Arthur K. Asbury, MD
Van Meter Professor of Neurology
Department of Neurology
University of Pennsylvania School of Medicine
    and Hospital of the University of Pennsylvania
Philadelphia, Pennsylvania, USA

and

R. W. Gilliatt, DM, FRCP
Professor of Clinical Neurology and Chairman
Department of Clinical Neurology
Institute of Neurology
The National Hospital
London, UK

Butterworths
London   Boston   Durban
Singapore   Sydney   Toronto   Wellington

First published 1984

© Butterworth & Co (Publishers) Ltd. 1984

British Library Cataloguing in Publication Data

Peripheral nerve disorders. – (Butterworths
  international medical reviews. Neurology,
  ISSN 0260-0137; 4)
  1. Nerves, Peripheral – Diseases
  I. Asbury, Arthur K.   II. Gilliatt, Roger W.
  616.8′7   RC409

  ISBN 0-407-02297-X

Photoset by Butterworths Litho Preparation Department
Printed and bound in England by Robert Hartnoll Ltd., Bodmin, Cornwall

Foreword

For almost a quarter of a century (1951–1975), subjects of topical interest were written about in the periodic volumes of our predecessor, *Modern Trends in Neurology*. Although both that series and its highly regarded editor, Dr Denis Williams, are now retired, the legacy continues in the present Butterworths series in Neurology. As was the case with *Modern Trends*, the current volumes are intended for use by physicians who grapple with the problems of neurological disorder on a daily basis, be they neurologists, neurologists in training, or those in related fields such as neurosurgery, internal medicine, psychiatry, and rehabilitation medicine.

Our purpose is to produce annually a monograph on a topic in clinical neurology in which progress through research has brought about new concepts of patient management. The subject of each monograph is selected by the Series Editors using two criteria: first, that there has been significant advance in knowledge in that area; and second, that such advances have been incorporated into new ways of managing patients with the disorders in question.

This has been the guiding spirit behind each volume, and we expect it to continue. In effect we emphasize research, both in the clinic and in the experimental laboratory, but principally to the extent that it changes our collective attitudes and practices in caring for those who are neurologically afflicted.

C. D. Marsden
A. K. Asbury
Series Editors

Preface

The guiding principle for this Butterworths series of monographic reviews is to focus on a particular neurological topic in which recent progress has altered the way in which patients are managed. It is with this principle in mind that the subject of peripheral nerve disorders was chosen. Intense interest in the peripheral nervous system and its pathophysiology at both fundamental and clinical levels has yielded an abundant harvest of new understanding. This in turn has been translated into new methods and approaches by which physicians are able to assess and manage individuals suffering from neuropathic disorders. Our purpose in this volume is to emphasize new diagnostic concepts and facts and to stress, in broadest terms, therapeutics. Modalities involved range from intensive care practices (Chapter 2) to genetic counselling and long-term care of insensitive limbs (Chapter 9). In sum, we dwell not upon recent research *per se*, but upon the fruits of that research.

A word is in order concerning the organization of this volume. The first chapter is intended to provide a framework of logic and a sequence of evaluation to guide the inquiring physician successfully through the maze of known peripheral neuropathies. Principles set forth in Chapter 1 are designed to create a conceptual context and to enhance understanding of subsequent chapters. Chapters 2–10 deal with the major groups and manifestations of peripheral neuropathies, often with a degree, by intention, of overlap. The final three chapters examine patterns of neuropathy experienced in parts of the world other than Europe and the United States.

Finally, we wish to signal our deep appreciation to all of the chapter authors for the rigor of their contributions and their timeliness. We are also indebted to the staff of Butterworths for unflagging support and pertinent advice.

A. K. Asbury
R. W. Gilliatt

Contributors

Otto Appenzeller, MD, PhD
Professor of Neurology and Medicine, University of New Mexico School of Medicine, Albuquerque, New Mexico, USA

Arthur K. Asbury, MD
Van Meter Professor of Neurology, University of Pennsylvania School of Medicine and Hospital of the University of Pennsylvania, Philadelphia, Pennsylvania, USA

Ruth Atkinson, MD
Associate Professor of Neurology and Pediatrics, University of New Mexico School of Medicine, Albuquerque, New Mexico, USA

Mark J. Brown, MD
Associate Professor of Neurology, University of Pennsylvania School of Medicine and Hospital of the University of Pennsylvania, Philadelphia, Pennsylvania, USA

R. W. Gilliatt, DM, FRCP
Professor of Clinical Neurology, University of London; and Chairman, Department of Clinical Neurology, Institute of Neurology, London, UK

Douglas A. Greene, MD
Associate Professor, Department of Medicine and Director, Clinical Research Unit, University of Pittsburgh School of Medicine and Presbyterian Hospital, Pittsburgh, Pennsylvania, USA

A. E. Harding, MD, MRCP
Lecturer in Neurology, Royal Postgraduate Medical School and Institute of Neurology, London, UK

Michael J. G. Harrison, DM, FRCP
Consultant Neurologist and Head of EEG/EMG Department, Middlesex Hospital;
Director of Research, Institute of Neurological Studies, Middlesex Hospital
Medical School, London, UK

Pamela M. Le Quesne, DM, FRCP
Member, MRC Toxicology Unit; Honorary Consultant, Middlesex Hospital,
London, UK

Arnold I. Levinson, MD
Assistant Professor of Medicine, University of Pennsylvania School of Medicine,
Philadelphia, Pennsylvania, USA

Robert P. Lisak, MD
Professor of Neurology, University of Pennsylvania School of Medicine,
Philadelphia, Pennsylvania, USA

James G. McLeod
Professor, Department of Medicine, Sydney University, New South Wales,
Australia

Akio Ohnishi, MD, DMedSci
Department of Neurology, Neurological Institute, Faculty of Medicine,
Kyushu University, Japan

B. O. Osuntokun, OFR, MB, BS(Lond), MD(Lond), DSc(Lond), PhD(Ibadan), FRCP(Lond),
FMCP(Nig), FWACP(Nig), FAS(Nig)
Professor of Neurology and Principal Investigator, WHO Collaborating Centre for
Research and Training in Neurosciences, Neurology Unit, Department of
Medicine, University of Ibadan, Nigeria

John D. Pollard
Department of Medicine (Neurology), Sydney University, New South Wales,
Australia

Allan H. Ropper, MD
Director, Neurological/Neurosurgical Intensive Care Unit, Massachusetts General
Hospital; Assistant Professor of Neurology, Harvard Medical School, Boston,
Massachusetts, USA

Bhagwan T. Shahani, MD, DPhil(Oxon)
Director, EMG and Motor Control Unit, Clinical Neurophysiology Laboratory;
Assistant Neurologist, Massachusetts General Hospital; Associate Professor of
Neurology, Harvard Medical School, Boston, Massachusetts, USA

Austin J. Sumner, MMedSc(NZ), MB, ChB, FRACP
Professor of Neurology, University of Pennsylvania School of Medicine,
Philadelphia, Pennsylvania, USA

P. K. Thomas, DSc, MD, FRCP
Professor of Neurology in the University of London at the Royal Free Hospital
School of Medicine and the Institute of Neurology, London, UK

Noshir H. Wadia, MD, FRCP(Lond), FAMS, FASc(India)
Director of Neurology, Jaslok Hospital and Research Centre, Bombay;
Consultant Neurologist, J. J. Group of Hospitals, Byculla, Bombay, India

Contents

1
The clinical approach to neuropathy
Arthur K. Asbury and Roger W. Gilliatt

INTRODUCTION

Currently the logic used to analyze and diagnose peripheral neuropathies, particularly polyneuropathies, is exceptionally cumbersome. First, a diagnosis of polyneuropathy is rendered, and second, a known association is sought. The process requires sifting through approximately 100 known associations (drugs, other toxins, metabolic disorders, dysimmune states, genetically-determined disorders), pinpointing one, and ruling out all the others. Sometimes the examiner is too successful and identifies two or three known associations (for example, diabetes, alcoholism and paraproteinemia). Third, one must decide how much, if any, each associated disorder contributes to the neuropathy. This scheme is at best unwieldy and frequently impossible to apply.

Part of the conundrum results from our lack of knowledge about the precise mechanism by which any given pathologic state, whether exogenous or endogenous, affects the nervous system to produce symptoms and signs of neuropathy. But more importantly, physicians have failed to take full advantage of recent advances in our understanding of clinical and electrophysiological phenomena. These improvements allow a more systematic stepwise approach.

In this chapter an effort is made to summarize the sum of our clinical knowledge and emphasize the logic and sequence of evaluation for the patient with neuropathy. Particular weight is placed on the role of electrodiagnosis.

PATHOLOGIC PROCESSES

Peripheral nerve has a limited repertoire of reactions to injury. When dealing with a particular patient with a neuropathy, it is helpful to ask which of the few known reactions of nerve is taking place. The major processes are:

(1) Wallerian degeneration (the response to transection);
(2) axonal atrophy and degeneration;

1

(3) segmental demyelination, and
(4) primary disorders of nerve cell bodies.

Other terms used to denote the latter three processes are axonopathy, myelinopathy and neuronopathy (Spencer and Schaumburg, 1976), their only advantage being a better degree of consistency with one another.

For Wallerian degeneration to occur, it must be preceded by physical interruption of an otherwise healthy axon or group of axons, as in a nerve trunk. If a nerve trunk is severed, the most obvious changes occur distal to the transection site. Paralysis and anesthesia in the distribution of the nerve trunk are immediate. Axons and myelin sheaths degenerate distal to the site of transection, conduction fails within days or weeks as the distal nerve becomes inexcitable, regeneration from the proximal stump begins early but proceeds slowly, and recovery is variable, but may be both incomplete and dysfunctional.

Quality of recovery depends upon the extent of Schwann tube, nerve sheath and surrounding soft tissue destruction. Other factors include the proximo-distal site of injury and the age of the individual. Although direct trauma to a nerve trunk is the usual cause of Wallerian degeneration, there are others. Nerve trunk ischemia, whether focal or multifocal, may produce extensive distal degeneration if blood flow is critically reduced. As a general rule, nerve trunk ischemia severe enough to produce focal axonal damage and distal Wallerian degeneration results from widespread pathological processes affecting small vessels and capillaries of the size of the vasa nervorum. Multifocal nerve trunk ischemia, as occurs with systemic vasculitis, is a frequent basis for mononeuropathy multiplex encountered clinically.

Segmental demyelination (myelinopathy) means damage to myelin sheaths with sparing of axons. Conduction block is the functionally important expression of demyelination. An axon which is blocked displays a functional deficit as severe as if the axon were transected. Although nerve transection and conduction block may show similar degrees of paralysis or sensory deficit acutely, they differ in terms of outlook, degree of wasting, tempo of recovery and electrophysiologic properties. For instance, in demyelinating neuropathies, conduction block is often transient and remyelination may be rapid, measured in days or weeks, and is frequently complete. This is much more favorable and rapid than the course of recovery expected with Wallerian degeneration.

In the past, often studied models of segmental demyelination in peripheral nerve were those produced by diphtheria toxin and lead salts. The lesion resulting from these intoxications was thought to be prototypical. Changes observed were widening of nodal gaps, paranodal retraction and breakdown of myelin, and eventual disintegration of whole internodes of myelin. But other ways have been described in which myelin sheath may be damaged as a primary event. For instance, with acute nerve compression, telescoping (intussusception) of myelin occurs at the nodes of Ranvier, representing a type of mechanical injury to myelin. With certain myelinotoxic agents such as hexachlorophene or triethyltin, striking edema occurs within the myelin sheath. In other demyelinating neuropathies such as the Guillain-Barré syndrome, peeling and engulfment of myelin by activated phagocytic cells both at the nodes of Ranvier and at other sites along the internode are the pathological hallmarks. In sum, a variety of recognizable morphological patterns may converge with a common result – demyelination. The electrophysiological counterpart of all of these is qualitatively the same.

Secondary segmental demyelination also occurs. Here primary axonal changes, usually chronic shrinkage and atrophy, are attended by recurrent myelin breakdown and reconstitution. Along atrophic axons, uniform demyelinative-remyelinative changes occur over many consecutive internodes, in contrast to primary demyelinating processes which tend to show a random hit-or-miss distribution. Protracted axonal atrophy eventually leads to progressive breakdown and resorption of the axon, back to and including the parent nerve cell body. Axonal atrophy and secondary demyelination occur in some chronic polyneuropathies such as that associated with uremia (Dyck *et al.*, 1971), in distal nerve fibers in chronic iminodiproprionitrile (IDPN) intoxication (Long *et al.*, 1980), in permanent axotomy (Dyck *et al.*, 1981) and in nerve fibers distal to a chronic constriction (Baba *et al.*, 1982).

Axonal degeneration (axonopathy) means a metabolic derangement within neurons which manifests as distal axonal breakdown. The clinical effect is that of a distal symmetrical 'stocking-glove' polyneuropathy with characteristic electrodiagnostic features which allow it to be distinguished from a demyelinating process. Although for years it has been said that the longest and largest fibers are at risk,

Table 1.1 Major pathological processes encountered in hereditary neuropathies (*see also* Tables 9.1 and 9.2)

I. *Axonal degeneration*
  Dominant
    Charcot-Marie-Tooth peroneal muscular atrophy*
    Hereditary amyloid neuropathies
    Porphyric neuropathy
  Recessive
    Analphalipoproteinemia (small sensory axons)
    Giant axonal neuropathy
    Ataxia-telangiectasia

II. *Demyelination*
  Dominant
    Charcot-Marie-Tooth peroneal muscular atrophy*
  Recessive
    Déjérine-Sottas hypertrophic neuropathy (HMSN-III)

III. *Neuronopathy*
  Dominant
    Hereditary sensory neuropathy I
  Sex-linked
    Fabry's disease (small DRG neurons)
  Recessive
    Hereditary sensory neuropathy II
    Abetalipoproteinemia (large DRG neurons)
    Friedreich's ataxia (large DRG neurons)

---

* Two major forms – one axonal ('neuronal') and the other demyelinating

this rule is frequently violated when the details of polyneuropathies are examined. Exogenous toxins and systemic metabolic disorders are the usual cause of axonal degeneration of peripheral nerve, but the exact sequence of events in nerve tissue which culminate in axonopathy remains obscure.

Neuronopathy signifies primary destruction of the nerve cell body. Either the lower motor neuron or the primary sensory neuron may be affected. When the anterior horn cell is the target of disease, as in poliomyelitis or motor neuron disease, motor neuronopathy is the result. Sensory neuronopathy means damage to dorsal root ganglion cells, often resulting in striking sensory syndromes. Examples include acute sensory neuronopathy (Sterman, Schaumburg and Asbury, 1980), inflammatory disorders of dorsal root ganglia and cranial ganglia, such as carcinomatous sensory neuropathy and herpes zoster, and toxic states such as experimental doxorubicin administration (Cho, Spencer and Jortner, 1980), pyridoxine hypervitaminosis (Schaumburg *et al.*, 1981), and experimental mercurialism (Jacobs, Carmichael and Cavanagh, 1977). Finally, several inherited disorders result in sensory neuronopathy (*Table 1.1*). Some of these have been recognized only recently as sensory neuronopathies. The point in distinguishing them from processes affecting myelin or peripheral axons lies in the observation that recovery in neuronopathies is usually poor.

In *Table 1.1* inherited neuropathies are used to illustrate categorization according to the predominant pathological process encountered in each. It is helpful to develop the habit of thinking in these terms for all neuropathies.

TYPICAL POLYNEUROPATHY

The prototypical polyneuropathy is a distal, symmetrical motor-sensory axonal process associated with exogenous intoxication (medications, alcohol, heavy metals, industrial organic chemicals) or endogenous metabolic derangement (nutritional disorder, uremia). Clinical manifestations of such a polyneuropathy are familiar to most readers, but are summarized in the following paragraphs to emphasize their full range. It should be noted that an acquired demyelinating polyneuropathy, given a similar temporal evolution, might also fit the same clinical description.

The first symptoms are frequently dysesthetic. Common dysesthesias consist of tingling, prickling, burning or band-like sensations in the balls of the feet, tips of the toes, or in a more generalized fashion over the soles of the feet. Symmetry of symptoms and findings in a distal graded fashion is the rule but, occasionally, dysesthesias appear in one foot. When this occurs, the examiner must take care to distinguish between polyneuropathy and mononeuropathy multiplex. If the polyneuropathy remains mild, i.e. confined to dysesthesias of the soles of the feet, no objective motor or sensory signs may be detectable.

As the neuropathy worsens, sensory deficit will creep over the dorsa of both feet, ankle jerks will be lost, and weakness of dorsiflexion of the toes, best demonstrated in the great toe, may appear. The only functional sign of weakness may be inability to walk on the heels, due to mild weakness of ankle dorsiflexion. With further worsening the sensory disturbance moves centripetally in a graded stocking manner. Patients may complain that their feet have a numb or 'wooden' feeling. Phrases used include, 'I feel as though I'm walking on stumps', or 'I feel there is a layer of something over my skin'. More difficulty walking on the heels is experienced during examination and the feet may slap while walking. Later, the knee jerk reflex disappears and foot drop results in a steppage gait. By the time sensory disturbance has reached the upper shin, dysesthesias will be noticed in the fingertips. The degree of spontaneous pain varies, but may be considerable. Light stimuli to hypesthetic areas, once perceived, may be experienced as searing burning pain, a phenomenon termed hyperpathia. Unsteadiness of gait out of proportion to muscle weakness may be due to proprioceptive loss.

Progression proceeds in a graded manner, creeping proximally, and equal on both sides of the body. Motor weakness is usually greater in the extensor muscles than in corresponding flexor groups and is accompanied by atrophy of weakened muscles, pansensory loss and areflexia. When the sensory disturbance reaches mid-thigh, a tent-shaped area of hypesthesia may be demonstrated on the lower abdomen. This will widen and the peak will extend rostrally toward the sternum as the neuropathy worsens. By this time, patients generally cannot stand or walk or hold objects in their hands.

In the most extreme cases ventilatory capacity may be reduced due to intercostal or diaphragmatic weakness. Rarely, sphincteric function may be involved. Hypesthesia at the crown of the scalp will be present, spreading radially into both the trigeminal and C2 distribution. From the foregoing description, it is apparent that nerve fibers are affected according to length of axon without regard to root or nerve trunk distribution, hence the aptness of the term stocking-glove hypesthesia.

Tempo of progression is usually smooth but, on occasion, may appear to increase in surges. The timing of acquired axonal polyneuropathies is subacute or chronic over weeks to months or several years. With this overall pattern of evolution of commonly encountered polyneuropathy in mind, our attention should now fasten upon the details of the history and examination.

SYMPTOMS

Preceding and concurrent events

Clues to diagnosis of peripheral neuropathies often lie in unnoted or readily forgotten events occurring weeks or months prior to the onset of symptoms. Inquiry should be made about recent viral illnesses; other systemic symptoms; institution of new medications; potentially toxic exposures to solvents, pesticides, or heavy metals; the occurrence of similar symptoms in family members or co-workers; habits concerning alcohol; and the presence of known underlying medical disorders. It is also useful to ask patients if they would otherwise feel well if free of their neuropathic symptoms, in order to obtain a sense of co-existing systemic illness.

Early symptoms

It is important to know how symptoms first appeared. Even with distal polyneuropathies, symptoms may appear in the sole of one foot a few days or a week or so before the other, but usually the patient will convey a sense of a distal graded process that moves evenly and symmetrically in centripetal fashion. Tingling dysesthesias will appear in the fingertips only when similar symptoms have reached the level of the knees. It is most important to determine whether symptoms first appeared in the distribution of individual digital nerves involving only one-half of a digit at a time and then gradually spread to become coalescent. This pattern of onset raises strong suspicions of a multifocal process (mononeuropathy multiplex) such as might be encountered with a systemic vasculitis or cryoglobulinemia.

Progression

Evolution of neuropathy ranges from a fulminant course of only a few days to an indolent process extending over many decades. For the most part, polyneuropathy with a slowly progressive course lasting more than 5 years is most likely to be genetically determined, particularly if the major manifestations are distal atrophy and weakness with few positive sensory symptoms. Exceptions are diabetic polyneuropathy and occasionally demyelinating neuropathies associated with monoclonal gammopathy, in which the progression may be slow and extend over many years. Axonal degenerations of toxic or metabolic origin tend to evolve over several weeks to a year or more, and the rate of progression of demyelinating neuropathies is highly variable, ranging from a few days in Guillain-Barré syndrome to many years in others.

If major fluctuations occur in the course of neuropathy it brings to mind two possibilites: (1) relapsing forms of demyelinating polyneuropathy, or (2) repeated toxic exposures. Other factors may also be responsible for fluctuation of symptoms; for instance, in catamenial sciatica endometrial implants on the sciatic nerve trunk in the pelvis produce symptoms only in relation to menses. Slow fluctuation in symptoms taking place over weeks or months (reflecting changes in the activity of the neuropathy) should not be confused with day-to-day variation or diurnal undulations of symptoms. The latter are common to all neuropathic disorders. An example is carpal tunnel syndrome in which dysesthesias may be prominent at night but absent during the day.

Nature of symptoms

Symptoms of neuropathic disorder, although numerous and heterogeneous, may be categorized as motor, sensory or autonomic. From a motor standpoint, the major symptom is weakness, the degree and distribution depending upon the nature and severity of the neuropathy. Dexterity is not disproportionately affected, as occurs in upper motor neuron lesions. In polyneuropathies, motor symptoms tend to be distal, thus events observed early in the illness may be undue tripping on rugs, doorsills and stair risers because of a degree of foot drop. A history may also be elicited of difficulty in winding an alarm clock, or removing lids from jars or turning a key in a lock. These tasks all require good strength of intrinsic hand muscles, which are generally the first to be affected in the upper extremities.

On the sensory side, the range and diversity of symptoms is impressive, and subsume both positive and negative phenomena. (For a recent discussion, *see* Gilliatt, 1982a). Positive symptoms include tingling and other dysesthesias, some of which are described as highly unpleasant or painful experiences. Hyperpathia (mentioned above) represents an extreme example of a positive symptom. Negative symptoms refer to numbness and other loss of sensation, such as loss of joint, muscle and tendon proprioception leading to imbalance and difficulty with stance and gait. This dysfunction is usually referred to as sensory ataxia, and its counterpart on examination is a positive Romberg sign. If there is severe large fiber

Table 1.2 Characteristics of two major forms of neuropathic pain

	Dysesthetic pain	*Nerve trunk pain*
Descriptors	Burning, tingling, raw, searing, crawling, drawing	Aching, occasionally knife-like
Recognition	Unfamiliar; never experienced before	Familiar; 'like a toothache'
Distribution	(1) Cutaneous or subcutaneous usually (2) Distal	(1) Deep (2) Relatively proximal
Constancy	Variable, may be intermittent, jabbing, lancinating, shooting	Usually continuous, but waxes and wanes
Better/worse	Little makes it better; worse following activity	Better with rest or optimal position; worse with movement, nerve stretch or palpation
Basis of pain (hypothetical)	Increased firing of damaged or abnormally excitable nociceptive fibers, particularly sprouting, regenerating fibers	Increased firing due to physiologic stimulation of endings of undamaged afferents from nerve sheaths themselves (nervi nervorum)
Examples	(1) Causalgia (2) Small fiber polyneuropathy	(1) Root compression (2) Brachial neuritis

(proprioceptive) deafferentation, the patient is usually unable to stand or walk unaided. Because of the lack of joint position sense, the patient may exhibit frequent involuntary-like movements of the fingers and hands when the arms are outstretched and the eyes closed. Pseudoathetosis is the descriptive term. Other negative symptoms include reduction of cutaneous touch-pressure sensitivity and hypalgesia.

Pain in neuropathy is a complex subject, but some general notions and ways of approaching neuropathic pain may be expressed. From a clinical descriptive standpoint, two major types of pain associated with neuropathy may be identified, dysesthetic pain and nerve trunk pain. Their features and distinguishing points are summarized in *Table 1.2* along with an hypothesis as to their separate bases. In addition to these two major types, patients with evolving poliomyelitis or Guillain-Barré syndrome may complain of muscle pain which they liken to having over-exercised (*see* Chapter 2 for further description).

Autonomic symptoms extend over an even broader range than sensory symptoms, and are dealt with in detail in Chapter 4. A subject often discussed in conjunction with autonomic symptoms, namely trophic changes, should be mentioned here. The array of observable changes in completely denervated muscle, bone and skin including hair and nails, is well described (*see* Chapter 4), if incompletely understood. It is unclear what portion of the changes are due purely to denervation versus those caused by disuse, immobility, lack of weight bearing and particularly recurrent, unnoticed painless trauma. Considerable evidence favors the view that ulceration of skin, poor healing, tissue resorption, neurogenic arthropathy and mutilation are simply the result of repeated heedless injury to insensitive parts. As such, this sequence of events is avoidable with proper care and monitoring (Brand and Ebner, 1969; Sabin and Swift, 1975; Harrison and Faris, 1976).

PATTERNS

Symmetry

In polyneuropathies, the findings can be expected to be quite symmetrical on both sides of the body. If one foot slaps when the patient walks, but the other does not, the examiner must take note that the process is not symmetrical. In addition, it is the muscles of extension and abduction which tend to be weakened to a greater extent in acquired symmetrical polyneuropathies. For example, the dorsiflexors tend to be weaker than the plantar flexors of the toes and ankles. To cite another example of how this principle operates in bilateral tarsal tunnel syndrome, an entrapment neuropathy of the posterior tibial nerve at the ankle, there may be painful dysesthesias and hypesthesia of the soles of the feet similar to some polyneuropathies, but the attendant motor weakness is restricted to the plantar flexors of the toes with normal strength of dorsiflexion. This finding helps distinguish bilateral tarsal tunnel syndrome from polyneuropathy, in which the dorsiflexors of the toes are weaker than the plantar flexors. Confirmation can usually be made electrodiagnostically. Management of the tarsal tunnel syndrome may include surgical release of the distal posterior tibial nerve (*see* Chapter 10).

Legs versus arms

In most polyneuropathies the legs are more severely affected than the arms. There are exceptions to this rule, as in lead neuropathy, in which manifestations of bilateral wrist drop may predominate, and occasionally in porphyric neuropathy, in which arms may be more affected than legs and proximal muscles more than distal.

Proximal versus distal

In some instances, even when the neuropathy is symmetrical and affects the legs more than the arms, the proximal limb muscles are more involved than distal ones. A demyelinating basis for the neuropathy should be suspected, and looked for on electrodiagnostic examination. Porphyric neuropathy may also behave in this fashion.

Nerve trunk or root versus graded findings

The anticipated pattern for most polyneuropathies is one in which the motor and sensory deficit and attenuation of reflexes is distal, symmetrical, and graded. Exceptions to this pattern raise the likelihood of a multifocal process affecting individual nerve trunks and roots. As an example, sensory disturbances extending as high as the head of the fibula on the lateral aspect of the leg but only extending above the malleolus on the medial aspect should suggest focal lesions of the L5 and S1 roots or the sciatic nerve trunk rather than polyneuropathy.

Plexopathy

Lesions affecting brachial plexus, usually unilaterally, are relatively common in neurological practice, and display characteristic signs quite different from those expected either in mononeuropathies of the upper limb or polyneuropathies (Mumenthaler, 1984). The usual causes are direct trauma to the plexus, brachial neuritis (neuralgic amyotrophy), cervical rib or bands (*see* Chapter 10), infiltration by malignant processes, and radiation therapy. When the upper portion of the plexus (arising from C5–7) is damaged, weakness and atrophy of shoulder and upper arm muscles ensues. Lower brachial plexus injury (arising from C8, T1) produces distal weakness, atrophy and sensory deficit in the forearm and hand. As an approximation, brachial neuritis, damage from radiation (greater than 6000 rad) and certain types of trauma (arm jerked downward) result in upper plexus findings; whereas malignant infiltration, cervical rib and bands, and other types of trauma (arm jerked upwards) cause lower plexus signs. Further detail may be found in Mumenthaler (1984), Kori, Foley and Posner (1981) and Tsairis, Dyck and Mulder, (1972).

SPECIFIC FEATURES

Features other than the distribution of the neurological deficit must also be considered.

Enlargement of nerve trunk

Palpation of the nerve trunk to detect enlargement is a frequently forgotten part of the neurological examination. In mononeuropathies, the entire course of the nerve trunk in question should be explored manually for focal thickening, the presence of neurofibroma, point tenderness, and Tinel's phenomenon (elicitation of a tingling sensation in the sensory territory of the nerve by tapping along the course of the nerve). In more generalized neuropathies, a good practice is for the examiner to assess the size of the common peroneal trunk in the popliteal fossa and the ulnar nerve at the elbow, following it more proximally into the medial upper arm. Care must be taken not to overinterpret findings on palpation of the ulnar nerve at the elbow, because epineurial sheaths of the ulnar nerve where it lies in the bicipital groove may normally be quite thick. Smaller cutaneous nerve trunks can also be readily felt, including the greater auricular nerve as it passes rostrally over the sternocleidomastoid muscle, and the branches of the radial cutaneous nerve as they pass over the extensor tendons of the thumb. In leprous neuritis, fusiform thickening of nerve trunks is frequent, and beading of nerve trunks may be encountered in amyloid polyneuropathy. Certain genetically-determined neuropathies of the hypertrophic variety (HMSN-I and HMSN-III) may be attended by uniform thickening of all nerve trunks, often to the caliber of a clothes line or larger.

Motor versus sensory deficits

In the Guillain-Barré syndrome, motor deficits tend to dominate the clinical picture, whereas in axonal polyneuropathies, distal dysesthesias and graded pansensory disturbances are most evident. A judgement should be reached in every instance as to the relative balance of motor and sensory findings.

Large fiber versus small fiber

All motor nerve fibers, except the gamma efferents to stretch receptors, are large myelinated axons, but peripheral afferent fibers are represented by the full size range of myelinated and unmyelinated axons. As a clinical approximation, temperature and painful sensations, including pinprick, are mediated by unmyelinated and small myelinated fibers, but proprioception, vibratory sense, and the afferent limb of the muscle stretch reflex arc are subserved by large myelinated fibers. Tactile sensibility is mediated by both large and small fibers, and autonomic functions are mostly carried out via unmyelinated fibers.

This information may be put to clinical use. In a polyneuropathy affecting mainly small fibers, diminished pinprick and temperature sensations, often with burning painful dysesthesias, may predominate along with autonomic dysfunction but with relative sparing of motor power, balance, and tendon jerks. Selected cases of amyloid and distal diabetic polyneuropathies fall into this category (Brown, Martin and Asbury, 1976; Dyck and Lambert, 1969). In contrast, large-fiber polyneuro-pathy is characterized by areflexia, imbalance, minimal distal numbness with few dysesthesias, and variable degrees of motor weakness.

Axonal versus demyelinating processes

It is not generally possible to make this distinction reliably on clinical examination alone, and it is in this category that electrodiagnostic analysis (*see below*), is often particularly useful. Nevertheless, the distinction in a neuropathic process between one which is primarily demyelinating from one which is primarily axonal is crucial because of the differing approaches to diagnosis and management. If, in a particular instance of progressive polyneuropathy of subacute or chronic evolution, the electrodiagnostic findings are those of an axonopathy, a long list of metabolic states and exogenous toxins (*see* Chapters 5, 6 and 8) come into consideration. A protracted course over several years raises the likelihood of the neuronal form of peroneal muscular atrophy (HMSN-II); family members must be examined and additional attention given to the family history (*see* Chapter 9).

Alternatively, if the electrodiagnostic findings are more indicative of primary demyelination of nerve, the approach is entirely different. The possibilities then include acquired demyelinating neuropathy, thought to be immunologically mediated, and genetically-determined neuropathies, some of which are marked by uniformly severe slowing of nerve conduction velocities (*see* Chapters 3 and 9).

With the preceding considerations in hand, one can construct a flow chart (*Figure 1.1*) which summarizes the clinical and electrodiagnostic approach to the evaluation and management of a neuropathic disorder. Using this scheme, the clinician determines for each patient the tempo, distribution, severity and functional impairment, and other features previously discussed, making a clinical judgement as to whether the problem represents a mononeuropathy, multiple mononeuro-pathies, or a polyneuropathy. Often this distinction is obvious. The next step is electrodiagnostic examination (*see below*). With the sum of clinical and electrodiagnostic information in hand, the differential diagnostic possibilities and management options will have been narrowed to only a few. The remainder of this monograph deals with the myriad details of this general formulation.

EFFECTS OF ISCHEMIA AND COLD ON NERVE

For peripheral nerve to be damaged by ischemia requires extensive compromise of blood flow to that region. This is true because of the richness of anastomotic connections within both the nutrient arterial supply and the vasa nervorum themselves (Lundborg, 1975). Extensive ligation of major arteries is required to produce experimental nerve ischemia (Hess *et al.*, 1979). From a clinical standpoint, therefore, widespread extensive involvement of blood vessels is necessary in order for neuropathic symptoms and signs to occur. Diseases which characteristically produce ischemic neuropathy are systemic vasculitides, which

12

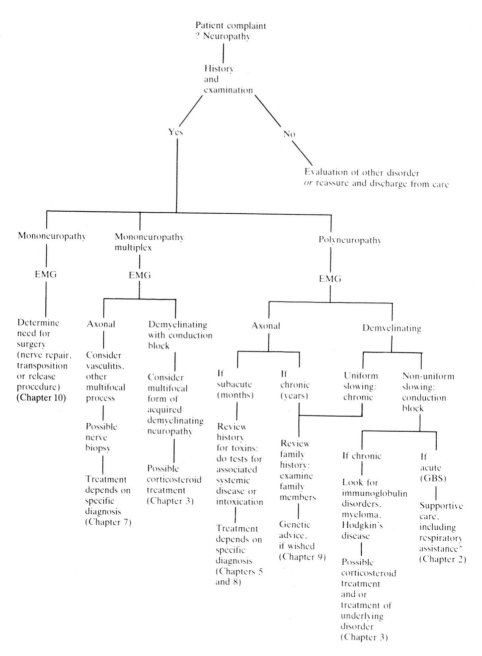

Figure 1.1 A schematic approach to the evaluation of a patient with peripheral neuropathy (modified from Asbury, 1983)

usually exhibit a penchant for vessels of the size range of vasa nervorum (small arteries and arterioles). Atherosclerosis severe enough to produce peripheral vascular insufficiency, including claudication and ischemic skin ulceration, may also cause mild neuropathy (Eames and Lange, 1967). The clinical pattern of nerve ischemia is frequently that of a mononeuropathy multiplex (*see* Chapter 7). A similar pattern follows acute non-compressible occlusion of a major limb artery (Wilbourn *et al.*, 1983).

Cold exerts deleterious effects on peripheral nerve directly without an intermediate step of ischemia being necessary. Cold injury to nerve occurs after prolonged exposure, usually of a limb or limbs, to moderately low temperatures, as with immersion of the feet in seawater; actual freezing of tissue is not required. Axonal degeneration of myelinated fibers is the pathological expression of cold injury (Peyronnard, Pedneault and Aguayo, 1977; Nukada, Pollock and Allpress, 1981). Frequently limbs affected by cold injury to nerve show persistent sensory deficit and dysesthesias, cutaneous vasomotor instability, painfulness and marked sensitivity to minimal cold exposure (Suri *et al.*, 1978). The pathophysiology of this phenomenon is uncertain.

CLINICAL ELECTRODIAGNOSIS (ELECTROMYOGRAPHY)

The requisites for evaluation of nerve and muscle disorders are the patient's history and a neurological assessment coupled with an electrodiagnostic examination. It must be emphasized that the electrodiagnostic evaluation is a physician-directed extension of the physical examination and not just a laboratory test. The term electromyography (EMG) is used here in the broadest sense and includes the evaluation of motor and sensory nerve function, the neuromuscular junction, sensory endings (by inference), and voluntary muscles.

Electrodiagnostic examination

For those unfamiliar with EMG, the following few paragraphs provide an overview. Specific detail may be found in more specialized volumes.

EMG examination of muscle may be carried out either by surface electrodes taped to the skin overlying a given muscle, or by needle electrodes inserted into the muscle belly. The latter is generally preferable. One must remember that electrodiagnostic testing of muscles is a sampling process that examines only those muscle fibers in the vicinity of the electrode. Conclusions must be drawn carefully, and only after multiple muscles and sites have been studied.

Normal resting muscle is ordinarily silent electrically once the needle electrode has been inserted. In myotonic disorders of muscle membrane, decrescendo bursts of electric activity are evident and form a basis for diagnosis. When the needle is in place and the patient is requested to make a voluntary contraction, increasing numbers of motor units fire. With primary disease of muscle, the amplitude of motor units during voluntary contraction is decreased. One sees frequent, polyphasic or short-duration, low-amplitude motor unit potentials during voluntary effort (Willison, 1967; Hayward and Willison, 1977). In myopathy, the important electrodiagnostic finding may be dissociation between the low force of contraction generated by voluntary activation of the muscle and the profuse electrical activity seen by simultaneous EMG.

Denervation presents a different picture in which individual muscle fibers discharge randomly at rest, producing fibrillation potentials, but during voluntary contraction the number of motor unit potentials is reduced although their amplitude is normal or increased. If, during the course of a slowly progressive denervating process, sprouting of new terminal neurites from surviving axons with collateral reinnervation occurs to a marked extent, giant motor unit potentials may be seen upon voluntary contraction. With the patient at rest, spontaneous activity of whole motor units is viewed as an indicator of anterior horn cell disease, particularly amyotrophic lateral sclerosis, and the phenomenon is referred to as fasciculation. Fasciculations may be visible to the clinician as fleeting longitudinal dimpling of the skin overlying a muscle. In contrast, fibrillations (contraction of individual muscle fibers) are not visible as muscular activity beneath the skin.

Determination of nerve conduction velocity and amplitude of evoked muscle and nerve action potentials provides essential information in investigating peripheral nerve dysfunction (Gilliatt, 1982b). This should be carried out routinely for both

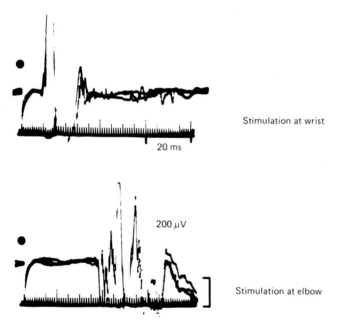

Stimulation at wrist

20 ms

200 µV

Stimulation at elbow

Figure 1.2 Reduced maximal conduction velocity with temporal dispersion of evoked muscle action potentials during recovery from acute inflammatory polyneuropathy. Co-axial needle recordings from abductor pollicis brevis with median nerve stimulation at the wrist and elbow. Three successive traces superimposed. The response latency was 9 ms with distal stimulation and 33 ms with proximal stimulation; conduction velocity in the forearm, 7.5 m/sec. (Courtesy of Dr R. G. Willison)

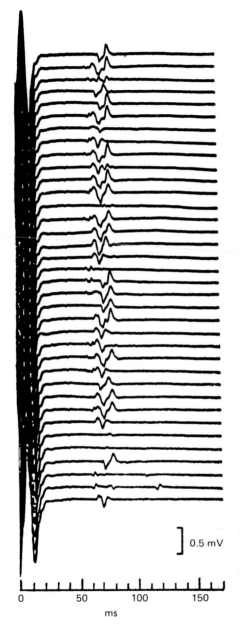

] 0.5 mV

Figure 1.3 Successive F waves recorded through surface electrodes from abductor digiti minimi following ulnar nerve stimulation at the wrist in a patient with chronic inflammatory polyneuropathy. Calibration 0.5 mV. F-wave latency is approximately 60 ms, which is double the expected normal value. (Courtesy of Dr K. R. Mills)

motor and sensory fibers. Nerve conduction velocity is a measure of only the fastest conducting fibers in a given nerve. Velocity is obtained by first measuring the latency (in milliseconds) of a muscle action potential after its motor nerve is stimulated close to the muscle (distal latency) and at some measured distance more proximally. From the difference in latency and distance between the two sites of stimulation, a velocity may be calculated. For most nerves, a normal velocity is

45–60 m/s. In axonal degenerations, conduction velocities are slowed only slightly, although amplitudes of nerve or muscle action potentials diminish progressively as more and more fibers fail completely. Segmental demyelination produces more striking slowing to 60% of normal or less (*Figure 1.2*). Other features characterize demyelination from an electrophysiological standpoint. These include desynchronization (dispersion) of evoked muscle action potentials, disproportionate prolongation of distal latencies (*see above*), slowing of F responses (the action potentials which have travelled to the spinal cord and back to the muscle) (*Figure 1.3*), and conduction block. Conduction block is determined by the finding of an abrupt fall in amplitude of the evoked muscle action potential when one stimulates the nerve at sites progressively more distant from (proximal to) the recording electrode.

In distinguishing peripheral nerve from anterior horn cell disease, reduction in amplitude of sensory action potentials (SAP) is a finding of particular importance because it places the lesion at or distal to the dorsal root ganglion cell. This finding indicates peripheral nerve involvement rather than spinal ventral horn disease. Motor conduction studies cannot be relied upon to make this distinction. It should be remembered that SAPs recorded through surface electrodes provide information only about large myelinated fibers. To study small myelinated fibers, intradermal histamine may be used to test for the flare of the triple response (*see* Chapter 4).

Uses of clinical electrodiagnosis

What is the type and specificity of information which may be gathered electrodiagnostically? As indicated in *Figure 1.1*, electrodiagnostic examination is useful in evaluating and managing virtally every patient with neuropathy, but the value of the examination to the referring clinician will depend on how well it is tailored to the specific problem. A well-tailored examination results only when the clinician informs the electromyographer of questions and suspicions raised by the clinical examination. Is there sensory involvement? Is the weakness neurogenic or is the process a primary myopathy? Is there evidence of disorder of neuromuscular transmission? How much Wallerian degeneration has occurred, and is the denervation on-going? Is this polyneuropathy demyelinating or axonal in character? In this neuropathy, is the pattern of chronic partial denervation in muscles most consistent with a radicular, a nerve trunk or a polyneuropathic distribution? These are the types of questions which should be posed to, and can be answered by, the electromyographer. It is not useful to request an electrodiagnostic examination simply to confirm the presence of a peripheral neuropathy which is clinically evident. Much more detailed and helpful information can be gleaned.

As mentioned, one should be able to distinguish between neurogenic and myopathic processes with high reliability. In a disorder which denervates muscle, the presence of sensory involvement helps distinguish neuropathy from pure anterior horn cell disease. Nerve root versus more distal nerve trunk lesions may be sorted out by patterns of nerve and muscle affection. More importantly, polyneuropathy may be separated from multifocal nerve trunk lesions which produce a clinical pattern resembling polyneuropathy. Axonal polyneuropathies are distinguishable from demyelinating polyneuropathies. In a given axonal polyneuropathy, an idea of its subclinical extent, its activity, and the degree of re-innervation may be gained. In demyelinating polyneuropathy, the extent of a secondary Wallerian degeneration may be estimated. Myotonia may be diagnosed and distinguished from continuous muscular activity of neuropathic origin. Cramp may be analyzed and clearly separated from physiological contracture, the latter being attended by electrical silence. Many other clinical uses of the electrodiagnostic examination may be made, but these are some of the major resolutions achievable.

CUTANEOUS NERVE BIOPSY

During the past 15 years, an extensive literature on peripheral neuropathy has accumulated which is based upon morphological findings in biopsied cutaneous nerve. As an investigational tool, nerve biopsy has proved to be informative, particularly through the application of techniques to tease and isolate nerve fibers, through semi-thin section and ultrastructural methods, and through morphometry. Sural nerve biopsy at the level of the lateral malleolus has usually been the procedure of choice.

Useful as nerve biopsy has been from a research standpoint, its role in clinical diagnosis is restricted. The main indication is in asymmetric and multifocal neuropathic disorders producing a clincial picture of mononeuropathy multiplex, the basis of which is still unclear after other less invasive laboratory investigations have been exhausted. Diagnostic considerations include vasculitis, amyloidosis, leprosy, and occasionally sarcoidosis. Additionally, nerve biopsy is helpful when one or more cutaneous nerves are palpably enlarged. Another clinical application is in establishing the diagnosis in some genetically-determined pediatric disorders such as metachromatic leukodystrophy, Krabbe's disease, giant axonal neuropathy, and infantile neuroaxonal dystrophy. In all of these recessively inherited diseases, both the central and peripheral nervous systems are affected.

There are very few if any other firm clinical indications for cutaneous nerve biopsy. As a generalization, distal symmetrical polyneuropathies, whether subacute or chronic, axonal or demyelinating, are not further clarified by nerve biopsy, once the less invasive evaluation scheme described above (*see Figure 1.1*) has been completed. Unfortunately, nerve biopsy tends to be carried out as part of the routine assessment of patients with neuropathy, often in the absence of adequate facilities or expertise to process and interpret the specimen. In this situation diagnostic yield is unacceptably low. Sural nerve biopsy is a highly invasive procedure which is not without complications. Wound infections, painful neuroma formation in the proximal stump, persistent dysesthesias in the heel and lateral foot, and local thrombophlebitis are all known to occur. Nerve biopsy should only be performed when there are strong indications, and when the diagnostic information cannot be obtained by other means. Further, it should be done only in centers where there is established experience with the technique.

RECAPITULATION

By using all the available clinical, electrodiagnostic and laboratory information, it is now possible to arrive at a satisfactory formulation in a large majority of patients with neuropathy. This is important because the key to effective management is correct diagnosis. Recently it has been estimated that approximately 50% of patients with neuropathy can be correctly diagnosed by the informed internist or neurologist without unusual investigation. For the remainder, if intensively studied at a center with special experience and interest in peripheral neuropathies, an acceptable explanation can be provided for almost three-quarters of these (Dyck and Oviatt, 1981). A significant fraction are familial, and require study of family members.

Many factors have converged to bring about recent progress with peripheral neuropathy, but perhaps the most important has been the development of electrodiagnosis.

References

Asbury, A. K. (1983) New aspects of disease of the peripheral nervous system. In *Harrison's Textbook of Internal Medicine*; Update IV, pp. 211–229. New York: McGraw-Hill

Baba, M., Fowler, C. J., Jacobs, J. M. and Gilliatt, R. W. (1982) Changes in peripheral nerve fibres distal to a constriction. *Journal of Neurological Science*, **54**, 197–208

Brand, P. W. and Ebner, J. D. (1969) Pressure sensitive devices for denervated hands and feet. *Journal of Bone and Joint Surgery*, **51A**, 109–116

Brown, M. J., Martin, J. and Asbury, A. K. (1976) Painful diabetic neuropathy: a morphometric study. *Archives of Neurology*, **33**, 164–171

Cho, E. S., Spencer, P. S. and Jortner, B. S. (1980) Doxorubicin. In *Experimental and Clinical Neurotoxicology*, edited by P. S. Spencer and H. H. Schaumburg, pp. 430–439. Baltimore: Williams and Wilkins

Dyck, P. J., Johnson, W. J., Lambert, E. H. and O'Brien, P. C. (1971) Segmental demyelination secondary to axonal degeneration in uremic neuropathy. *Mayo Clinic Proceedings*, **46**, 400–431

Dyck, P. J. and Lambert, E. H. (1969) Dissociated sensation in amyloidosis. *Archives of Neurology*, **20**, 480–507

Dyck, P. J., Lais, A. C., Karnes, J. L. *et al.* (1981) Permanent axotomy, a model of axonal atrophy and secondary segmental demyelination and remyelination. *Annals of Neurology*, **9**, 575–583

Dyck, P. J. and Oviatt, K. F. (1981) Intensive evaluation of referred unclassified neuropathies yields improved diagnosis in neuropathies. *Annals of Neurology*, **10**, 222–228

Eames, R. A. and Lange, L. S. (1967) Clinical and pathological study of ischemic neuropathy. *Journal of Neurology, Neurosurgery and Psychiatry*, **30**, 215–226

Gilliatt, R. W. (1982a) Paraesthesiae. In *Abnormal Nerves and Muscles as Impulse Generators*, edited by W. J. Culp and J. Ochoa, pp. 477–489. Oxford: Oxford University Press

Gilliatt, R. W. (1982b) Electrophysiology of peripheral neuropathies – an overview. *Muscle and Nerve*, **5**, S108–S116

Harrison, M. J. G. and Faris, I. B. (1976) The neuropathic factor in the etiology of diabetic foot ulcers. *Journal of Neurological Science*, **28**, 217–223

Hayward, M. and Willison, R. G. (1977) Automatic analysis of the electromyogram in patients with chronic partial denervation. *Journal of Neurological Science*, **33**, 415–423

Hess, K., Eames, R. A., Darveniza, P. and Gilliatt, R. W. (1979) Acute ischaemic neuropathy in the rabbit. *Journal of Neurological Science*, **44**, 19–43

Jacobs, J. M., Carmichael, N. and Cavanagh, J. B. (1977) Ultrastructural changes in the nervous system of rabbits poisoned with methylmercury. *Toxicology and Applied Pharmacology*, **39**, 249–260

Kori, S. H., Foley, K. M. and Posner, J. B. (1981) Brachial plexus lesions in patients with cancer: 100 cases. *Neurology*, **31**, 45–50

Long, R. R., Griffin, J. W., Stanley, E. F. and Price, D. L. (1980) Myelin sheath responses to alterations in axon caliber. *Neurology*, **30**, 435 (abstract)

Lundborg, G. (1975) Structure and functions of the intraneural microvessels as related to trauma, edema formation and nerve function. *Journal of Bone and Joint Surgery*, **57A**, 938–948

Mumenthaler, M. (1984) Brachial plexus neuropathy. In *Peripheral Neuropathy*, 2nd edition, edited by P. J. Dyck, P. K. Thomas, E. H. Lambert and R. P. Bunge. Philadelphia: W. B. Saunders (in press)

Nukada, H., Pollock, M. and Allpress, S. (1981) Experimental cold injury to peripheral nerve. *Brain*, **104**, 779–811

Peyronnard, J. M., Pedneault, M. and Aguayo, A. J. (1977) Neuropathies due to cold: quantitative studies of structural changes in human and animal nerves. From *Proceedings of the 11th World Congress of Neurology, Amsterdam*. Excerpta Medica International Congress Series No. 434, Neurology, pp. 308–329. Amsterdam: Excerpta Medica

Sabin, T. D. and Swift, T. R. (1975) Leprosy. In *Peripheral Neuropathy*, edited by P. J. Dyck, P. K. Thomas and E. H. Lambert, pp. 1166–1198. Philadelphia: W. B. Saunders Co.

Schaumburg, H., Kaplan, J., Rasmus, S. and Vick, N. (1982) Pyridoxine megavitaminosis produces sensory neuropathy in humans. *Annals of Neurology*, **12**, 107 (abstract)

Spencer, P. S. and Schaumburg, H. H. (1976) Central and peripheral distal axonopathy – the pathology of dying-back polyneuropathies. In *Progress in*

Neuropathology, edited by H. M. Zimmerman, pp. 253–295. New York: Grune and Stratton

Sterman, A. B., Schaumburg, H. H. and Asbury, A. K. (1980) Acute sensory neuronopathy – a distinct clinical entity. *Annals of Neurology*, **7**, 354–360

Suri, M. L., Vijayan, G. P., Puri, H. C., Barat, A. K. and Singh, N. (1978) Neurological manifestations of frost-bite. *Indian Journal of Medical Research*, **67**, 292–299

Tsairis, P., Dyck, P. J. and Mulder, D. W. (1972) Natural history of brachial plexus neuropathy. Report on 99 cases. *Archives of Neurology*, **27**, 109–117

Wilbourn, A. J., Furlan, A. J., Hulley, W. and Ruschhaupt, W. (1983) Ischemic monomelic neuropathy. *Neurology*, **33**, 447–451

Willison, R. G. (1976) Analysis of electrical activity in healthy and dystrophic muscle in man. *Journal of Neurology, Neurosurgery and Psychiatry*, **27**, 386–394

2
Diagnosis and management of acute areflexic paralysis with emphasis on Guillain-Barré syndrome

Allan H. Ropper and Bhagwan T. Shahani

INTRODUCTION

Several developments in the last decade, and in particular respiratory intensive care, have dramatically changed the management and outcome in acute Guillain-Barré syndrome (GBS). Advances in electrophysiologic diagnosis have clarified the pathophysiology of GBS, and other forms of acute areflexic paralysis have been identified, some the result of modern forms of therapy. Much of the specialized care of these patients has unfortunately been delegated to non-neurologists. It is our view that the major decisions affecting these patients are best handled by neurologists and that this leads to further understanding of the disease processes causing generalized paralysis. This chapter reflects our experience in the Neurological/Neurosurgical Intensive Care Unit of the Massachusetts General Hospital with 45 GBS patients from 1978–1983, and a retrospective review from 1962–1979 of 157 patients with GBS (collected mostly by Dr Bradley Truax). Important features in the medical management of the severely paralyzed patient and modern diagnostic electrophysiologic techniques are emphasized. Our recent experience with plasma exchange for acute GBS in over 30 patients is also reviewed.

CLINICAL CONSIDERATIONS IN THE DIAGNOSIS OF GUILLAIN-BARRÉ SYNDROME

Guillain-Barré syndrome is the most common acute areflexic quadriparesis and it is generally not difficult to establish the diagnosis (Asbury, 1981). A summary of the clinical features in our patients with acute GBS from 1962–1979 is presented in *Table 2.1* (Ropper, 1983a). Typically, about two-thirds of patients give a history of recent acute infection, usually a mild respiratory syndrome. A number of cases follow other well defined episodes such as mononucleosis (Gautier-Smith, 1965), acute exanthemas or, rarely, surgery (Arnason and Asbury, 1968). We have

21

recently seen three cases following a mild mononucleosis-like illness with slightly elevated liver enzymes that were apparently due to cytomegalovirus. Two of these patients were nurses exposed to blood products. Postsurgical GBS occurs 2–3 weeks after an operation and has been reported after intracranial, abdominal, thoracic and orthopedic operations as well as after spinal anesthesia. Eight of 157 patients (5%) in our retrospective study had recent surgery.

The outstanding early clinical sign of GBS is weakness, usually appearing symmetrically in the legs, and more often proximal than distal. Ascending paralysis is a misnomer for GBS since foot drop is rarely seen as the initial sign. In our series,

Table 2.1 Experience with GBS at Massachusetts General Hospital

Number of cases	157
Average age	39 years
Age range	8–81 years
Prior illness	Upper respiratory infection (approximately 70%)
Onset to maximal deficit and plateau	Average 17 days
	40% by first week
	77% by second week
	89% by third week
Mortality	1.25%
Respiratory failure requiring endotracheal tube	29%
Average hospitalization	61 days
Average intubation	51 days
Residual deficits at 1 year	23% (severe in 8%)

56% of patients initially had more lower than upper extremity weakness, 12% more upper than lower extremity weakness and in 32% the limbs were affected about equally. Sensory symptoms (numbness) with only mild sensory signs may be prominent early in the illness and are initially distal. Only 65% of our retrospective group had definite sensory signs early in the illness but paralysis was rare. Muscle, back, or neuritic pain occurs in approximately 50% of patients initially, but develops in up to another 25% later in the illness (*see below*). Weakness usually evolves over 2–17 days but may continue to worsen for up to one month and does not remit until a plateau of maximal weakness is reached. Symmetric facial weakness occurs in more than 50% of cases (57% in our retrospective study), particularly if limb paresis is severe. About 6% in our series had partial ophthalmoplegia and another 3% complete ophthalmoplegia. Virtual quadriplegia can rarely occur without any facial weakness. Respiratory muscle weakness is the most serious complication of GBS and occurs in about one-third of patients (33% in our series). Sphincter symptoms are unusual, but do occur transiently early, most commonly as urinary retention for 1–2 days. Many patients with sphincteric disturbances also complain of sacral paresthesias. Urinary retention occurred in 23% of our retrospective series. Some patients complain of orthostatic dizziness as part of an early associated autonomic neuropathy.

GBS variant illnesses are well known, the most striking being the polyneuropathy with ophthalmoplegia and ataxia described by Fisher (1956). Others include 'descending paralysis' with ocular, facial and pharyngeal paresis occurring before limb paresis which simulates botulism or early diphtheria; instances of early and almost purely respiratory failure, and the pure pandysautonomic illness described by Young *et al.* (1975). The latter is likely to be a variant of inflammatory neuropathy but this remains unproved and the connection to GBS rests largely on an elevated CSF protein level. Instances of GBS without any sensory signs or symptoms, i.e. a 'pure motor' inflammatory neuropathy, are more common than generally appreciated (34% in our study).

Patients with GBS initially exhibit few objective signs besides weakness. Sensory signs are usually confined to mild or moderate glove and stocking paneuropathy that may worsen over the first 3 weeks. About 15% of patients will have a severe vibration and position sense loss early in the illness and virtually all of these will have ataxia if their weakness allows its demonstration. Substantial degrees of pinprick or moderate vibration sense loss early in the illness should raise the suspicion of an illness other than GBS or another superimposed neuropathy such as diabetes. A persistent sensory level excludes GBS, though transient graded loss on the trunk that simulates a level has been seen rarely (2 out of 157 patients). Areflexia is almost always present in paretic limbs, and the persistence of more than slight (1/4) reflex activity in a region that has been weak for more than 3 days makes the diagnosis questionable. We have seen exceptional cases with preserved but diminished reflexes for up to 8 days after leg weakness began. Many of the oculomotor signs in GBS, particularly in the Fisher variant, have been proposed to represent examples of central nervous system inflammation, but pathology in these cases shows only peripheral disease (Grunnet and Lubow, 1972) and alternative explanations have been forwarded (Ropper, 1983b; Ropper and Shahani, 1983). Arguments center predominantly around the conjugate nature of recovery of ophthalmoplegia, recovery of upgaze before horizontal versions, and preservation of the Bell's phenomenon with impaired voluntary upgaze, all alleged to be supranuclear in origin (Jampel and Haidt, 1972). It is our opinion that most putative central nervous system signs in GBS can be explained on a peripheral nerve basis, although there may be very rare instances of scattered inflammation in the spinal cord or brainstem. There are a number of unexplained seizures that occur in GBS patients but in our experience these have been related to hyponatremia or other metabolic abnormalities.

Autonomic dysfunction, of particular interest in the intensive care unit, is common in GBS (Appenzeller and Marshall, 1963; Lichtenfield, 1971). It ranges from fixed tachycardia and reduced sweating to sudden shock with loss of cardiac filling pressure (Weintraub, 1979). An alteration in beat to beat (R–R) interval on the electrocardiogram in many patients has been said to reflect an autonomic neuropathy (Frison *et al.*, 1980). but this may be an artifact of tachycardia (Smith and Smith, 1980). Ileus, bladder dysfunction (particularly retention as noted above), idioventricular arrhythmia (Pace, 1976) and transient hypertension are all rare but probably occur as part of the autonomic neuropathy of GBS. Dangerous arrhythmias seem to be more common in children. Renin levels have been said to be raised in hypertensive GBS patients (Lauffer *et al.*, 1981). Interesting and dramatic parasympathetic discharges may occur, with flushing, chest tightness and profuse bronchorrhea. In one such patient we observed associated dermatographia suggesting that histamine release was related to the episode. It has become clear that GBS patients (and probably those with other generalized paralyses) should not receive succinylcholine since it may cause ventricular arrhythmias (Ferguson *et al.*, 1981). The drug does not seem to produce myonecrosis as it may in some myopathies.

A number of GBS-associated derangements in other organs should be mentioned. Mild or asymptomatic glomerulonephritis is present early in the course of many cases (Rodriguez-Iturbe *et al.*, 1973). About one-third of our cases have had transient proteinuria in the first week. This is an important observation because it adds credibility to the humoral theory of GBS pathogenesis. The syndrome of inappropriate antidiuretic hormone secretion is frequently reported.

Pseudotumor cerebri with papilledema has drawn much attention (Morley and Reynolds, 1966). It occurred in 5 of 157 (3%) consecutive patients seen at our institution. The most commonly proposed explanation for this syndrome is an absorption block created by elevated CSF protein levels. Reports of CSF flow studies and ventricular volume further suggest that this is the mechanism, but others have pointed out that cervical, cisternal and ventricular CSF protein is often low, and that GBS associated pseudotumor has occurred in patients with only slightly elevated CSF protein (Arnason, 1975). It appears to us that a prolonged illness with persistently raised CSF pressure is necessary for pseudotumor. We recently studied a patient with GBS pseudotumor by using CSF infusion and withrawal methods (Shapiro, Marmarou and Shulman, 1980) and found that CSF production rate was normal, but resistance to outflow was slightly elevated, as observed in idiopathic pseudotumor (Hussey, Schanzer and Katzman, 1970). However, it is clear that the magnitude of this elevation is not sufficient to explain raised CSF pressure. Instead, raised venous pressure parallels the rise in CSF pressure and it is likely that the mechanism of pseudotumor in GBS has to do with venous outflow pressures rather than an abnormality on the CSF side of the absorption apparatus.

The course of GBS is lengthy, but 80–90% of patients recover with little or no disability (Loeffel *et al.*, 1977; Ravn, 1967). About 5% have relapses; the rest are monophasic. In the modern intensive care unit era mortality is 1–3%, but hospital stays are frequently measured in months and complicated by intubation or tracheostomy (10–35%), pneumonia, phlebitis, pulmonary embolus and severe psychological depression. The residual effects of GBS understandably increase with the severity and duration of illness, the commonest protracted problem being nerve pressure palsies (Ravn, 1967), rather than direct inflammatory nerve damage.

Apart from the examination of cerebrospinal fluid and electrophysiologic testing (*see below*), laboratory findings are of little value. An increased level of CSF protein is helpful in making the diagnosis, but occurs only after 3–10 days of illness. Occasionally, CSF protein is normal throughout the illness. In our group of 157 patients studied retrospectively only 2 had normal CSF protein after day 14, and 7 were normal between days 10 and 14. The average protein in the whole group was

1.57 g/l determined at various times. The absence of cells in the CSF is said to be necessary for the diagnosis of GBS, but it is only supportive and about 5–10% of cases have 3–100×10^6 lymphocytes/l, with rare cases exceeding 200×10^6 cells/l. Transient elevations of liver function tests are not uncommon during the first 2 weeks of illness and creatine phosphokinase (CPK) is elevated in about 20%, especially if there is pain.

SPECIAL DIAGNOSTIC PROBLEMS

Despite listing GBS in most texts along with a slew of rare neuropathies, such as porphyria and heavy metal poisoning, few of these oddities, with the exception perhaps of tick paralysis, have a clinical presentation similar enough to cause confusion. More interesting problems occur when unusual features of GBS simulate non-neuropathic illnesses such as brainstem vascular disease or myopathy. Major difficulties arise when the bulbar and/or ocular muscles are affected first, and deep tendon reflexes are diminished but nevertheless present. Below are some points derived from experience that may be helpful to neurologists with problematic cases.

The diagnosis of ophthalmoplegia and quadriparesis

When ophthalmoplegia is a prominent feature of GBS and the illness evolves rapidly, there may be some difficulty distinguishing it from basilar artery occlusion with the 'locked in syndrome'. We have seen three such patients who had had cerebral arteriograms performed because of these similarities. One was found to have basilar occlusion and two had GBS. In these few difficult cases detailed electrophysiologic studies (abnormalities of F waves particularly) will confirm the diagnosis of GBS, but these are not always immediately available. Helpful distinguishing clinical features in favor of basilar occlusion are truly normal or increased ankle and knee reflexes, though these are often not found in the age group with occlusive vascular disease, many of whom have diabetes. Babinski signs are the most dependable sign of basilar occlusion, but the toes are frequently silent in early basilar occlusion and rare patients with GBS have transient extensor plantar responses. Unreactive pupils in an awake patient indicate GBS rather than stroke. Asymmetry of limb movements, relative preservation of vertical or horizontal gaze, conjugate ocular movements, nystagmus, ptosis or ataxia may occur in both processes.

Distinguishing myasthenia from GBS may be a problem, particularly in the presence of severe ophthalmoplegia. Though most patients with GBS will have ptosis, its absence favors GBS over myasthenia. The single most helpful differential feature is the relative preservation of jaw power compared with facial muscles in GBS, whereas the jaw is invariably slack, often hanging open, when there is severe facial weakness in myasthenia. Severe facial weakness out of proportion to limb weakness usually indicates GBS but this has not been as consistently helpful as the jaw sign.

When GBS obliterates the pupillary light response it may appear similar to advanced botulism. Ataxia, hyporeflexia and ophthalmoplegia may occur in both illnesses. Botulism is identified by the early loss of the near accommodation response. In addition, bradycardia is one of the most consistent features of botulism, in contrast to the regular and frequently fixed rate tachycardia in most patients with severe GBS.

Acute quadripareses due to tick paralysis or porphyria

The clinical features of tick paralysis simulate typical GBS. Early in the illness, before CSF protein is consistently elevated in GBS, there is virtually no way to distinguish the two diseases by signs or symptoms unless the tick is found. Both may begin with mild paresthesias and an ascending areflexic paralysis eventually involving bulbar muscles. Prominent distal paresthesias or pain occurring prior to severe weakness is much more typical of GBS. Sensory signs are absent in tick paralysis, but there may be ataxia similar to some cases of GBS. Early in the illness the CSF protein is normal in GBS but persistently normal CSF is indicative of tick paralysis. Electrophysiologic studies may be similar to GBS, particularly early slowing of motor nerve conduction. In patients with possible tick exposure it is reasonable to inspect the scalp and pubic hairline upon admission.

Acute intermittent porphyria can also simulate GBS but in virtually all cases other signs of the illness precede the motor neuropathy. CSF protein is normal and unusual patterns of sensory loss should raise the suspicion of porphyria.

Pain as an early or initial symptom

The most common pain in GBS is an aching 'muscular pain' in the thighs or shoulders that is eventually present in about one-half of patients and may occur up to 1 week before weakness. The description of pain is most often likened to the soreness experienced a day after heavy exercise and it is invariably worse at night. It is similar to some descriptions of the limb pain which occurs in polio. Severe pain may lead to the erroneous diagnosis of polymyositis or rheumatologic disorders. The correct diagnosis becomes evident within a few days as weakness progresses. Pain occurs in GBS even without other sensory symptoms or signs. In a prospective study of 26 consecutive patients, 13 with pain, we found no consistent relationship between the characteristic muscular pain and either clinical signs or electrophysiologic abnormalities. Most patients with pain, however, will have elevated serum CPK levels suggesting that some degree of myonecrosis may be related to the pain. Radicular pain, usually asymmetric bilateral sciatica, may rarely precede or occur simultaneously with distal paresthesias in GBS and 2 of our 13 patients with 'muscular' limb pain had sciatic pain elicited by straight leg raising. Bilateral hamstring weakness demonstrated by the Barré prone-flexed-knee maneuver, or quadriceps weakness evident on arising from a chair, should raise the suspicion of GBS in patients complaining of unusual sciatica.

Early GBS mistaken for hysteria

A mistake occasionally made in emergency rooms is to dismiss early GBS as hysteria. The usual history is one of worsening rubbery feeling and weakness in the legs over several hours to 2 days. Knee and ankle jerks may only be minimally reduced at this early stage of GBS, and the CSF protein level, if measured, would almost certainly be normal. This clinical situation can be misread as hysterical weakness, particularly if the patient is unfortunate enough to have a background of psychiatric difficulties. Awareness of GBS as an explanation for acute 'rubber legs' is the best way to avoid this diagnostic pitfall.

Ataxia

The most intriguing occasional neurological findings in GBS are limb and gait ataxia with little or no loss of joint position sense. These occur in otherwise typical cases (Richter, 1962) as well as in the Fisher variant, and cannot be distinguished from cerebellar ataxia. In our retrospective series it occurred in 13% of patients, usually disappearing as weakness was progressed. A mechanism for this cerebellar ataxia based solely on peripheral nerve mechanisms has been proposed (Ropper and Shahani, 1983). The hypothesis is based on the findings of normal joint position sense with abnormal spindle afferents as detected by a study of 'silent periods'. The mismatching of these two afferent signals or simply disruption of cerebellar afferents could cause a cerebellar ataxia. This is consistent with Richter's pathological findings (Richter, 1962). There is also a slightly different sensory ataxic tremor associated with obvious joint position sense loss (Sobue *et al.* 1983).

ELECTROPHYSIOLOGICAL STUDIES IN GBS

Diagnosis of GBS is normally made on the basis of characteristic history, physical examination and laboratory findings of increased CSF protein with low cell count. It is claimed by many authors that during early phases of the disease electrophysiological studies may not show any abnormality. However, our experience suggests that both early in the course of the disease, and thereafter with sequential electrophysiological studies, one can document characteristic changes that are helpful in the diagnosis and monitoring of GBS. These studies are also useful in excluding alternative diagnoses such as myasthenia or botulism. Moreover, we believe that electrophysiologic studies are the most sensitive laboratory test in GBS and abnormalities of nerve conduction are usually detected prior to elevation of CSF protein (Shahani, Lachman and Young, 1975; Shahani and Sumner, 1981). Despite their sensitivity, it should be noted that conventional electrophysiological studies only grossly, or not at all, parallel clinical signs in GBS (Shahani *et al.*, 1980).

A number of physiological studies must be performed in order to fully characterize the illness in an individual patient. These include conventional motor and sensory nerve conduction studies, needle electromyography and, most importantly, late response studies including H reflex, F response and blink reflex studies (Shahani and Young, 1983; Shahani, Lachman and Young, 1975). In some instances single fiber EMG, nerve conduction in different diameter fibers using collision techniques, and repetitive stimulation tests are useful to further elucidate pathophysiological mechanisms underlying GBS, but these are currently of mainly research interest. Finally, pathophysiologic data on ataxia, as in the Fisher variant of GBS, have been obtained through tremor analysis using surface EMG recordings and accelerometric tracings as well as 'silent period' studies in different muscles (Ropper and Shahani, 1983).

Early changes in GBS

Conventional motor nerve conduction studies may be initially normal in many patients. However, careful analysis of the compound muscle action potential (CMAP) evoked by electrical stimulation of peripheral nerves is frequently abnormal. The CMAP becomes more asynchronous as the site of stimulation is moved more proximally. Sometimes the shape and amplitude of the CMAP improves within days during the early course of clinical recovery in GBS (Shahani et al., 1980). These findings suggest that the early changes of asynchrony and reduced amplitude may be due to reversible physiological blockage of motor impulses in distal segments of the nerve. In nearly 20% of patients the sensory nerve action potentials will initially be abnormal. Needle electromyography usually shows reduced recruitment patterns without evidence of active denervation, i.e. fibrillations and positive sharp waves. The presence of early fibrillations and positive sharp waves indicates axonal degeneration and in our experience the prognosis for early recovery in these patients is not as good as in patients who show severe abnormalities of nerve conduction but no denervation.

   The most sensitive electrophysiologic tests during early phases of GBS are late response studies. H reflexes are either absent (corroborating absent ankle jerks) or have a prolonged latency. In some patients the H reflex becomes very asynchronous. F responses which can be recorded from several different muscles may show abnormalities in the distribution of some peripheral nerves and not in others. When patients have severe clinical weakness, F responses are frequently difficult to elicit. The absence or abnormality of F responses with simultaneously normal motor and sensory conduction suggests a block at the level of the roots, plexus or proximal segments of the nerve. We have seen a number of patients who have severe clinical weakness with normal conventional motor and sensory conduction and absent F responses. As the patient improves clinically the F responses reappear, although with increased latencies. Presumably this means that weakness in some patients is due to proximal 'blockage' of motor impulses, mediated by reversible nodal and paranodal changes rather than by more long-lasting changes of complete demyelination and subsequent remyelination of whole internodes. In fact, changes produced by segmental demyelination-remyelination such as prolonged latencies (more than 40% increase in latencies) of late responses, and extreme slowing of nerve conduction can be seen at a time when the patient is recovering. Early changes in F responses include:

(1) prolonged minimal latency,
(2) increased minimal–maximal latency difference,
(3) decreased persistence or absence of F responses (Shahani, Lachman and Young, 1975).

Blink reflex studies should also be performed in many patients because when they are absent, or latencies are abnormally prolonged, they may be the most easily detectable electrophysiologic abnormality in the first few days of illness. We have seen several patients in whom GBS is superimposed on a previously existing axonal neuropathy, such as uremic or diabetic neuropathy, and prolonged latencies of blink reflex components were helpful in detecting a demyelinating neuropathy (Shahani and Young, 1983). Blink reflexes and F response abnormalities are also the quickest way to corroborate GBS when ocular signs suggest basilar artery thrombosis as an alternative diagnosis. It must be emphasized that GBS may affect different nerve segments and different peripheral nerves asymmetrically and therefore it is important to test many segments (proximal, intermediate and distal) and several peripheral nerves.

Electrophysiological studies later in GBS and correlation with clinical signs

When sequential electrophysiological studies are performed as the illness advances there are several stereotyped changes in conventional motor and sensory conduction. Most patients show significant slowing of motor conduction 2–3 weeks after the onset of illness. Sensory potentials are absent in some patients even when it is difficult to document clinical loss of sensory function. There are a number of possible reasons for this. There may be an asynchrony of responses rather than significant blockage of impulses or the clinical examination may be too crude a test for evaluation of sensory deficit (sensory loss may not be detected even after losing function of up to 40% of sensory fibers). With regard to motor conduction studies, there appears to be no consistent correlation between slowing of nerve conduction and clinical weakness. The electrophysiological study that does appear to correlate to some extent with the clinical state of GBS is the persistence of F responses. When F responses are absent or have decreased persistence they indicate a 'block' at a proximal site and these patients usually have significant weakness (Kimura and Butzer, 1975; Shahani *et al.*, 1980). F responses during the chronic phase of the disease show increased minimal latency and minimal–maximal latency difference rather than the decreased persistence that is seen during the acute illness.

In some variants of GBS, particularly Fisher's syndrome, special studies have suggested possible physiological mechanisms underlying cerebellar ataxia. Tremor tests performed with surface EMG electrodes placed on pairs of antagonistic muscles and accelerometers attached to the fingers show the characteristic patterns of a cerebellar ataxic-tremor. In two patients silent periods recorded from proximal and distal muscles of the arm showed absence of proprioceptive silent periods in parts of the limb where joint position sense was intact. In contrast 'proprioceptive' silent periods were normal where joint position sense was diminished. We believe that mismatching of information from muscle spindles and joint position receptors may be responsible for ataxia in some patients with GBS, rather than a lesion in the central nervous system (Ropper and Shahani, 1983).

Our preliminary studies with collision techniques suggest that there may be a conduction block in smaller diameter fibers well before large diameter motor fibers are affected. The presence of large amplitude motor unit potentials with minimal effort, seen on conventional needle EMG within a few days of the onset of the disease, may also indicate that smaller units are blocked early in the illness. The findings of selective early involvement of smaller diameter nerve fibers correlates well with some experimental studies.

GENERAL CARE AND MEDICAL COMPLICATIONS OF ACUTE GENERALIZED PARALYSIS

Attention to the mundane details of daily care more than any specific therapy provides the best chance of a good outcome in GBS patients (Griswold, Guanci and Ropper, 1983). The comments below generally pertain to severely paralyzed patients being cared for in an intensive care unit but they apply to all forms of generalized limb and respiratory paralysis.

Positioning and skin care

Patients indicate they are most comfortable supine and least comfortable prone. The major determinant of comfort seems to be the position of the face, with pressure on the chin being most distressing. For this reason the lateral decubitus and slightly head down position, which is favorable for lung drainage, is not well tolerated for more than a few minutes. The lateral decubitus position with the head slightly elevated (10–20°) is a reasonable compromise between comfort and pulmonary drainage. Frequent turning and positional changes to relieve pressure on skin cause great discomfort to most awake paralyzed patients. A water mattress and lamb's wool covering minimizes this discomfort. The use of 'Roto-beds' and similar special care beds may be helpful but a simple and dedicated nursing routine will prevent decubiti in almost all patients. Skin emollients twice daily are helpful in preventing breakdown, and powdering of the groin daily prevents both dyshydrotic rash and candidiasis.

Bladder and bowel care

If the patient is able to communicate the need to void then a Foley catheter is rarely necessary after the first few days of illness. (About 10–20% of patients will have urinary retention initially.) A condom or 'Texas' catheter may be used for immobile males and is preferable to an indwelling catheter from the point of view of infection and to occasional accidental incontinence with regard to comfort and skin care. The skin under the strap of the condom catheter must be dressed frequently and the catheter removed regularly to allow drying. If penile skin breakdown occurs then a urinal bottle may be left loosely around the penis. In older men with prostatism, prolonged supine bedrest may cause painless obstructive uropathy and an indwelling catheter then becomes necessary. Intermittent catheterization every 6–8 hours may eventually be used in place of the catheter.

No entirely satisfactory method for female bladder care exists. Women patients who are unable to consistently communicate that the bladder is full have a tendency to urinary retention with associated reflex hypertension and tachycardia. This response is not blunted even in patients with severe autonomic neuropathy (nor does it appear to be excessive). If an adequate bed pan routine cannot be established, or if it is clear that a patient is dilating the bladder from persistent urinary retention, then intermittent Foley catheterization is recommended. Urinary irrigants are of unproven value in continuously catheterized patients and prophylactic urinary antibiotics only lead to the development of resistant organisms (*see below*).

Constipation is a problem in the first week of illness but rarely requires treatment beyond milk of magnesia, and a rectal suppository. Ileus is rare (2% of our retrospective series) but does occur, particularly in diabetics. Once nasogastric feeding begins, diarrhea is common and laxatives should therefore generally be avoided if not clearly necessary.

Eye and mouth care

The severe bifacial palsy frequently present in acute areflexic paralysis causes corneal dessication. This is painless until a lash hair or other object causes an abrasion. Methylcellulose artificial tears should be instilled into each eye every 2–6 hours depending on the extent of deficiency in eyelid closure. Taping the lids closed during sleep or taping one closed during waking is reserved for complete lid paralysis and then only to prevent dessication. The sensory deprivation caused by lid closure must be coordinated with appropriate psychological support.

The oral cavity should be swabbed twice daily and clean dentures kept in place if possible in order to maintain proper jaw articulation. Suctioning the posterior oropharynx regularly, particularly prior to cuff deflation, adds to patient comfort.

Fluid and nutrition

The stress of a severe illness such as GBS generally increases metabolic needs, but complete immobility reduces caloric requirements as well as CO_2 production. Feeding is not necessary for the first week of paralysis but further undernutrition leads to poor skin condition and hypoalbuminemia. Severe hypoalbuminemia occurred in 2% of our retrospective series and was usually associated with skin edema. If previous nutrition was adequate and the bowel has peristalsis then a small caliber mercury-tipped feeding tube should be inserted before the end of the first week. The major complication of these small tubes is inadvertent transbronchial passage, sometimes through to the pleural space. They are also expensive. Large gauge nasogastric tubes, however, should be avoided because their size offers no advantage and they cause gastric wall erosion and favor aspiration. We have also found directly placed transabdominal gastric feeding tubes cause more iatrogenic problems than their convenience justifies.

Any of the low residue high calorie feeding mixtures may be used, beginning at half-strength (i.e. mixed with an equivalent amount of water) intermittently, 50 ml every 1–2 hours. The volume is advanced over 3–7 days to approximately 75–125 ml of full strength formula hourly. The usual preparations supply approximately 1 kcal/ml (4.2 J/ml) at full strength but are relatively protein deficient. A general range of 1600 kcal (6720 J)/day for basal energy expenditure in paralyzed patients is desirable. Diarrhea may be abated by simultaneous adminstration of opiates or codeine, 30–45 mg administered with every fourth feeding. Some of the more concentrated formulations cause mild hypernatremia and dehydration.

Infected or septic patients require 2200–2800 kcal (9240–11 760 J)/day and therefore need parenteral alimentation. This requires a central venous catheter placed under sterile conditions. Several medical problems are associated with hyperalimentation including hyperglycemia, hyperosmolarity and catheter-related sepsis and this technique should be performed by an experienced individual. There is also a well described acute areflexic paralysis which results from hypophosphatemia due to hyperalimentation (Furlan *et al.*, 1975). Peripheral hyperalimentation (through a peripherally placed intravenous catheter) is a safer way of supplementing fat and proteins with a lower infection risk. However, in critically ill patients it does not provide enough nutrition alone and may lead to overhydration. Its use in paralyzed but stable patients is controversial since a nasogastric tube is able to provide more nutrition.

Fluid management in the paralyzed patient, particularly with GBS, is designed to balance the need for adequate hydration with varying degrees of excessive ADH secretion which occur in many patients. Mechanically ventilated patients are notably prone to hyponatremia. Dextrose 0.5% in normal saline with potassium supplementation is administered at a rate of approximately 100 ml/hour before tube feedings begin. More fluid is required if there is fever but serum hypo-osmolarity should be avoided.

The stress of acute illness generally increases potassium losses. Once feeding begins, the typical urinary potassium losses in a bedridden patient are initially replaced with 80–120 mmol KCl intravenous supplementation each day. It should be noted that the level of serum potassium, when above approximately 3.2 mmol/l, does not accurately reflect total body potassium. Chloride and CO_2 are better indications of intracellular potassium. Therefore, if hypochloremic alkalosis develops after the first week, then KCl can be added to the tube feedings or diet. A serum chloride of 96 and CO_2 of 32 is associated with a total body K deficit of approximately 300 mmol, irrespective of serum potassium level.

Other electrolytes generally do not require replacement in the first weeks and are adequately supplemented in commercial formulas. Oral or nasogastric tube iron supplementation is desirable to replace loss from phlebotomy, but it often causes nausea and poor tolerance of tube feedings and then must be stopped. Thus, patients over age 55, or younger patients with sepsis, may be transfused when their hematocrit reaches approximately 30% or below. Some authorities recommend intramuscular vitamin K once or twice weekly in order to prevent the elevation in prothrombin time associated with formula feeding or starvation. It is fairly common for latent or mild diabetics to become transiently but severely hyperglycemic due to the stress of generalized paralysis. Insulin may be required to keep blood sugars below 180 mg/100 ml but it can usually be discontinued after 2 weeks if there was no previous insulin requirement. Oral hypoglycemic drugs are not useful in the acute stages of illness.

Nosocomial infections

Pneumonia occurred in 25% and urine infections in 20% of our retrospective GBS group. Virtually all infections acquired in the hospital are due to local nosocomial organisms and therefore can be anticipated. For this reason culture surveillance of the sputum and urine once or twice a week provides useful information should an infection arise. After 3–5 days in hospital most patients will have their sputum colonized by local organisms, frequently pseudomonas species. It is best to treat only bona fide infections rather than beginning antibiotics whenever a fever appears. Many fevers lower than 100.5°F (38°C) are related to pulmonary atelectasis and are better treated with aggressive chest physical therapy than with antibiotics. In bedridden patients with difficulty clearing pulmonary secretions and emptying the bladder there are usually several infections during the course of illness and excessive antibiotic use only leads to resistant organisms. An infiltrate seen on the chest X-ray or more than 10 white blood cells per high power field in the urine are good indications of infection. One common exception is tracheitis. This is identified by fever, a clear chest X-ray, a report from the nurses that the sputum has become more purulent in character, and frequently by the appearance of a new organism compared with previous surveillance cultures. We have also seen several instances of sepsis related to acquired sinusitis or otitis in intubated patients. This is presumably related to impaired sinus or ear drainage from an endotracheal tube.

Urinary irrigants and prophylactic antibiotics are not recommended for routine use. Care in keeping urinary bladder drainage systems closed at all times is the best defence against nosocomial urinary infections. After 5 days, all patients with catheters will have nosocomial colonization of the urinary tract but as already noted only patients with significant pyuria need treatment. One point in regard to treatment of enterococcal urinary tract infections is worth mentioning because this organism has appeared so commonly in our GBS patients. Culture sensitivities may indicate resistance or intermediate sensitivity to most antibiotics. Nevertheless, at this time, ampicillin in adequate doses (2–4 g/day) usually produces urinary concentrations high enough to be bactericidal.

The single most important measure in preventing infections in these patients is handwashing by physicians and nurses.

Pain

In our experience pain control has been the most difficult intermediate-term management problem in patients with GBS. Over half of those weak enough to be bedridden have pain during the second to the fifth weeks of illness. Symptoms occur in three varieties. The more common one is a deep 'aching', 'charley-horse' or strain in areas of large fleshy muscles, mainly the buttocks, anterior thighs, calves and trapezii. This pain is worse in the evening and at night and interferes with sleep. In about one-half of patients the pain is worsened by squeezing the muscle and improved by passive movement. The second most common pain is a sharp localized discomfort near large joints, especially the hips and knees. This occurs at rest and is worsened with movement. A few patients have a hot-burning sensation perceived as just under the skin in the thighs, calves and feet. A night-time restless leg syndrome may be associated with any of these. Those without voluntary leg movement strong enough to resist gravity do not usually complain of a need to move the limbs.

Despite a report of its effectiveness, we have not found that quinine relieves any of these pains. Mild narcotics are very effective at night and have not caused dependence in our experience. Codeine, Percodan or Percocet seem best. Non-steroidal anti-inflammatory agents are inconsistently successful for a few days in some patients. Antidepressants have not had a clear effect. The most dramatically effective treatment for severe pain has been a single injection of methylprednisolone (Solumedrol) 20–40 mg i.m. This reduces pain for several days in many patients.

Psychological support

Even the most severely affected patients with acute areflexic paralysis have a good chance of recovery and independence. We are told by patients that continuously stressing this optimistic outlook is of great importance to them. Many physicians do not perceive the progress made by a patient unless they compare functional ability with 1 or 2 weeks previously. We have seen four patients who were quadriparetic and bedbound at 6 months but who made satisfactory recoveries at 18–24 months. There is much to be gained from having former patients visit and emphasize the potential for recovery. Depression becomes a regular feature of GBS if quadriparesis persists for more than one month. It is also difficult for nurses to care for these patients for many consecutive days but learning each patient's individual needs are important. Rotating nurses on each shift for 3 days at a time keeps the staff empathetic but many patients prefer to have one primary nurse who is familiar with their idiosyncracies.

Fear of being left alone and without aid plagues all of these patients. Those most severely disabled with quadriplegia and blepharoptosis can frequently open their jaw and push an electronic switch to turn on an alarm. We have also used surface EMG electrodes to trigger an alarm. As soon as thumb movement is possible a switch should be positioned within reach. The most valuable psychological support to the partially ventilated patient is a 'talking trach' which allows communication. When thumb power is adequate the patient can control the flow of air through the larynx using this device. Most find this preferable to a letter board or lip reading.

Physical therapy

No organized or controlled study has been made of the effects of physical therapy on GBS. Some have suggested that premature therapy is detrimental but with an illness as variable as GBS it is unlikely that this question will be satisfactorily resolved. It is our impression that overly-aggressive treatments seem to worsen night-time pain. On the other hand there is also a clear indication from patients that keeping the limbs flexible quickens the time to when they are able to walk with help. A program organized by a physical therapist allows the patient and physician to gauge functional progress. For this reason we encourage a uniform and fairly aggressive physical therapy approach after pain has subsided with an attempt to have one therapist closely associated with each patient. Passive motion of all joints is attempted twice daily for 2–3 weeks. In patients who are able, active motion and motion against resistance is then attempted. When hip flexion and knee extension are better than 3/5 in power (able to resist gravity for several seconds), the patient is allowed to stand and then walk to a chair with assistance for brief periods. Many patients become orthostatically dizzy and should spend 30 minutes sitting or preferably in a reclining chair before arising.

Prevention of leg vein thrombosis and pulmonary embolus

Venous thromboembolic disease (along with sepsis) is cause of serious morbidity in GBS. It occurred in 5% of our retrospective group. Intermittent pneumatic calf compression is a convenient and inexpensive way of prevention, but we feel that the device may injure the inflamed peroneal nerve. We therefore use subcutaneous heparin instead, 5000 U every 12 hours. Pneumatic plethysmographic testing may be used weekly for surveillance of leg vein thrombosis. There have been no instances of leg vein or pulmonary thrombosis in over 40 consecutive GBS patients receiving this 'mini-heparin' regimen although occasional patients with other illnesses, such as stroke, have had emboli. We perform nuclide ventilation-perfusion scans liberally for the diagnosis of pulmonary embolus but unfortunately false positive or equivocal tests are frequent with atelectasis.

Phlebotomy and operations

Virtually all of these severely ill patients become anemic from blood drawing and undernutrition. A schedule that limits phlebotomy to 2 or 3 days in each week minimizes the anemia. As mentioned above, iron supplementation causes severe constipation in these supine, immobilized patients and we prefer to use transfusion when necessary.

There is a theoretical objection to performing surgical procedures in patients with GBS because neural antigens may be released and exacerbate the illness. This is the putative mechanism for post-surgical GBS. However, among patients having a tracheostomy and/or gastrostomy during the first 3 weeks of illness we have found no evidence of an increase in limb or respiratory weakness. Several other minor procedures including nerve biopsies have also been free of adverse effect.

RESPIRATORY CARE

Mechanisms of mechanical ventilatory failure in acute generalized paralysis

An understanding of the mechanism of mechanical or 'bellows' respiratory failure allow prevention of most pulmonary complications. Although it is generally assumed that the hallmark of mechanical ventilatory failure is hypercarbia, this is a very late finding and treatment should be instituted prior to its occurrence.

Mechanical respiratory failure in GBS is distinguished from parenchymal pulmonary failure, such as pneumonia, by two major features: atelectasis and respiratory muscle fatigue. The usual sequence of events in mechanical failure is as shown in *Figure 2.1*. As weakness progresses, the ability to make intermittent large

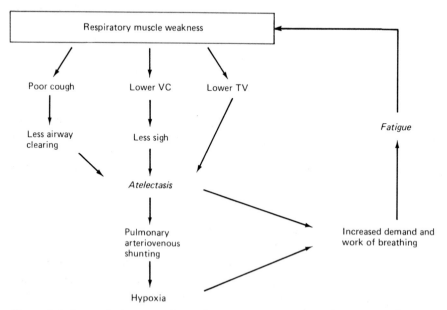

Figure 2.1 As respiratory muscle weakness progreses atelectasis occurs and leads to mild hypoxia as the earliest sign. Muscle fatigue plays a dynamic role in worsening respiratory failure and atelectasis. The chest X-ray is normal during this cycle

volume sighs is lost. Sighs are negative pressure pleural based breaths that keep the peripheral alveoli open. There is also a loss of the force and effectiveness of coughing and this prevents adequate airway clearing. The loss of sigh and cough together cause progressive miliary atelectasis in the periphery of the lung; this is not visible radiographically. When miliary atelectasis begins the patient is usually asymptomatic and the blood gases are normal or minimally hypoxic. As weakness progresses and tidal volume breaths diminish, more and more alveoli collapse for longer portions of the respiratory cycle. The respiratory rate increases slightly to compensate for this so that PCO_2 initially remains normal. Because atelectatic alveoli are still being perfused, a 'shunt' is created in which under-oxygenated blood returns to the left heart and lowers the arterial oxygen tension. Therefore, the earliest laboratory sign of subacute mechanical ventilatory failure in evolving GBS is mild hypoxia due to atelectasis, not hypercarbia (Ringel and Carroll, 1980). In acute ventilatory failure occurring over minutes to hours, hypercarbia and hypoxia occur simultaneously but, as a general rule, mild hypoxia is the first laboratory sign of mechanical bellows failure. We emphasize again that during this early state the chest X-ray is normal.

There is another very significant feature of bellows failure which many clinicians do not appreciate – the dynamic contribution of respiratory muscle fatigue. In patients who are slowly weakening there is a drive to maintain CO_2 exchange as tidal volume decreases. Already weakened respiratory muscles, particularly the diaphragm, quickly fatigue when stressed in this way (Roussos and Macklem, 1982; *Figure 2.1*). Thus, even with no further deterioration of the underlying process in GBS, myasthenia or botulism there may be very rapid respiratory failure from muscle fatigue. Fatigue is easily detected by physical examination. In most patients the stress of increased work of breathing is reflected by brow sweating and mild tachycardia. Once diaphragm fatigue has occurred, abdominal breathing becomes paradoxical with abdominal inversion during inspirations. This is soon followed by respiratory arrest. The reason for emphasizing the early appearance of fatigue and hypoxia in mechanical ventilatory failure is because of the need for intubation and positive pressure ventilation at this point, prior to the occurrence of a spiral of increased ventilatory demand and severe fatigue. This turning point is somewhere near a vital capacity of 15 ml/kg (*Figure 2.2*), but may be higher if fatigue is just beginning or there is already significant hypoxia. The clinical signs of increased work of breathing should always be heeded. Fatigue is also the reason for some late deteriorations in vital capacity after weakness has reached a plateau.

Monitoring respiratory and bulbar function

Several sophisticated measurements of the power generated by the respiratory bellows are available, such as airway occlusion pressures, but they are not practical for routine use (Black and Hyatt, 1969; Tanner, 1980). The methods generally used for monitoring mechanical respiratory function are inspiratory vital capacity, expiratory vital capacity and maximum inspiratory force. Expiratory pressure is said to reflect limb muscle power more closely than expiratory vital capacity

(Griggs *et al.*, 1981) but the former measurement tends to be less consistent from test to test. The results of any of these tests performed consecutively may vary as much as 25% especially at low lung volumes, and bellows spirometers consistently underestimate vital capacity compared with other devices. The most important contributing factor to consistent measurements is having the same examiner. For the expiratory vital capacity maneuver the patient is exhorted to take as large a breath as possible over 2 seconds (not longer) and to exhale over 2–5 seconds (not longer) and then vice versa for inspiratory vital capacity. The patient's nose is held closed to avoid volume loss due to bulbar weakness. If there is facial weakness the lips are sealed around the mouthpiece by holding them closed. An error may be introduced by changing meters between tests. The most commonly used Wright spirometer is somewhat insensitive at the low flow rates typical in these patients. Air loss through the nose and around the mouthpiece, and the insensitivity of some devices, all combine to underestimate vital capacity, but so long as these deficits are minimized and the test is performed in a consistent manner, the measurements are useful in a longitudinal way. It is exceedingly important to have a patient perform inspiratory exercises after the vital capacity maneuver in order not to promote atelectasis.

Respiratory measurements must be combined with observation of physical signs. As noted above, incipient respiratory muscle fatigue is indicated by brow sweat, tachycardia and inspiration in the middle of brief spoken sentences. Later, paradoxical diaphragmatic respirations appear. Because intubation should be performed well before severe respiratory failure occurs, there is generally no need for hourly or 2-hourly determinations of vital capacity. At night it is preferable to allow patients to sleep for at least 4 hours and to avoid awakening for pulmonary function tests since rest enhances performance.

Bulbar dysfunction is difficult to quantify, but its severity generally follows facial and respiratory weakness more closely than limb or oculomotor weakness. As a rule, aspiration of saliva is more frequent than observation of the gag reflex suggests. Therefore, intubation without mechanical ventilation is justified as a precautionary measure in many GBS patients. Large nasogastric tubes increase pharyngeal dysfunction and aspiration. The use of methylene blue mixed with custard or jelly and its recovery from tracheal aspirates is an undependable guide to aspiration. A physician observing the patient for coughing and sputtering after each swallow is the best means of gauging the ability to swallow. Feeding should not be attempted for at least 24 hours after extubation because of depressed pharyneal reflexes. Patients with tracheostomies who have apparently good bulbar function may be fed soft solids carefully.

Respiratory care plan and respirators

With the above notions of mechanical ventilatory failure and airway protection in mind, a reasonable and conservative respiratory care plan is outlined in *Figure 2.2.* The major points are:

(1) A need for aggressive chest physical therapy and inspiratory exercises when the cough and sigh are diminished
(2) Intubation for airway protection from bulbar weakness or if there is a need for positive pressure ventilation (VC = 15 ml/kg)
(3) Varying degrees of positive pressure ventilation as CO_2 exchange fails, ending in full mechanical ventilation when vital capacity is below about 5 ml/kg.

A few points about ventilators should be familiar to neurologists caring for these patients. A large tidal volume is required in order to prevent atelectasis. This essentially replaces the normal sigh mechanism. As opposed to the normal 5–8 ml/kg tidal volume, mechanical breaths of 15 ml/kg are used. Generally,

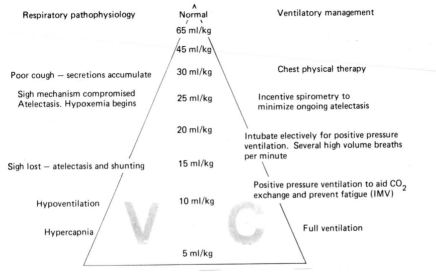

Respiratory pathophysiology | Normal 65 ml/kg | Ventilatory management

Poor cough — secretions accumulate — 30 ml/kg — Chest physical therapy

Sigh mechanism compromised Atelectasis. Hypoxemia begins — 25 ml/kg — Incentive spirometry to minimize ongoing atelectasis

20 ml/kg — Intubate electively for positive pressure ventilation. Several high volume breaths per minute

Sigh lost — atelectasis and shunting — 15 ml/kg

Positive pressure ventilation to aid CO_2 exchange and prevent fatigue (IMV)

Hypoventilation — 10 ml/kg

Hypercapnia — Full ventilation

5 ml/kg

Figure 2.2 The management of patients with mechanical-bellows ventilatory failure is guided by an understanding of respiratory pathophysiology. Approximate vital capacity levels are shown corresponding to each event during deterioration. The central value is approximately 12–15/kg at which point most patients should soon be intubated and ventilated. (From Ropper, 1983a, courtesy of the Publishers, *Neurological and Neurosurgical Intensive Care*)

5–10 cm H_2O of positive end expiratory pressure (PEEP) are applied to replace the end expiratory pressure usually provided by the closed mouth and lips. Initially, only 2–3 breaths per minute are required in order to prevent ongoing atelectasis and respiratory muscle fatigue, but as mechanical failure proceeds, full ventilation at 6–9 breaths is required. The therapeutic goals are to maintain an arterial Po_2 of 100 torr and Pco_2 of 40 torr, but at the same time, allow the patient to use as much of the normal respiratory apparatus as possible without fatiguing. As a rule of thumb, normal lungs require 90 ml/kg/min of ventilation to provide a Pco_2 of 40 torr (at normal body temperature). Many patients experience dyspnea at the lower than normal ventilator rates of 6–9 per minute. Reassurance and checking blood gases and endotracheal tube position are all that is necessary. Humidification should be provided with mechanical ventilation, and the air temperature must be kept close to 37°C to prevent mucus inspissation and endotracheal drying.

Volume cycled ventilators are the only type used because they are more dependable and far more comfortable for the patient than pressure cycled machines. We feel strongly that synchronized intermittent mandatory ventilation (IMV) is preferable to controlled or unsynchronized ventilation. In the synchronized IMV mode the machine assures that the preset rate and volume of gas will be exchanged each minute, but it will do so simultaneously with the patient's efforts. This allows for an optimal ventilator rate and keeps the patient working without producing the excessive drive that leads to fatigue. It also avoids ill-timed ventilator breaths that fight the patient or superimpose breaths at end-inspiration. IMV greatly facilitates weaning.

Negative pressure or curass ventilators derived from the iron lung have a theoretical advantage in mechanical ventilatory failure. They have not been used because of their unreliability and awkwardness and because many patients with generalized paralysis require endotracheal intubation for bulbar paresis and pulmonary toilet.

Weaning

Weaning from the ventilator requires a great deal of judgement from the neurologist. Weaning begins with the use of the IMV ventilator mode rather than totally controlled ventilation, since the IMV rate may be adjusted to allow the patient to use his own muscles as much as possible. It is generally stated that successful weaning is associated with a spontaneous vital capacity of greater than 15 ml/kg, an inspiratory force of greater than -20 cm H_2O, and an arterial PO_2 of greater than 100 torr with an inspired oxygen tension of 40%. These criteria, however, were designed for patients with parenchymal pulmonary disease and do not fully take into account the prominent mechanical fatigue of patients with neuromuscular problems. It has been suggested that a more dynamic measure such as the ability to voluntarily double the resting minute ventilation (amount of air moved in one minute) or maximum flow rates (Tanner, 1980) are better tests of the ability to wean. We have found that the best way to handle weaning is to attempt to lower slowly the IMV rate once the vital capacity has reached about 8 ml/kg. If the patient fatigues or blood gases show hypoxia then the rate is again raised. Mild hypercarbia (less than 50 torr) is tolerated if the patient is comfortable. Weaning is generally held to a decrease of 1 or 2 breaths per day and may proceed by one-half breath per minute increments in patients with vital capacity between 8 and 10 ml/kg. It is well to rest patients at night with one or two extra breaths per minute. Most patients will wean totally when vital capacity exceeds 18 ml/kg and many are successfully weaned at 14–16 ml/kg because they do not fatigue as they did when the illness was initially progressing.

Some patients with GBS who are expected to wean as indicated by respiratory measurements do not tolerate lowering the ventilator rate. Prolonged ventilation occasionally produces a neurological dependence on the machine, wherein the nervous system seems incapable of producing normal, well-coordinated, spontaneous breaths. In this 'dyscoordination syndrome' the abdominal muscles and diaphragm move inwards during inspiration (paradoxical respiration) and breathing is ineffective. The patient appears to be struggling against an airway obstruction but investigation does not demonstrate a block. Dyscoordination of some degree is very frequent in GBS and may be related to autonomic neuropathy and/or vagal disturbance. Time and continued attempts at weaning with IMV eventually restore normal breathing.

Marginally ventilating patients who can be weaned to an IMV rate of 1–2 breaths/minute can frequently be weaned off the ventilator simply by switching from a modern machine to an older model such as the Emerson. This is because newer models have an electronic switch for IMV that closes off the ventilator circuit when the patient breathes spontaneously. This requires the patient to first pull open the switch and then suck air from a compartment in which pressure drops as the patient inspires. Older machines have a large reservoir bag into which air flows at high rates and precludes the need for opening a switch or sucking gas under low pressures. These amenities decrease the work of breathing and prevent fatigue. One problem with older respirators is that they have inadequate alarm systems for mechanical failure and apnea.

Other factors such as hypokalemia with alkalosis, poor nutritional state and particularly fever, may interfere with weaning and should be considered if a GBS patient fails to wean. Insensitivity to CO_2 or sleep apnea has not been a problem in our patients.

SPECIFIC THERAPY FOR GBS

Although corticosteroids are theoretically an attractive treatment for GBS, there is no convincing evidence beyond anecdote that they are effective. The major randomized study by Hughes *et al.* (1978) suggested that prednisolone had no beneficial effect in acute GBS. In addition to previous criticisms on Hughes' study (the small sample size and differing entry times between treated and control groups) it should be emphasized that the statistical power of this study is very low, i.e. the chances of a Type II, or false negative error, are large. It probably can be stated that if there is a beneficial effect, it is not likely to be very strong. There is a suggestion in the Hughes study, seconded by others, that steroid use contributes to relapses. There are, however, enough instances of dramatic improvement after steroid or ACTH administration (McQuillen and Swick, 1978) to leave this question unresolved.

Following the report by Brettle *et al.* (1978) of apparent improvement in acute GBS after plasma exchange, other anecdotal reports have followed (Ropper, Shahani and Huggins, 1980). There have even been reports of improvement after hemodialysis (Vital *et al.*, 1980). A large multicentered trial of plasma exchange is almost completed at the time of writing. If the results are unfavorable, then the same problems that plagued the interpretation of steroid trials may pertain. An opinion can only be offered based on our experience in which virtually every measure of outcome has been better in the treated group (*Table 2.2*). A larger cohort than is available from our hospital is necessary to make firm conclusions but we feel that, on balance, the treatment is effective if used with attention to the details below. This is subject to revision as the results of larger trials become available. There have been many patients who undergo plasma exchange early in the course of weakness and continue to deteriorate. Others have stopped worsening, and yet others have improved substantially within 48 hours of beginning a series of exchanges. These results may approximate to the expectations of a large group of GBS patients, but those few in whom quadriplegia and complete ventilatory failure quickly reverse exceed our previous experience.

Table 2.2 MGH patients (unable to walk without assistance-grade 3) randomized to plasma exchange compared with conventional therapy as of 12/82

	Treated	*Conventional*
No. of patients	10	10
Grade at protocol	4.0 ± 0.8	3.9 ± 0.6
Age	42 ± 18	45 ± 14
CSF protein/g/l	1.09 ± 0.64	0.71 ± 0.44
CSF cells/μl	1.4 ± 2.2	3.5 ± 8.7
Days hospitalized	27 ± 11	52 ± 44
Days in intensive care unit	13 ± 9 (9)	26 ± 25 (8)†
Days on ventilator	12 ± 11 (5)	74 ± 54 (4)†
Days to one grade improvement	20 ± 25	45 ± 45
Deaths	0	1 (sepsis)
Grade 2 in < 100 days*	10/10	6/10
Grade 0 or 1 at 6 months	10/10	6/10
Relapse	0	1

* Able to walk independently but weak. † Numbers in parenthesis refer to number of patients requiring intensive care unit care or mechanical ventilation

If plasma exchange proves to be useful, then several points are worth mentioning. Virtually all of our apparently excellent responses were in patients exchanged within the first 10 days of symptoms and with 170–200 ml/kg removed over one week in three to four exchanges. Smaller exchanged volumes or starting later seem to be less effective. About one-half of patients, whether they have sustained improvement or not, experience a brief improvement in power and vital capacity a few hours after the exchange. The side effects of plasma exchange have been minor and subcutaneous heparin administration to prevent thromboembolism has not caused untoward difficulties. Acral and peri-oral paresthesias are very common and reversed by calcium infusion. Patients may become hypotensive and in some this appears to be related to an autonomic neuropathy. It has been suggested that replacement of removed plasma with fresh frozen plasma is effective where albumin and saline are not.

The final word on diagnosis and specific therapy for GBS awaits the identification of those immunologic factors responsible for inciting demyelination. Even if the disease process can be stemmed, we believe that attention to the pertinent details of neurological intensive care will continue to provide the best overall program for patients with GBS and other generalized paralytic illnesses.

Acknowledgements

The authors wish to thank Dr Bradley Truax of the Department of Neurology at the State University of New York at Buffalo for allowing the use of patient data from the MGH retrospective series, and the plasma exchange group at the Massachusetts General Hospital for their interest and support: Drs Charles Huggins, Rita Addison, Kathy Kosinski and Jettie Hunt.

References

Appenzeller, O. and Marshall, J. (1963) Vasomotor disturbances in Landry-Guillain Barré syndrome. *Archives of Neurology*, **9**, 368–372

Arnason, B. (1975) Inflammatory polyradiculoneuropathies. In *Peripheral Neuropathy*, edited by P. J. Dyck, P. K. Thomas and E. H. Lambert, pp. 1110–1148. Philadelphia: W. B. Saunders

Arnason, B. and Asbury, A. (1968) Idiopathic polyneuritis following surgery. *Archives of Neurology*, **18**, 500–507

Asbury, A. K. (1981) Diagnostic considerations in Guillain-Barré syndrome. *Annals of Neurology*, **9**(Suppl.), 1–5

Black, L. F. and Hyatt, R. E. (1969) Maximal static respiratory pressures in generalized neuromuscular disease. *American Review of Respiratory Diseases*, **99**, 696–702

Brettle, R., Gross, M., Legg, N., Lockwood, M. and Pallis, C. (1978) Treatment of acute polyneuropathy by plasma exchange. *Lancet*, **2**, 1100

Fergusson, R. J., Wright, D. J., Willey, R. F., Crompton, G. K. and Grant, I. W. (1981) Suxamethonium is dangerous in polyneuropathy. *British Medical Journal*, **282**, 298–299

Fisher, C. M. (1956) An unusual variant of acute idiopathic polyneuritis (syndrome of ophthalmoplegia, ataxia and areflexia). *New England Journal of Medicine*, **255**, 57–65

Frison, J., Sanchez, L., Garnacho, A., Bolfill, J., Olivero, R. and Miquel, C. (1980) Heart rate variations in the Guillain-Barré syndrome. *British Medical Journal*, **281**, 694

Furlan, A., Hanson, M., Cooperman, A. and Farmer, R. (1975) Acute areflexic paralysis. Association with hyperalimentation and hypophosphatemia. *Archives of Neurology*, **32**, 706–707

Gauthier-Smith, P. C. (1965) Neurological complications of glandular fever (infectious mononucleosis.). *Brain*, **88**, 323–334

Griggs, R., Donohue, M., Utell, M., Goldblatt, D. and Moxley, R. (1981) Evaluation of pulmonary function in neuromuscular disease. *Archives of Neurology*, **38**, 9–12

Griswold, K., Guanci, M. and Ropper, A. (1983) Care of the patient with Guillain-Barré syndrome. *Heart and Lung* (in press)

Grunnet, M. and Lubow, M. (1972) Ascending polyneuritis and ophthalmoplegia. *American Journal of Ophthalmology*, **74**, 1155–1160

Hughes, R., Newsom-Davies, J., Perkins, G. and Pierce, J. (1978) Controlled trial of prednisolone in acute polyneuropathy. *Lancet*, **2**, 750–753

Hussey, F., Schanzer, B. and Katzman, R. (1970) A simple manometric test for measurement of CSF absorption. II. Clinical studies. *Neurology*, **20**, 605–680

Jampel, R. and Haidt, S. (1972) Bell's phenomenon and acute idiopathic polyneuritis. *American Journal of Ophthalmology*, **74**, 145–153

Kimura, J. and Butzer, J. (1975) F-wave conduction velocity in Guillain-Barré syndrome. *Archives of Neurology*, **32**, 524–529

Lauffer, J., Passwell, J., Kern, G. *et al.* (1981) Raised plasma review activity in the hypertension of the Guillain-Barré syndrome. *British Medical Journal*, **282**, 1272–1273

Lichtenfield, P. (1971) Autonomic dysfunction in the Guillain-Barré syndrome. *American Journal of Medicine*, **50**, 772–780

Loeffel, N., Rossi, L., Mumenthaler, M., Luetsch, J. and Ludintt, P. (1977) The Landry-Guillain-Barré syndrome. Complications, prognosis and natural history in 123 cases. *Journal of Neurological Sciences*, **33**, 71–79

McQuillen, M. and Swick, H. (1978) ACTH in Guillain-Barré syndrome. *Lancet*, **2**, 1209

Morley, J. and Reynolds, E. (1966) Papilloedema and the Landry-Guillain-Barré syndrome. Case reports and a review. *Brain*, **89**, 205–222

Pace, N. L. (1976) Cardiac monitoring and demend pacemaker in Guillain-Barré syndrome. *Archives of Neurology*, **33**, 374

Ravn, .H. (1967) The Landry-Guillain-Barré syndrome. *Acta Neurologica Scandinavica*, **30**, 8–64

Richter, R. B. (1962) The ataxic form of polyradiculoneuritis. *Journal of Neuropathology and Experimental Neurology*, **21**, 171–184

Ringel, S. P. and Carroll, J. E. (1980) Respiratory complications of neuromuscular disease. In. *Respiratory Dysfunction in Neurologic Disease*, edited by W. J. Weiner, pp. 113–115. Mt. Kisco: Futura Press

Rodriguez-Iturbe, B., Garcia, R., Rubiro, L., Zabala, J., Moros, G. and Torres, R. (1973) Acute glomerulonephritis in the Guillain-Barré-Strohl syndrome. *Annals of Internal Medicine*, **78**, 391–395

Ropper, A. H. (1983a) Management of Guillain-Barré syndrome. In *Neurological and Neurosurgical Intensive Care*, edited by A. H. Ropper, S. K. Kennedy and N. T. Zervas, pp. 163–174. Baltimore: University Park Press

Ropper, A. H. (1983b) The CNS in Guillain-Barré syndrome. *Archives of Neurology*, **40**, 397–398

Ropper, A. H. and Shahani, B. T. (1983) Proposed mechanisms of ataxia in Fisher's syndrome. *Archives of Neurology*, **40**, 537–538

Ropper, A. H., Shahani, B. T. and Huggins, C. (1980) Improvement in four patients with acute Guillain-Barré syndrome after plasma exchange. *Neurology*, **30,** 361

Roussos, C. and Macklem, P. T. (1982) The respiratory muscles. *New England Journal of Medicine*, **307,** 786–797

Shahani, B. T., Domingue, J., Potts, F. and Ropper, A. (1980) Serial electrophysiological studies in patients with acute Guillain-Barré syndrome undergoing plasmapheresis. *Muscle and Nerve*, **8,** 440

Shahani, B. T., Lachman, T. and Young, R. R. (1975) Late responses as an aid to diagnosis in peripheral neuropathy. *Journal of Postgraduate Medicine*, **21,** 7–19

Shahani, B. T. and Sumner, A. J. (1981) Electrophysiological studies in peripheral neuropathy: early detection and monitoring. In *Clinical Neurophysiology*, edited by E. Stalberg and R. R. Young, pp. 117–144. London: Butterworths

Shahani, B. T. and Young, R. R. (1983) The blink reflex. In *Electrodiagnosis of Neuromuscular Disease*, edited by J. Goodgold and A. Eberstein, pp. 258–263. Baltimore: Williams and Wilkins

Shapiro, K., Marmarou, A. and Shulman, K. (1980) Characterization of clinical CSF dynamics and neural axis compliance using the pressure-volume index: I. The normal pressure-volume index. *Annals of Neurology*, **7,** 508–514

Smith, S. A. and Smith, S. E. (1980) Heart rate variations in the Guillain-Barré syndrome. *British Medical Journal*, **281,** 1009

Sobue, G., Senda, Y., Matsuoka, Y. and Sobue, I. (1983) Sensory ataxia: a residual disability of Guillain-Barré syndrome. *Archives of Neurology*, **40,** 86–89

Tanner, C. M. (1980) Respiratory dysfunction in peripheral neuropathy. In *Respiratory Dysfunction in Neurologic Disease*, edited by W. J. Weiner, pp. 83–112. Mt. Kisco: Futura Press

Vital, C., Aparicio, M., Brechenmacher, C. and Laurentjoye, L. (1980) Improvement of Guillain-Barré syndrome by hemodialysis. *Annals of Neurology*, **7,** 496

Weintraub, M. (1979) Autonomic failure in Guillain-Barré syndrome: value of Swan-ganz catherization. *Journal of the American Medical Association*, **242,** 513–514

Young, R. R., Asbury, A. K., Cobett, J. L. and Adams, R. D. (1975) Pure pandysautonomia with recovery: description and discussion of diagnostic criteria. *Brain*, **98,** 613–636

3
Chronic demyelinating neuropathies

Austin J. Sumner

INTRODUCTION

The chronic demyelinating polyneuropathies form a distinctive group which presents particular problems in diagnosis and treatment. Because of their protracted course and unpredictable response to known therapies, these patients are usually referred to specialized centers, where they have been the subject of intensive study in the last decade. A classification of these neuropathies is proposed in *Table 3.1*. The hereditary demyelinating neuropathies will also be addressed elsewhere (*see* Chapter 9), but are included here because of the difficulties which

Table 3.1 Classification of chronic demyelinating neuropathies

---

Hereditary
    (1) Hypertrophic Charcot-Marie-Tooth disease (HMSN, I)
    (2) Dejerine-Sottas disease
    (3) Refsum's disease
    (4) Leukodystrophies with neuropathy
        (a) metachromatic
        (b) globoid cell
        (c) Cockayne's syndrome

Acquired
    (1) Chronic inflammatory demyelinating polyneuropathy
        (a) relapsing
        (b) chronic progressive
        (c) monophasic
        (d) multifocal with persistent conduction block
        (e) Schwann cell inclusions with persistent muscle fiber activity
    (2) Chronic demyelinating polyneuropathy with paraproteinemia
        (a) benign gammopathies
        (b) multiple myeloma (especially osteosclerotic form)
        (c) Waldenstrom's macroglobulinemia

---

sometimes arise in clinical practice in differentiating hereditary from acquired forms of the disease. The demyelinating neuropathies associated with paraproteinemia are also covered in the section on neuropathy associated with systemic disease (*see* Chapter 5), but they are included here because they require special recognition and treatment. All patients with chronic demyelinating polyneuropathies share the diagnostic features of progressive neuropathy involving all four extremities, electrodiagnostic studies demonstrating slowed conduction velocities, and nerve biopsy findings of segmental demyelination and remyelination, usually leading to onion-bulb formations. The differentiation between hereditary and acquired forms of the disease is important in prognosis, genetic counselling, and in planning rational therapy.

Hereditary chronic demyelinating polyneuropathies

Demyelinating form of Charcot-Marie Tooth disease (hypertrophic peroneal muscular atrophy, hereditary motor-sensory neuropathy, type I)

Charcot and Marie (1886) in France, and Tooth (1886) in England, gave the first systematic descriptions of a slowly progressive hereditary disease characterized by wasting and flaccid weakness of the intrinsic muscles of the feet, and the muscles innervated by the peroneal nerve. With the introduction of motor conduction velocity studies, severe slowing of conduction velocity along peripheral nerve trunks was noted in some cases (Lambert, 1956; Gilliatt and Thomas, 1957; Gilliatt and Sears, 1958; Dyck, Lambert and Mulder, 1963; Amick and Lemmi, 1963). A few studies reported normal or near normal conduction velocities (Gilliatt, Goodman and Willison, 1961; Earl and Johnson, 1963). These differences were reconciled when Dyck and Lambert (1968) recognized that the results of nerve conduction studies allowed a separation of this clinical entity into two main types, the hypertrophic or demyelinating type, subsequently called hereditary motor sensory neuropathy type I (HMSN, I) in which there is marked conduction velocity slowing together with nerve biopsy findings of hypertrophic onion-bulb formation, and the neuronal type (HMSN, II) in which nerve conduction velocity is normal or near normal and nerve biopsy findings indicate only axonal degeneration. It is with the former type that we are concerned here.

CLINICAL FEATURES
Clinical symptoms are typically noticed before the age of 10 years, in contrast to the neuronal form in which symptoms often begin in middle life. The initial complaint is of fatigue during walking. Motor impairment is usually symmetrical. Marked weakness and atrophy is found in extensor digitorum brevis and other intrinsic foot muscles, and in anterior compartment muscles. Pes cavus is almost invariably present. Plantar extension is mildly affected in comparison with plantar flexion and clinically significant weakness of knee flexion or extension is only found late in the course of the disease. Ankle jerks are typically absent and knee jerks are depressed or absent. Upper extremity involvement is usually restricted to weakness and atrophy of the intrinsic hand muscles, the extent of which is not related to the

severity of lower extemity involvement. Occasionally patients have atrophy and weakness of scapular muscles (scapulo-peroneal form), (Harding and Thomas, 1980b), some have weakness of neck flexion and other patients have kyphoscoliosis.

Some degree of sensory involvement is usually present but it is seldom prominent, consisting typically of diminished light touch, vibration, and pinprick in feet and hands. The disease, although restricted in distribution, is progressive with a marked increase in distal weakness becoming apparent over 5-year intervals.

FAMILY HISTORY

This disease has a dominant inheritance but diagnostic problems often arise because of the heterogeneity of expression in affected kin or because a family history is not available due to adoption or for some other reason. Dyck, Oviatt and Lambert (1981) found that this was the most common chronic neuropathy that had previously gone undiagnosed; this usually occurred because of a failure to recognize affected kin. Index cases seldom had the classical well developed clinical features described above, and in some genetically affected kin the only indications of involvement were reduced motor conduction velocities and abnormal nerve biopsy findings. Dyck, Oviatt and Lambert (1981) stress the importance of clinical examination of relatives, including limited nerve conduction studies, if a hereditary etiology is suspected.

ELECTRODIAGNOSIS

In all the demyelinative neuropathies the demonstration of altered nerve conduction is the key to clinical diagnosis. This is particularly true of the hypertrophic form of Charcot-Marie-Tooth (CMT) disease where nerve conduction velocities are always slowed to less than 60% of normal values in each nerve examined. Buchthal and Behse (1977) studied the sural nerve sensory responses and compared them with the biopsy findings. In practice, motor conduction studies on an upper extremity nerve often prove more useful than motor or sensory studies on a lower extremity nerve. Denervation of extensor digitorum brevis is often complete, or so advanced that severe axon loss contributes to the reduced velocity recorded. In studies using the median nerve, a median motor conduction velocity of 38 m/s was the cut off value between the demyelinating and axonal forms of CMT disease. There was good concordance of motor conduction velocity within affected kinships (Thomas and Calne, 1974; Harding and Thomas, 1980a). Recently, the uniformity of the conduction slowing along the whole length of a nerve, the close correlation of values in two adjacent nerves in the same extremity, and the lack of differential dispersion, or conduction block, have been emphasized as electrodiagnostic features typical of hereditary demyelinating neuropathies. These features often allow a distinction between hereditary and acquired types (Lewis and Sumner, 1982).

PATHOGENESIS

The nature of the underlying metabolic defect responsible for hypertrophic CMT is unknown. Recent studies have shown that the genetic defect in this disease is linked to the Duffy locus on chromosome 1 (Guiloff *et al.*, 1982). The caliber of intermediate and large diameter axons of sural nerve is small relative to myelin thickness, to the number of myelin lamellae and to the length of the myelin spiral. This has been interpreted to mean that axonal atrophy is the primary pathologic change and that segmental demyelination and remyelination may be secondary in this disease. There is, however, evidence from grafting human sural nerve biopsies on mouse sciatic nerve to indicate that CMT Schwann cells are defective since they fail to myelinate regenerating mouse sciatic nerve fibers normally (Aguayo *et al.*, 1978).

TREATMENT

No specific treatment is known, and therapy is palliative. Foot elevating splints are helpful as foot drop becomes severe. Orthopedic procedures for tendon lengthening or transfer, and joint arthrodeses are sometimes indicated.

Refsum's disease (heredopathia atactica polyneuritiformis)

This is a recessively inherited disorder. Its clinical manifestations are a chronic peripheral neuropathy and retinitis pigmentosa (sine pigmentum) together with sensory-neural hearing loss, icthiotic skin changes, skeletal abnormalities and cardiac manifestations. These associated clinical features usually clearly distinguish Refsum's disease from the more common forms of chronic demyelinating neuropathy. Age of onset varies from early childhood to the third decade. A specific metabolic abnormality leading to accumulation of phytanic acid in nerve and other tissues is an essential finding for its diagnosis (Refsum, 1975).

Motor and sensory impairment occur in many degrees and combinations. Motor conduction velocity (MCV) in the majority of cases is substantially reduced, and this is directly related to prominent segmental demyelination. Other cases, however, show only mild slowing (Ulrich *et al.*, 1965; Sahgal and Olsen, 1975; Barolin *et al.*, 1979; Flament-Durand *et al.*, 1971) suggesting that the degree of segmental demyelination is not a primary feature of the metabolic abnormality, but perhaps an expression of its severity. There is some evidence that, unlike the other hereditary demyelinating neuropathies discussed in this chapter, in Refsum's disease the degree of peripheral nerve demyelination may vary greatly among affected members in the same family, and may even be more pronounced in proximal (roots and caudal equina) than in distal portions of peripheral nerves (Flament-Durand *et al.*, 1971).

Chronic inflammatory-demyelinating polyneuropathies (CIDP)

These disorders are considered to be a chronic variant of the Guillain-Barré syndrome (GBS). They share the histological features of scattered inflammatory lesions distributed in roots, plexi, trunks and nerve terminals, with associated distinctive electrophysiological features reflecting this variable multifocal distribution of demyelinating lesions. Other than the time course of evolution, the clinical features of the two entities (acute GBS and this chronic neuropathy) are similar. It is generally accepted that both disorders have an immunological basis largely from evidence gained from animal studies of experimental allergic neuritis induced by whole peripheral nerve myelin or purified antigens such as P2, or galactocerebro-side (*see* Whitaker, 1981; Saida *et al.*, 1980; Iqbal, Oger and Arnason, 1981; Cook and Dowling, 1981). The relevance of these models to a precise understanding of the human diseases remains uncertain (Zweiman *et al.*, 1983). It is well established, however, that some cases show a good response to immunosuppressive therapies. The diagnosis depends on recognition of non-hereditary chronic polyneuropathy with demyelinating features demonstrated by nerve conduction studies and inflammatory-demyelinating changes confirmed by nerve biopsy. Diagnosis also depends on eliminating other systemic diseases or toxic exposure associated with neuropathy.

CLINICAL FEATURES

The disease is seen in all age groups from childhood to late adult life with a peak incidence in the fifth and sixth decades. In most large series it is significantly more common in males than females. The course is steadily progressive, stepwise progressive or relapsing (Thomas *et al.*, 1969; Dyck *et al.*, 1975). Occasionally after an acute or subacute onset a chronic monophasic illness is encountered (Sobue *et al.*, 1983). In rare patients there is a history of preceding infection, immunization or receipt of biologic materials (sting or injection) within a few weeks of the onset of symptoms, or associated with relapses. Muscle weakness and sensory symptoms occur equally. Involvement is typically symmetrical, but cases presenting with a mononeuritis multiplex are recognized (Lewis *et al.*, 1982). Unlike the axonal polyneuropathies, proximal limb weakness is almost as pronounced as distal weakness, leading to complaints of difficulty in rising from a chair or lifting objects from overhead, as well as the familiar tripping or weakness of grip. Sensory symptoms of glove and stocking distribution usually implicate large fiber damage, at least initially during the process. This is described as numbness ('asleep' or 'tingling') while pain in hands and feet is much less common. Intercostal weakness and bulbar weakness are present in some patients. Additional occasional findings are papilledema, and palpable thickening of peripheral nerve trunks. A focal thickening associated with Tinel's phenomenon has been described in the multifocal form of this disease (Lewis *et al.*, 1982). This is often located in the median and ulnar nerve trunks of the upper arm and can be associated with focal conduction block which persists at the same site for months or years.

Approximately one-half of patients show a progressive course, one-third relapsing, and the remainder monophasic with the peak deficit persisting 6 months or more after onset. In the Mayo Clinic series of 53 patients followed for a mean of 7.4 years, 4% recovered, 68% remained ambulatory, 28% were confined to bed or a wheelchair, and in this group the death of six patients could be attributed to the disease (Dyck *et al.*, 1975).

ELECTRODIAGNOSIS

There is a pattern of nerve conduction changes that strongly suggests acquired demyelinating neuropathy, and allows a distinction between this and the chronic familial demyelinating neuropathies. These patients have differential slowing of conduction velocity when proximal velocities and distal latencies and equivalent segments of two nerves in the same limb are compared. Marked differential dispersion of the compound motor action potential is always present, and conduction block is frequently encountered (Lewis and Sumner, 1982). These latter features are particularly prominent in the subgroup identified as multifocal demyelinative neuropathy with clinical features suggesting a chronic mononeuritis multiplex. Here focal conduction block, which is usually identified in the upper arm, may persist for months or years, suggesting a focal area of demyelination with a persistent failure to remyelinate. The recognition of focal sites of conduction block in multiple nerves not located at regions of nerve entrapment is the key to diagnosis. This subgroup, in which the clinical deficits can be related closely to well localized sites of conduction block, offers particular advantages in studying efficacy of various therapies because objective electrophysiological measurements can be used to document response to treatment.

SPINAL FLUID

Spinal fluid lymphocyte count is usually normal although a few patients show an elevated cell count on at least one occasion.

CSF protein in excess of 45 mg/100 ml is found in most patients on at least one occasion. Protein levels are often elevated to several hundred mg/100 ml but an elevated protein level is not essential for the diagnosis, and may relate to the presence or absence of radicular inflammatory lesions.

NERVE BIOPSY

In clinical practice, cutaneous nerve biopsy is occasionally necessary for the diagnosis. Biopsy involves a choice of sural, superficial peroneal or superficial radial nerves. Electrodiagnostic evidence of involvement is important in selecting the biopsy site.

Histological abnormalities as recognized on paraffin and epon sections consist of mononuclear cell infiltrations, endoneural edema and onion-bulb formations. Mononuclear infiltrations are perivascular, or can be more diffuse in the endoneurium. They are found in about 50% of cases. Segmental demyelination is best recognized in teased fiber preparations (Dyck *et al.*, 1975; Asbury and Johnson, 1978). Myelinated fiber loss is usually obvious, but can be confirmed by axon counts per square millimeter of fascicular area.

TREATMENT

Corticosteroids

Since 1958 when Austin reported a case of recurrent polyneuropathy responding dramatically to corticosteroids, several reports indicate beneficial effects of corticosteroids in CIDP (Austin, 1958; DeVivo and Engel, 1970; Matthews *et al.*, 1970; Dyck *et al.*, 1978; Oh, 1978; Prineas and McLeod, 1976; Dalakas and Engel, 1981). Treatment is usually started with high single doses of prednisone 100 mg/day (1.5 mg/kg in children). After an initial 4 weeks of therapy, this dose is tapered over

3 months to a daily maintenance dose of 20–40 mg/day. Some authors favor alternate day therapy at this point, giving 100 mg on alternate days. This form of administration is said to minimize the side effects of cushingoid appearance, diabetes, osteoporosis and avascular neurosis. On either therapy a 'breakthrough' relapse is often encountered during the tapering period. Should this occur, an increase in dosage is usually required to bring the disease under control again. After a period of stabilization, the dose is again gradually reduced but this time more slowly as an optimal maintenance level is approached.

Side effects from this therapy are significant. Osteoporosis, especially in females, and cataracts are the most common. Avascular necrosis of the femoral or humoral head, gastric perforation or hemorrhage, and the activation of pulmonary tuberculosis are well known serious side effects. Hyperglycemia and hypertension develop in some apparently predisposed individuals.

Azathioprine
To date, there have been no reports of controlled clinical trials of azathioprine in CIDP. There are, however, several reports of small numbers of patients in which this agent has been useful (Yuill *et al.*, 1970; Cendrowski, 1977; Prusinski *et al.*, 1978; Walker, 1979; Dalakas and Engel, 1981; Portland *et al.*, 1982). In these series, azathioprine has been used in a dose of 2–3 mg/kg/day, often in combination with prednisone 1 mg/kg/day. It has usually been employed in seriously disabled patients who have failed a trial of corticosteroid therapy. It is also used in responders who require high maintenance doses of corticosteroids with its inherent risks. Azathioprine is a potentially hazardous drug and patients need careful follow-up with frequent monitoring of blood and platelet counts. Complications include lymphopenia, hepatotoxicity, increased rate of lymphoma, and increased susceptibility to infections.

Plasmapheresis
The role of plasma exchange in treating CIDP is as yet undetermined. Some cases show consistent response to this therapy (Tindall, 1982; Gross *et al.*, 1982; Toyka *et al.*, 1982; Server *et al.*, 1979). In a double blind trial in progress at the Mayo Clinic (Dyck *et al.*, 1982), some patients showed responses in both the treated and sham-treated groups, and it was considered too early in the trial to draw any conclusion, other than that a double-blind study is feasible and necessary.

Other therapies
There are a number of other therapies being employed in experimental clinical trials. These include antilymphocytic globulin (ALG), cyclosporin A, whole body irradiation and PolyICLC. None can be recommended at this time.

CIDP with paraproteinemia

An interesting group of patients with the clinical, electrophysiological, spinal fluid and histological features of CIDP have a circulating paraprotein, usually IgMk. In several instances the IgM has shown specific binding to a species-restricted myelin component, myelin associated glycoprotein (MAG). Although it is tempting to speculate that this antibody is responsible for the peripheral nerve demyelination, it has yet to be proven. One recent study has reported that intraneural injection of a patient's serum and of the purified IgM produced focal demyelination in cat sciatic nerve (Hays *et al.*, 1983). One aspect of the clinical findings that seems to be a prominent feature in many of these cases is the presence of sensory limb ataxia and tremor (Smith *et al.*, 1983). No consistent effect from lowering the serum levels of paraprotein by plasma exchange or other immunosuppressive therapy has been reported (Latov *et al.*, 1980; Abrams *et al.*, 1982; Dalakas and Engel, 1981b; Bosch *et al.*, 1982).

CIDP with osteosclerotic myeloma

The osteosclerotic form of multiple myeloma is uncommon. When it does occur, 50% of patients develop CIDP. Most of these patients have detectable levels of monoclonal serum proteins, all with lambda light chains, but the results of other laboratory studies are usually normal. Most patients also have organomegaly, endocrine abnormalities, or both (*see* Chapter 12). Treatment of solitary lesions with tumoricidal irradiation usually improves the neuropathy. Chemotherapy for multiple osteosclerotic lesions is less helpful (Kelly *et al.*, 1983).

References

Abrams, G. M., Latov, N., Hays, A. P. *et al.* (1982) Immunocytochemical studies of human peripheral nerve with serum from patients with polyneuropathy and paraproteinemia. *Neurology (NY)*, **32**, 821–826

Aguayo, A. J., Perkins, S., Duncan, I. and Bray, G. (1978) Human and animal neuropathies studied in experimental nerve transplants. In *Peripheral Neuropathies*, edited by N. Caval and G. Pozza, pp. 37–48, Amsterdam: Elsevier/North-Holland Biomedical Press

Amick, L. D. and Lemmi, H. (1963) Electromyographic studies in peroneal muscular atrophy. *Archives of Neurology*, **9**, 273–284

Asbury, A. K. and Johnson, P. C. (1978) *Pathology of Peripheral Nerve*, pp. 130–132. Philadelphia: W. B. Saunders Co.

Askanas, V., Engel, W. K., Berginer, V., Odenwald, W. F. and Galdi, Al. (1981) Lyosomal abnormalities in cultured Schwann cells from a patient with peripheral neuropathy and continuous muscle fiber activity. *Annals of Neurology*, **10**, 238–242

Austin, J. H. (1958) Recurrent polyneuropathies and their corticosteroid treatment. *Brain*, **81**, 157–194

Barolin, G. S., Hodkewitsch, E., Horfinger, E., Scholtz, H., Berneheimer, H. and Molzer, B. (1979) Klinisch-biochemische Verlaufsuntersuchungen bei Heredopathia atactica polyneuritiforms (Morbus Refsum). *Fortschritte der Neurologie und Psychiatrie*, **47**, 53–66

Bosch, E. P., Ansbacher, L. E., Goeken, J. A. and Cancilla, P. A. (1982) Peripheral neuropathy associated with monoclonal gammopathy. Studies of intraneural injections of monoclonal immunoglobulin sera. *Journal of Neuropathology and Experimental Neurology*, **41**, 446–459

Buchthal, F. and Behse, F. (1977) Peronseal muscular atrophy and related disorders, I. Clinical manifestations as related to biopsy findings, nerve conduction and electromyography. *Brain*, **100**, 41–66

Cammermeyer, J. (1975) Refsum's disease. Neuropathological aspects. In *System Degenerations and Atrophies*, edited by P. J. Vinken, G. W. Bruyn and J. M. B. V. DeJong, **21**, pp. 231–261. Amsterdam: Elsevier Scientific Publishing Company

Cendrowski, W. (1977) Treatment of polyneuropathy with azathioprine and adrenal steroids. *Acta Medica Polona*, **18**, 147–156

Charcot, J. M. and Marie, P. (1886) Sur une forme particuliere d'atrophie progressive souvent familiale debutant par les pieds et les jambes et atteignant plus tard mains. *Revue Medicale* (Paris), **6**, 97–138

Cook, S. and Dowling, P. (1981) The role of autoantibody and immune complexes in the pathogenesis of Guillain-Barré syndrome. *Annals of Neurology*, **9**, 70–79

Dalakas, M. and Engel, W. K. (1981) Chronic relapsing (dysimmune) polyneuropathy: pathogenesis and treatment. *Annals of Neurology*, **9**, 134–145

Dalakas, M. and Engel, W. K. (1981b) Polyneuropathy with monoclonal gammopathy: studies of 11 patients. *Annals of Neurology*, **10**, 45–52

DeVivo, D. C. and Engel, W. K. (1970) Remarkable recovery of a steroid-responsive recurrent polyneuropathy. *Journal of Neurology, Neurosurgery and Psychiatry*, **33**, 330–337

Dyck, P. J., Lais, A. C., Ohta, M., Bastron, J. A., Okazaki, H. and Groover, R. V. (1975) Chronic inflammatory polyradiculoneuropathy. *Mayo Clinic Proceedings*, **50**, 621–637

Dyck, P. J. and Lambert, E. H. (1968) Lower motor and primary sensory neuron diseases with peroneal muscular atrophy. I. Neurologic, genetic, and electrophysiologic findings in hereditary polyneuropathies. *Archives of Neurology*, **18**, 603–618

Dyck, P. J., Lambert, E. H. and Mulder, D. W. (1963) Charcot-Marie-Tooth disease: nerve conduction and clinical studies of a large kinship. *Neurology*, **13**, 1–11

Dyck, P. J., O'Brien, P. C., Oviatt, K. F. *et al.* (1978) Suggestive preliminary evidence from controlled 3 month clinical trials that prednisone improves chronic inflammatory polyneuropathy. *Annals of Neurology*, **4**, 165 (abstract)

Dyck, P. J., Oviatt, K. and Lambert, E. H. (1981) Intensive evaluation of referred unclassified neuropathies yields improved diagnosis. *Annals of Neurology*, **10**, 222–226

Dyck, P. J., Pineda, A., Swanson, C., Low, P., Windebank, A. and Daube, J. (1982) The Mayo Clinic experience with plasma exchange in chronic inflammatory-demyelinating polyneuropathy (CIDP). *Progress in Clinical Biological Research*, **106**, 197–204

Earl, W. C. and Johnson, E. W. (1963) Motor nerve conduction velocity in Charcot-Marie-Tooth disease. *Archives of Physical Medicine*, **44**, 247–252

Flament-Durand, J., Noel, P., Rutsaert, J., Tiussaint, D., Malmendier, C. and Lyon, G. (1971) A case of Refsum's disease. Clinical, pathological, ultra-structural and biochemical study. *Pathologia Europaea*, **6**, 172–191

Gilliatt, R. W., Goodman, H. V. and Willison, R. G. (1961) The recording of lateral popliteal nerve action potentials in man. *Journal of Neurology, Neurosurgery and Psychiatry*, **24**, 305–318

Gilliatt, R. W. and Sears, T. A. (1958) Sensory nerve action potentials in patients with peripheral nerve lesions. *Journal of Neurology, Neurosurgery and Psychiatry*, **21**, 109–118

Gilliatt, R. W. and Thomas, P. K. (1957) Extreme slowing of nerve conduction in peroneal muscular atrophy. *Annals of Physical Medicine*, **4**, 104–106

Gross, M. L., Legg, N. J., Lockwood, M. C. and Pallis, C. (1982) The treatment of inflammatory polyneuropathy by plasma exchange. *Journal of Neurology, Neurosurgery and Psychiatry*, **45**, 675–679

Guiloff, R. J., Thomas, P. K., Contreras, M., Armitage, S., Schwarz, G. and Sedgwick, E. M. (1982) Evidence for linkage of type I hereditary motor and sensory neuropathy to the Duffy locus on chromosome I. *Annals of Human Genetics*, **46**, 25–27

Harding, A. E. R. and Thomas, P. K. (1980a) The clinical features of hereditary motor and sensory neuropathy. Types I and II. *Brain*, **103**, 259–280

Harding, A. E. R. and Thomas, P. K. (1980b) Distal and scapuloperoneal distributions of muscle involvement occurring within a family with type I hereditary motor and sensory neuropathy. *Journal of Neurology*, **224**, 17–23

Hays, A. P., Takalsu, M., Latov, N. and Sherman, W. H. (1983) Focal demyelination of cat sciatic nerve induced by intraneural injection of serum from patients with polyneuropathy and monoclonal IgM reactive with myelin associated glycoprotein. *American Association of Neuropathologists*, June 9–12, Abstract 134

Iqbal, A., Oger, J. and Arnason, B. (1981) Cell-mediated immunity in idiopathic polyneuritis. *Annals of Neurology*, **9**, 65–69

Kelly, J. J. Jr., Kyle, R. A., Miles, J. M. and Dyck, P. J. (1983) Osteosclerotic myeloma and peripheral neuropathy, *Neurology (NY)*, **33**, 202–210

Lambert, E. H. (1956) Electromyography and electric stimulation of peripheral nerves and muscle. In *Clinical Examinations in Neurology*, pp. 237–317. Philadelphia: W. B. Saunders Co.

Latov, N., Gross, R. B., Kastelman, J. *et al.* (1980) Plasma cell dyscrasia and peripheral neuropathy with a monoclonal antibody to peripheral nerve myelin. *New England Journal of Medicine*, **303**, 618–621

Lewis, R. A. and Sumner, A. J. (1982) The electrodiagnostic distinctions between chronic familial and acquired demyelinative neuropathies. *Neurology (NY)*, **32**, 592–596

Lewis, R. A, Sumner, A. J., Brown, M. H. and Asbury, A. K. (1982) Multifocal demyelinating neuropathy with persistent conduction block. *Neurology (NY)*, **32**, 958–964

Matthews, W. B., Howell, D. A. and Hughes, R. C. (1970) Relapsing corticosteroid dependent polyneuritis. *Journal of Neurology, Neurosurgery and Psychiatry*, **33**, 330–337

Oh, S. J. (1978) Subacute demyelinating polyneuropathy responding to corticosteroid treatment. *Archives of Neurology*, **35**, 509–516

Pentland, B. (1980) Azathioprine in chronic relapsing idiopathic polyneuropathy. *Postgraduate Medical Journal*, **56**, 734–735

Pentland, B., Adams, G. G. W. and Mawdsley, C. (1982) Chronic idiopathic polyneuropathy treated with azathioprine. *Journal of Neurology, Neurosurgery and Psychiatry*, **45**, 866–869

Prineas, J. W. and McLeod, J. G. (1976) Chronic relapsing polyneuritis. *Journal of Neurological Science*, **27**, 427–458

Prusinski, A., Szulc-Kuberska, J. and Zawadzki, Z. (1978) A case of chronic Guillain-Barré syndrome treated successfully with azathioprine. *Wiadomosci Lekarskie*, **31**, 1545–1547

Refsum, S. (1975) Refsum's Disease. In *System Degenerations and Atrophies*, edited by P. J. Vinken, C. W. Bruyn and J. M. B. V. DeJong, **21**, 181–229. Amsterdam: Elsevier Scientific Publishing Company

Sahgal, V. and Olsen, W. O. (1975) Heredopathia atactica polyneuritiformis (phytanic acid storage disease). A new case with special reference to dietary treatment. *Archives of Internal Medicine*, **135**, 585–587

Saida, T., Saida, K., Silberberg, D. and Brown, M. (1980) Experimental allergic neuritis induced by galactocerebroside. *Annals of Neurology*, **9**, 87–101

Server, A. C., Lefkowith, J., Braine, H. and McKhann, G. M. (1979) Treatment of chronic relapsing inflammatory polyradiculoneuropathy by plasma exchange. *Annals of Neurology*, **6**, 258–261

Smith, I. S., Kahn, S. N., Lacey, B. W. *et al.* (1983) Chronic demyelinating neuropathy associated with benign IgM paraproteinaemia. *Brain*, **106**, 169–195

Sobue, G., Senda, Y., Matsuoka, Y. and Sobue, I. (1983) Sensory ataxia. A residual disability of Guillain-Barré syndrome. *Archives of Neurology*, **40**, 86–89

Thomas, P. K. (1975) Peripheral neuropathy. In *Recent Advances in Clinical Neurology*, edited by W. B. Matthews, pp. 253–283. Edinburgh: Churchill Livingstone

Thomas, P. K. and Calne, D. B. (1974) Motor nerve conduction in peroneal muscular atrophy. Evidence for genetic heterogeneity. *Journal of Neurology, Neurosurgery and Psychiatry*, **37**, 68–75

Thomas, P. K., Lascelles, R. G., Hallpike, J. F. and Hewer, R. L. (1969) Recurrent and chronic relapsing Guillain-Barré polyneuritis. *Brain*, **92**, 589–606

Tindall, R. S. (1982) The role of therapeutic apheresis in acute, relapsing and chronic inflammatory demyelinating polyneuropathy. *Progress in Clinical and Biological Research*, **106**, 205–217

Tooth, H. H. (1886) The peroneal type of progressive muscular atrophy. Thesis, Cambridge

Toyka, K. V., Augspach, R., Wietholter, H. *et al.* (1982) Plasma exchange in chronic inflammatory polyneuropathy: evidence suggestive of a pathogenic humoral factor. *Muscle and Nerve*, **6**, 479–484

Ulrich, J., Esslen, E., Regli, F. and Bishoff, A. (1965) Die Beziehungen der Nervenleitgeschwindgkeit sum histologischen Befund and peripheren Nerven. *Deutsche Zeitschrift für Nervenheilkunde*, **187**, 770–786

Walker, G. L. (1979) Progressive polyradiculoneuropathy. Treatment with azathioprine. *Australia and New Zealand Journal of Medicine*, **9**, 184–187

Whitaker, J. N. (1980) The protein antigens of peripheral nerve myelin. *Annals of Neurology*, **9**, 56–64

Yuill, G. M., Swinburn, W. R. and Liversedge, L. A. (1970) Treatment of polyneuropathy with azathioprine. *Lancet*, **2**, 854–856

Zweiman, B., Rostami, A., Lisak, R. P., Moskovitz, A. R. and Pleasure, D. E. (1983) Immune reactions to P2 protein in human inflammatory demyelinative neuropathies. *Neurology (NY)*, **33**, 234–237

4
Autonomic disorders: assessment and management
Otto Appenzeller and Ruth Atkinson

INTRODUCTION

The recognition of the clinical importance of autonomic accompaniments of peripheral nerve disease has been given impetus by the recent advent of simple objective tests to assess autonomic nervous system involvement. Many of these tests are now considered reliable, reproducible, simple and quick to carry out and, above all, non-invasive. Such criteria for values of tests of autonomic function are mainly fulfilled by those that test cardiovascular reflexes. Whether these tests reflect damage elsewhere in the autonomic nervous system is not definitively established, but suggestive evidence supports this view. It is of clinical and prognostic importance to assess autonomic damage in peripheral nerve disease, particularly in patients with diabetes mellitus, but the tests may be used to diagnose autonomic dysfunction caused by other disorders.

BASIC PRINCIPLES

The integrative activity of the autonomic nervous system is best seen in syndromes of autonomic failure which provide an opportunity to observe clinically the extensive ramifications of autonomic dysfunction. Although most patients with autonomic failure associated with peripheral nerve disease suffer from chronic autonomic insufficiency, there are some rare exceptions in which acute devastation of autonomic functions occurs and the normal adaptability of the nervous system has not yet restored partial function (Appenzeller, 1982).

AUTONOMIC ANATOMY

Visceral functions are regulated by peripheral and central neurons comprising the autonomic nervous system. In the past, it was thought that voluntary control of this system was totally absent, but it is now clear that volitional influences can affect autonomic function.

The autonomic nervous system includes all neurons lying outside the central nervous system that innervate viscera except the sensory neurons in posterior root ganglia and in some cranial nerve ganglia. Spinal cord, brainstem, and brain neurons that connect with peripheral autonomic neurons are also part of the autonomic nervous system, which is then subdivided functionally into sympathetic and parasympathetic divisions. Because the gut is richly innervated with autonomic neurons and may function without central control, a third division has been proposed – the enteric nervous system. This division contains ganglionated plexuses housing up to 10^8 neurons, which approaches the neuronal number within the spinal cord (Furness and Costa, 1981).

The neuroendocrine system, which regulates and releases hormones, is also included in the autonomic nervous system by some, and the hypothalamus or 'head ganglion' of the autonomic nervous system has a major role in endocrine function. The autonomic dysfunction discussed here relates to autonomic neurons lying outside the central nervous system. Those disorders of central autonomic pathways usually associated with other chronic neurologic syndromes are not included.

Acute disorders of autonomic function

Autonomic dysfunction may be acute or chronic. In acute pandysautonomia, autonomic activity throughout the body ceases acutely. Symptoms and signs include postural hypotension, fixed heart rate, absent sweating, dry eyes, nasal and oral mucus membranes, mid-position non-reactive pupils, absent bowel motility and hypotonic bladder. Laboratory studies are normal in this condition. The disease is self-limiting, at least symptomatically, and most patients eventually recover. The glucose tolerance curve may be diabetic and protein may be elevated in the cerebrospinal fluid. During this severe multisystem failure, mental function, extra-ocular motility, muscle strength and coordination, sensation, and deep tendon and superficial reflexes remain normal. The condition has been attributed to an immunologic insult against peripheral unmyelinated fibers. In the chronic stage of the disorder when clinical recovery is already present, nerve biopsies show many smaller than normal unmyelinated axons, suggesting regeneration of such fibers (Appenzeller and Kornfeld, 1973).

Chronic disorders of autonomic function

Cardiovascular deconditioning is an example of chronic, primary autonomic dysfunction and occurs in persons exposed to prolonged weightlessness or in patients bedridden for a time. Symptoms, primarily dizziness, may appear after resumption of normal daily activities and often take several days to disappear.

A primary affection of autonomic function, perhaps not exclusively related to the peripheral vegetative nervous system, occurs after drug therapy that interferes with autonomic activity. Examples include postural hypotension associated with antihypertensive therapy and the hyperthermia resulting from drugs which interfere with temperature regulation (sweating and vasomotor function).

Secondary disorders of autonomic function

These are associated with other diseases, but symptoms of autonomic failure may overshadow those caused by the underlying condition. Examples include diabetic neuropathy and severe postural hypotension, impotence, sweating abnormalities, and changes in pupillary reactivity. Similar changes plus sphincter dysfunction occur in patients with amyloid neuropathy.

Positive autonomic phenomena

Autonomic dysfunction can also manifest with positive phenomena. In tetanus, for example, hyperhidrosis accompanies hypertension and tachycardia and, in autonomic hyperreflexia due to spinal cord transection, bouts of hypertension, sweating, bradycardia, pupillary changes, and outpouring of catecholamines occur in response to non-specific stimuli of bladder filling stretch or peristaltic movements. Alternatively, autonomic paralysis may be associated with compensatory hyperactivity in normally innervated areas; for example, facial hyperhidrosis in patients with diabetic neuropathy and the segmental hyperhidrosis in partial peripheral nerve injuries. Autonomic function may be impaired in the paraspinous area when lung tumors invade the pleura, but hyperhidrosis occurs in such areas associated with tumor invasion of intercostal nerves.

Negative autonomic phenomena

These are common and include dizziness due to orthostatic hypotension, heat illness or heat stroke, susceptibility to accidental hypothermia, particularly in the elderly, anhidrosis in parts of the body, and sphincter dysfunction.

Special aspects of autonomic dysfunction

Because of the pervasive influence of the autonomic nervous system on all body systems, its failure affects the whole body and may seriously influence disease of other systems. The autonomic nervous system, in turn, can also compensate to some extent for dysfunction of other systems helping to preserve the body's functional integrity. This compensatory capacity declines with advancing age. Thus, thermoregulation may be reasonably intact under ordinary circumstances in patients with anhidrosis due to skin disease, for example. If the system is additionally stressed by excessive ambient temperatures, the compensatory abilities (vasodilatation) may not be sufficient to maintain normal body temperature. Similarly, with advancing age and decreasing cerebral blood flow secondary to atherosclerosis, slight postural falls in blood pressure (orthostatic hypotension) may result in transient neurologic deficits.

In the past, medical thinking has completely separated volitional from autonomic activity. More recently, however, it is clear that volitional changes in autonomic activity are possible with training, resulting in the widespread practice of biofeedback conditioning. Body temperature, heart rate, blood pressure, and sphincter control, to name a few, can be changed with this method, but its role in modifying autonomic activity and in treating disease is uncertain.

PATHOLOGY OF AUTONOMIC NEUROPATHIES

Autonomic nervous system pathology associated with peripheral neuropathies has been studied extensively in patients with diabetic neuropathy, and specific findings are few. Peripheral autonomic structures show change in a variety of patients with peripheral neuropathy and autonomic dysfunction, and the degree of alteration varies from case to case and at different sites. The major autonomic ganglia, the unmyelinated visceral fibers, the vagus nerve and smooth muscles are principally involved.

Changes in sympathetic ganglion cells

Abnormal neurons, found scattered throughout the sympathetic ganglia, are considerably larger than normal (giant sympathetic neurons), and often have rounded outlines and a peripheral nucleus; empty spaces are seen where ganglion cells have disappeared (Duchen *et al.*, 1980). Abnormal argyrophilic masses are frequently apposed to ganglion cells in the chain ganglia and occasionally continue along the axons and dendritic processes. Their origin is not known. Lymphocytic infiltrations, macrophages, and plasma cells are found along autonomic nerve bundles and ganglia. Unmyelinated axon tangles are occasionally found in Schwann cells in perivascular areas or abdominal organs. These nodules are contiguous with nerve bundles, resemble neuromas histologically, and may represent aberrant axonal regeneration.

Cell counts of spinal cord intermediolateral cell columns are reduced in patients with diabetic or alcoholic autonomic neuropathy.

The vagus nerve can be severely demyelinated in patients with diabetic and alcoholic neuropathies, attributed to a common demyelinating factor previously demonstrated in diabetic patients with peripheral nerve disease (Low *et al.*, 1975a, 1975b). Because of the heterogeneity of the findings (both degenerative and inflammatory) many etiologic factors must be considered in peripheral autonomic neuropathy, including toxic and immunologic insults.

CARDIAC DENERVATION IN AUTONOMIC NEUROPATHIES

Cardiac denervation has important clinical consequences although transplanted hearts function within limits without autonomic modulation. Heart transplants usually have a high resting heart rate without sinus arrhythmia because of the absence of vagal tone. During exercise, heart rate increases slowly and peak rates are achieved only after about five minutes; slowing of the heart rate on cessation of activity is comparably delayed. The heart rate changes are attributed to alterations in circulating catecholamines with exercise and not to autonomic activity. The denervated human heart function depends on the Frank Starling mechanism (the force of contraction is related to the stretching of heart muscle), and it therefore functions well enough, but the lack of sympathetic drive limits exertional increase in stroke volume, and the absence of vagal tone results in resting tachycardia. Most activities undertaken by heart transplant recipients are performed well, and circulatory needs are met by adjustments of stroke volume and by effects mediated by circulating catecholamines (*British Medical Journal*, 1980). Cardiac denervation due to autonomic neuropathy, particularly in diabetics where it has been most extensively studied, is a similar situation. Measurement of heart rate variation during deep breathing (sinus arrhythmia) has been used diagnostically as a test of autonomic function. In normal subjects the heart rate varies considerably during deep breathing, but these variations are absent in patients with autonomic neuropathy (*Table 4.1*), indicating parasympathetic damage.

Blackouts, faintness, and dizziness or visual obscuration on standing are frequent complaints of patients with autonomic neuropathy and reflect the effects of postural hypotension on brain perfusion. These symptoms are similar to those of hypoglycemia in insulin-treated diabetics but, if blood pressure is measured during the episodes, the postural hypotension leaves little doubt about the cause of the symptoms.

In managing patients with postural hypotension, one needs to consider the possible deleterious effects on blood pressure of a variety of drugs including hypotensive agents, diuretics, tricyclic antidepressants, phenothiazines, vasodilators and glyceryl trinitrate. Insulin can also aggravate postural hypotension, tentatively attributed to decreased venous return, altered capillary endothelial permeability and reduced plasma volume, or a direct insulin effect on the neurovascular junction. The advent of congestive heart failure or the nephrotic syndrome often improves existing postural hypotension.

Postural hypotension is generally attributed to lesions in the efferent part of the baroreflex arcs and the damaged fibers are thought to be in the sympathetic vasoconstrictors of the splanchnic bed, skeletal muscles and skin. Nevertheless, renal denervation may be associated with a diminished plasma renin response to standing and potentiation of the postural fall in blood pressure. Decreased basal and reflex outpouring of plasma norepinephrine on standing is also contributory. Occasional patients with diabetic autonomic neuropathy have elevated norepinephrine levels on standing and postural hypotension. The mechanism of this paradoxic situation is not known.

Resting tachycardia

In patients with postural hypotension a resting heart rate of 90–100 beats per minute has often been found, and rates up to 130 beats per minute occur (Watkins and Mackay, 1980). The explanation of this tachycardia was deduced from heart rate measurements in those with autonomic blockade or in patients with orthotopic cardiac transplants suggesting this to be due to parasympathetic denervation.

Table 4.1 Some useful tests of vegetative nervous function in man (from Appenzeller, 1982, courtesy of the Publishers, *The Autonomic Nervous System. An Introduction to Basic and Clinical Concepts*, 3rd Edn)

Test	Methods	Expected normal response	Lesion	Clinical signs or symptoms	Abnormal responses
Postural change in BP; Valsalva's maneuver; Lower body negative pressure	Sphygmomanometer; intra-arterial BP recording	No change in BP; 'overshoot' at end of Valsalva's maneuver or after release of negative pressure	Afferent, central or efferent baroreceptor reflex pathways	Symptomatic fall in blood pressure in acute stage, only rarely thereafter	Fall in BP on standing or tilt-up; no 'overshoot'
Radiant heating of trunk	Hand or forearm plethysmography or calorimetry	Vasodilatation, increase in blood flow	Skin receptors; afferents; central structures; efferents or blood vessels	?Sensory loss on heated area	No increase in blood flow
Application of cold to feet	Plethysmography of hand; BP recording	Reflex fall in blood flow within seconds; it accommodates increase in BP	Skin receptors; afferents; central structures; efferents or blood vessels	?Sensory loss on cooled area	No change in blood flow; no increase in blood pressure
Measurement of oral, rectal or external auditory canal temperature	Heating or appropriate weather conditions	Normal temperature	Central thermoregulatory mechanism, sudomotor or vasomotor fibers; skin disease	Confusion, coma, absence of sweating, dry hot skin	Hyperthermia
	Cooling or appropriate weather conditions	Normal temperature	Central thermoregulatory structures or efferent vasoconstrictor connections; metabolic disorders	Confusion, coma, cold skin, rigidity, absence of shivering	Hypothermia
	IV pyrogen	Fever	Central thermoregulatory structures or efferent vasomotor connections, ?hypothalamic or cord above sympathetic outflow		No fever

Table 4.1 continued

Prolonged heating of limb	Plethysmography or calorimetry of hand or forearm	Vasodilatation, increase in blood flow	Central thermoregulatory structures, efferent vasomotor connections or abnormalities in vessels	No change in blood flow
Body heating, monitor temperature in external auditory canal	Measurement of electrical skin resistance or observation	Fall in skin resistance, sweating	Central thermoregulatory structures, efferent sympathetic sudomotor connections or sweat glands	?Skin disease; heat intolerance · No change in skin resistance, no sweating
Mental arithmetic, noise, pain	Plethysmography of hand, intra-arterial BP recording	Fall in hand blood flow, rise in BP	Efferent constrictor fibers to skin vessels	No change
Passive elevation of legs in recumbent subjects, negative pressure breathing, squatting	Forearm plethysmography	Increase in forearm blood flow (decrease in constrictor tone)	Sympathetic vasoconstrictor fibers to vessels in skeletal muscle or blood vessels	No change in blood flow
Tilting from horizontal to standing, positive pressure breathing, Valsalva's maneuver, radial acceleration, hypercapnia, exercise of legs	Same	Decrease in forearm blood flow (increase in constrictor tone)	Same	No change in blood flow
Emotional stimuli, fright, mental arithmetic, pain	Same	Increase in forearm blood flow	Sympathetic cholinergic vasodilator fibers to skeletal muscle or blood vessels	No change
Observation of hairs on skin	Intradermal injection of acetylcholine	Piloerection	Postganglionic sympathetic nerves	No change

Table 4.1 continued

Test	Methods	Expected normal response	Lesion	Clinical signs or symptoms	Abnormal responses
Infusion of ephedrine or methylamphetamine into brachial artery, 50–500 µg/min	Plethysmography of hand	Fall in hand blood flow	Same	Hot, dry hand	No change
Measurement of finger temperature or heat elimination during cooling of fingers	Immersion in cold water	Alternating vasodilatation and constriction, Lewis's shunting reaction	Blood vessels	Evidence of blood vessel disease	No change
Intra-arterial (brachial artery) or intravenous norepinephrine, 30–10 µg/min	Plethysmography of hand or intra-arterial BP	Fall in blood flow, rise in blood pressure			No change
Intra-arterial (brachial artery) acetylcholine, 300–500 µg/min	Plethysmography of hand; observation	Rise in blood flow or flush			No change
Heart rate	IV atropine	Increase in heart rate	Vagus nerve or nuclei	Tachycardia	No change
Gastric acidity	0.01 U insulin/kg body weight	Increase in gastric acidity	Same		No change
Resting heart rate	Electrocardiogram	60–80 beats/min	Parasympathetic damage	Tachycardia 90–100 beats/min	
Beat-to-beat (R–R interval) heart rate variation during deep breathing	Deep breaths (6/min) record on instantaneous heart rate monitor; difference between max. and min. heart rates	≥15 beats/min	Parasympathetic damage		≤10 beats/min

Table 4.1 continued

30/15 Ratio	ECG recording; measure R–R intervals at beat 15 and 30 after standing	>1.03	Vagus nerve		≤1.00
Valsalva ratio	Blow into mouthpiece connected to manometer; maintain at 40 mmHg for 10 s (tubing has small leak) Longest R–R intervak after Valsalva/shortest R–R interval during Valsalva	≤1.21	Afferent, central or efferent baroreceptor reflex pathways	Symptomatic fall in blood pressure on standing acute stage; rare thereafter	1.11–1.20 (borderline) ≤1.10
Diving reflex	Facial immersion (cool water)	Bradycardia; apnea; increase in BP	Trigeminal nerve sensory distribution; carotid bodies; vagal reflexes (pulmonary); brainstem (inspiratory neurons; cardioinhibitory center); vagus efferents	Reflex cardiac arrest during intubation or respiratory toilet; asthma; dental procedures; chronic respiratory insufficiency; sleep apnea; Pickwickian syndrome; Ondine's curse; apnea-stridor-bradycardia syndrome	Tachycardia or no change in heart rate; no change or fall in BP

Cardiovascular reflex impairment in autonomic neuropathy

Valsalva's maneuver

Valsalva's maneuver is associated with tachycardia and peripheral vasoconstriction during the period of increased intrathoracic pressure which is then followed by an overshoot in the blood pressure and bradycardia after release of the high intrathoracic pressure. Measurement of intra-arterial blood pressure has hitherto been the standard method for assessing responses to Valsalva's maneuver, but is invasive. Heart rate changes are also reliable guides to the hemodynamic events during Valsalva's maneuver, are not invasive, and can be used to evaluate the response in those with suspected abnormalities of cardiovascular reflex function.

The standard technique for performance of Valsalva's maneuver is to ask the subject to blow into a mouthpiece connected to a manometer and to hold the pressure at 40 mmHg for 10 s. The mouthpiece has a slight leak to make it difficult to maintain inflation with a closed glottis without the pressure being transmitted to the intrathoracic structures. The subject is connected to an electrocardiogram which records continuously before, during, and after the maneuver. A 'Valsalva ratio' has been calculated from the ratio of the longest pulse interval (R–R interval) after the maneuver that reflects the overshoot bradycardia to the shortest R–R interval during the maneuver that reflects the tachycardia during the strain. A Valsalva ratio of 1:21 or greater is normal, 1:11 to 1:20 is borderline, and less than 1:10 is abnormal (*Table 4.1*). Accuracy of this test depends on the patient's effort and cheating is possible, but if this is excluded it gives reliable evidence of reflex abnormalities. Other methods of non-invasive assessment of cardiovascular reflex function in autonomic neuropathy include heart rate variation during deep breathing, during standing with measurements of the standard deviation, during lying with measurements of mean square successive differences, and after a single deep breath. The methods and their interpretations are given in *Table 4.1*. Additional measures of cardiovascular reflex function in autonomic disturbances include heart rate and blood pressure responses to standing and to sustained muscular exercise (*Table 4.1*).

DIVING RESPONSE

The diving response (not reflex) consists of apnea, peripheral vasoconstriction, hypertension, and bradycardia. It occurs in humans and in most air-breathing vertebrates during breath-holding while immersed in water. The response results from a number of reflexes and their interactions arising from stimulation of trigeminal receptors, and is partly volitional. Apnea causes arterial hypoxemia and hypercapnia which stimulate carotid and aortic body chemoreceptors to support and reinforce the cardiovascular reflexes. Stimulation of other body areas can produce similar responses. Reflexes arising in the upper airways protect against inhalation of noxious agents, and cardiac arrest may result from an exaggerated response during airway suctioning of patients on artificial ventilators.

Studies of this response in animals and man indicate negative inotrophic effects on the ventricles. The cardiac output falls proportional to the bradycardia, but blood pressure is maintained by increased peripheral resistance. In man, the vasoconstriction is predominantly in the trunk and limbs, and the cardiac output is diverted to the brain. The hemodynamic responses are most prominent in diving mammals and probably account for their ability to remain submerged at great depths for long periods. The nasal mucosa is another site capable of initiating the same reflexes via trigeminal receptors. Weak stimuli cause sneezing, but stronger stimuli can initiate the typical cardiovascular reflexes of the diving response. Stimulation of receptors in the larynx also results in redistribution of blood flow with maintenance of brain perfusion. Laryngeal reflexes are very potent in newborns and their activation may produce bradycardia and death.

The diving response plays a role in the capacity of professional divers to breath-hold at depths and also in survival in fetal asphyxia. Recovery after prolonged cold water immersion has been attributed to redistribution of blood to the brain in victims who were found apneic, bradycardic, cyanotic and hypothermic.

In normal individuals the temporary apnea of the diving response, together with central or reflexly induced asphyxia and consequent carotid body excitation, increases the risk of serious cardiac arrhythmias, bradycardia, cardiac arrest and sudden death (de Burgh Daly and Angell-James, 1979).

When the diving reflex is used to test autonomic function (*Table 4.1*) certain conditions are necessary. Immersion of the face into a pan filled with water which is below skin temperature is important in eliciting the proper reflex responses. Water must make contact with the face. Testing the diving response in patients with peripheral neuropathy and autonomic dysfunction may be dangerous.

CATECHOLAMINE LEVELS IN POSTURAL HYPOTENSION

Postural hypotension may be a symptom of several disorders that impede blood pressure maintenance against gravity. The specific mechanisms resulting in postural hypotension should be identified for successful therapy that is usually independent of the pathogenesis, but is effective if properly directed. Among the many possible causes of postural hypotension are abnormalities in catecholamine release to appropriate stimulation, specifically, norepinephrine. The primary neurogenic component of the circulatory response to orthostasis or exercise is an increase in sympathetic tone mediated by norepinephrine release, and this release may be seriously affected in a variety of patients with peripheral autonomic neuropathies. The finding of low circulating norepinephrine levels sometimes allows an educated guess about the pathogenesis of postural hypotension. For example, in patients with idiopathic orthostatic hypotension who have isolated autonomic dysfunction, norepinephrine is markedly depleted in peripheral neurovascular bundles. Such patients do not respond to tyramine, known to release norepinephrine from its stores, with the normally expected rise in blood norepinephrine, and during recumbency norepinephrine levels are low, reflecting the depleted tissue stores. On standing, the blood pressure drops; there is no associated increase in heart rate, and plasma norepinephrine is unchanged. Exercise also is not associated with increased circulating norepinephrine in these patients.

In patients with peripheral neuropathy and orthostatic hypotension, norepinephrine secretion is also less than normal in response to orthostasis and low levels are found during recumbency. In some neuropathies, particularly diabetic and uremic, intravascular volume changes are important in producing symptomatic orthostatic hypotension. If plasma volume effects are dominant, then the sympathetic response to standing may be greater than normal, a situation characteristically found in those with orthostatic hypotension due solely to volume depletion. In diabetics and uremics with mild neuropathy, norepinephrine levels may be high in response to orthostasis, and postural hypotension can occur in the presence of considerable tachycardia when the patient stands. In this situation, treatment is aimed at volume expansion only. A similar mechanism of postural hypotension exists in otherwise normal individuals, particularly during or immediately after physical activity in hot ambient conditions. Normal autonomic function results in norepinephrine release on standing and blood pressure falls due to volume depletion. In such individuals, high resting plasma norepinephrine and further increases in norepinephrine to very high values on standing occur without adequate maintenance of blood pressure and brain perfusion. Concurrent thorough neurologic examination, including the autonomic nervous system, gives useful information on the cause of the postural hypotension, whether it is related to drug therapy, diseased peripheral autonomic structures, abnormal autonomic integration, or perhaps volume depletion (Ziegler, 1980).

BLADDER DYSFUNCTION IN PERIPHERAL NEUROPATHY

Physiology and anatomy of the bladder and urethra

The urinary tract is innervated by the sacral parasympathetic nerves, the thoracolumbar sympathetic nerves, and sacral somatic nerves (predominantly the pudendal nerves). The parasympathetic sacral preganglionic fibers, the major excitatory input into the bladder, travel in the pelvic nerve and project on ganglion cells in the bladder wall. These cholinergic and/or purinergic (perhaps ATP) cells excite detrusor smooth muscle.

The sympathetic preganglionic fibers originate in the thoracolumbar spinal cord segments (eleventh thoracic to the second lumbar) and via the presacral and hypogastric nerves pass through the inferior hypogastric ganglion to peripheral adrenergic neurons to innervate the bladder and urethra. Stimulation of postganglionic sympathetic nerves causes norepinephrine release and excites the bladder trigone and urethral smooth muscle, but inhibits the vesical parasympathetic ganglia and detrusor muscles. The bladder afferent impulses travel via both somatic and autonomic fiber types in the pelvic nerves to the sacral cord and signal distention, which is primarily responsible for reflex activation of the detrusor muscle. Pain, on the other hand, travels in the pelvic and hypogastric nerves to the sacral and thoracolumbar spinal cord segments.

The somatic innervation of the external urethral sphincter (striated muscle) is via the pudendal nerve from the anterior horn cells in the third and fourth sacral segments. The pudendal nerve also carries efferent impulses to pelvic floor muscles and proprioceptive afferent signals from these muscles. Sensory input from the urethra is also via fibers in the pudendal nerve. Affection of both autonomic and somatic fibers in peripheral nerves may result in bladder dysfunction.

The motor neurons innervating the external urethral sphincter and pelvic floor muscles have a tonic activity which is inhibited by bladder filling and by urethral urine flow. Normal interaction between the urethra and bladder require relaxation of the urethral sphincters at the appropriate time during micturition. However, inappropriate contractions or failure of external or internal urethral sphincter relaxation, simultaneous with detrusor contraction, result in dysfunction termed detrusor-urethral sphincter dyssynergia, a feature of diabetic peripheral neuropathy. The treatment of this condition includes the use of centrally or peripherally acting muscle relaxants if excessive external sphincter activity (striated muscle) is the cause of the problem. On the other hand, if it results from internal sphincter (smooth muscle) dysfunction, adrenergic blockade is more appropriate.

Intact sympathetic supply to the lower urinary tract does not appear to be essential for micturition. Nevertheless, transection or pharmacologic blockade of sympathetic innervation reduces urethral outflow resistance, increases frequency of micturition, and causes a reduced bladder capacity in some persons. Animal experiments suggest that vesical sympathetic reflexes provide negative feedback in normal bladder activity. Thus, increased bladder pressure tends to increase the inhibitory input to vesical ganglia and smooth muscle, allowing the bladder to distend and accommodate to larger volumes. Sympathetic firing to the trigone and urethra complements the inhibitory mechanisms by increasing outflow resistance. For complete bladder emptying, these reflexes must be overcome by supraspinal controls. Use of phenoxybenzamine, an alpha-adrenergic receptor blocker, has, therefore, some value in decreasing urethral resistance in patients with bladder-sphincter dyssynergia and alpha receptor stimulation with ephedrine may decrease incontinence.

The autonomic ganglia on the bladder surface have unusual physiologic characteristics suggesting a potential for modulation of autonomic impulses. They contain adrenergic, cholinergic, and purinergic ganglion cells and adrenergic small intensely fluorescent cells. Animal studies suggest that the ganglion synapses function as gating circuits ('filters') that suppress excitatory input to the bladder when the intravesical pressure and preganglionic firing rates are low, but facilitate the neural input during micturition when preganglionic electrical activity is high. The electrical transmission characteristics of vesical ganglia seem appropriate for maintaining continence and for producing sustained, strong detrusor contractions during micturition.

Histochemistry of bladder ganglia shows that they receive dense innervation from adrenergic small intensely fluorescent cells that are predominantly directed at cholinergic ganglion cells. Exogenously and endogenously administered norepinephrine depresses transmission in the ganglia, primarily due to decreased acetylcholine release from preganglionic fibers and forms an important part of the vesical sympathetic negative feedback circuit.

Spontaneous activity has been recorded experimentally from isolated vesical ganglion cells. This activity may function in regional circuits and modulate peripheral reflexes.

The pathology of neurogenic bladder

Pathologic alterations in the bladders of diabetics closely resemble those described in sympathetic ganglia of patients with the same disease. Axon thickening and vacuolation of the thickened areas with spindle-shaped beaded appearances visualized by silver impregnation techniques have been described in severe cases of diabetic neuropathy. The changes were unrelated to inflammatory or vascular alterations which sometimes accompany the disease in patients with diabetic bladder dysfunction. Similar abnormalities were seen in the corpora cavernosa in impotent diabetic males and in the myenteric plexuses, particularly of the esophagus. The bladder wall ganglion cells show changes previously described including giant sympathetic neurons, shrunken nerve cells, hypochromatic ganglion cells and occasional empty spaces previously occupied by neurons (Mastri, 1980).

Neurogenic bladder involvement in diabetics (diabetic cystopathy) begins insidiously, and symptoms usually appear when the disease is advanced. Diabetic cystopathy and peripheral neuropathy occur together in 75–100% of patients, and some consider the presence of peripheral neuropathy a *sine qua non* for the diagnosis of diabetic cystopathy. On the other hand, in those who have peripheral nerve dysfunction, 83% have diabetic cystopathy on cystometric examination. Symptoms and signs of neurogenic bladder include residual urine from 90 to over 1000 ml (the definition of residual urine depending upon the investigator). The absence of the desire to void when the bladder contains over 500 ml and increased bladder capacity are indications of diabetic cystopathy. An obstructed bladder neck should be ruled out in the presence of the above abnormalities.

Characteristically, the patient with a diabetic neurogenic bladder has residual urine, infection, pyelonephritis, sepsis and azotemia. He may present with the complaint of increasing intervals between voiding, and urination may occur once or twice a day only. This is often accompanied by the need for straining to initiate and maintain voiding, weakness of the stream, dribbling, and a sensation of incomplete emptying. Many patients are oblivious to the symptoms and a proper history can be obtained only by direct questioning. Some present with abdominal or pelvic tumor, and differential diagnosis includes peritoneal metastasis, prostatic hypertrophy or intestinal obstruction. The diagnosis can be established by abnormal cystometric studies and a large amount of residual urine. The cystometrogram shows a long low pressure curve and no sensation of filling when bladder capacity is tested until bladder distention is greater than normal. Ureteral orifices are often incompetent, showing reflux during radiographic studies.

The treatment of diabetic cystopathy includes use of an indwelling catheter for 10 days together with appropriate antibiotics. Thereafter, the patient should void every 3 hours, aided by manual compression of the suprapubic area (Credé maneuver) and receive parasympathomimetic drugs. About 40% of patients respond to this therapy, at least temporarily, until urinary tract infection recurs. Transurethral surgery and bladder neck resection in those without obvious mechanical obstruction may also be useful. Initially, the parasympathomimetic drug can be given parenterally, for example, bethanechol twice weekly, and may be continued orally in a dose of 40–50 mg every 6 or 8 hours. Cholinergic treatment is withdrawn when residual volumes are less than 100 ml for at least a week (Ellenberg, 1980a).

SEXUAL DYSFUNCTION IN PERIPHERAL NEUROPATHIES

The sacral parasympathetic and thoracolumbar sympathetic nerves are efferent vasodilator nerves for penile vessels and are responsible for erection produced by arterial dilatation and increased blood flow to the erectile tissues. Erection is reflexly initiated by visual or olfactory stimuli, or by imagery that affect supraspinal centers, but it can also be achieved by gentle stimulation that reflexly activates spinal mechanisms. The parasympathetic nerves also stimulate secretion from the seminal vesicles and prostate including Cowper's glands during the plateau phase of the sexual response. Emission of semen, ejaculation, and the accompanying sensations occur during orgasm. Emission depends on sympathetic innervation of the urethra which initiates contraction of smooth muscles in the vas deferens, seminal vesicles and prostate. The rhythmic contractions of striated muscles including the bulbocavernosus and ischiocavernosus innervated by the pudendal nerves eject semen from the urethra. It is clear, therefore, that peripheral neuropathies involving the nerves controlling any phase of the sexual response in males or females lead to sexual dysfunction. Diabetic autonomic neuropathy of the pelvic parasympathetic nerves (nervi erigentes) accounts for about 60% of impotence in diabetic males, and diabetic men tend to become impotent at an earlier age than others. Psychologic factors are by far the commonest cause of impotence in the general population, but this is usually of sudden onset in contrast to diabetic impotence which progresses slowly. Neurogenic impotence is characterized by absence of erection at any time under any circumstances and is often associated with decreased testicular sensitivity, whereas in psychogenic impotence testicular sensation is unimpaired.

Many medications may cause impotence. These include estrogens used for the treatment of carcinoma of the prostate, alcohol, phenothiazines, antidepressants, and some of the antihypertensive agents, all drugs frequently used in patients with diabetes.

When the diabetes is poorly controlled, impotence can reflect malnutrition, wasting, and weakness and may improve with proper diabetic management. If psychogenic factors are associated with the decreasing potency, these should be appropriately managed and drugs affecting sexual function should be withdrawn. In many cases, however, the neurogenic nature of diabetic sexual dysfunction leaves no useful therapy and the prognosis is poor. Mechanical devices have been proposed and used, but their efficacy is difficult to evaluate (Karacan, 1980).

The diagnosis of erectile impotence can be aided by monitoring nocturnal penile tumescence; this can provide evidence of erectile capacity or lack thereof and establish the organic nature of impotence. Penile blood pressure in organic impotence is low and bulbocavernosus reflex response latencies are delayed, but the plasma concentrations of testosterone and prolactin are normal in such patients. These tests should be performed together with behavioral evaluation before penile prostheses for diabetic autonomic impotence are considered.

Sexual dysfunction in female patients with diabetic neuropathy

While the autonomic nervous system is similarly involved in females with diabetes mellitus, there is little to suggest that sexual dysfunction in females is common or troublesome. Careful studies indicate that diabetes has no effect on sexual performance in women. So far, no anatomic, neurologic, or physiologic differences have been identified to explain the observed differences in sexual function between the two sexes. Perhaps it is a psychologic aspect of sexual behavior that accounts for the remarkable differences in the effect of autonomic neuropathy in the two sexes (Ellenberg, 1980b).

SWEATING

Two types of sweating are recognized:

(1) Thermoregulatory sweating, which occurs over the whole body in response to environmental temperature changes or exercise;
(2) Emotional sweating, which is confined to palms, axillae, soles, and some parts of the face.

It is not entirely clear whether thermoregulatory sweating always depends on a rising blood temperature that activates central structures responsible for thermoregulation or whether a peripheral heat-sensitive receptor reflexly activates these central structures. Under certain circumstances, either of these mechanisms alone or combined may produce sweating and may be differentially affected in disease. An example of reflex peripheral regulation of sweating is the temporary inhibition of sweat secretion in a hot environment, achieved by applying ice to the skin, but sweating induced by the action of pilocarpine on sweat glands is not inhibited by cooling.

Microelectrode recordings from human cutaneous nerves show that sudomotor impulses occur in periods with intervals of about 0.6 seconds. The rhythmic sudomotor nerve activity corresponds to changes in electrodermal responses that measure skin conductance, which, in turn, depends upon sweat secretion. Therefore, sweat periodicity, well-documented in humans, is governed by sympathetic nervous activity. Evaporation rates correlate closely with discharge periodicity from cutaneous nerves.

Normal postural influences related to pressure on the skin affect the sweating rate reflexly. When a subject lies on his back in a hot environment, sweating occurs equally over the body. Lying on one side, however, increases sweating remarkably on the uppermost side and inhibits sweat gland activity on the other. Standing after recumbency induces sweating on the upper part of the body and inhibits it in the legs (Takagi and Sakurai, 1950). These hemihidrotic reactions can be activated readily by pressing the axillae or adjacent pectoral region, and the responses are limited either to the upper or lower half of the body separated by an ill-defined border adjacent to the iliac crests.

Faradic stimulation initiates reflex sweating; although it is not a physiologic stimulus to sweat glands, its peripheral mechanism induces sweating by the same means as normal innervation of the glands. Faradic-stimulation-induced sweating can be inhibited by atropine and augmented by prostigmine. It depends on a local axon reflex mediated by postganglionic sympathetic fibers involving many overlapping axonal systems.

The relationship of sweat secretion to cutaneous blood flow is complicated and varies from one body part to another. In some parts of the body, vasodilatation of skin vessels may depend on vasodilator substances in the sweat, and both of these thermoregulatory modalities occur concurrently. However, cutaneous vasodilatation in the hand in response to increased central temperature may be abolished in patients with the Landry-Guillain-Barré syndrome and yet sweating occurs normally in response to heat loads (Appenzeller and Marshall, 1963). In freshly amputated limbs without circulation, direct electrical stimulation of peripheral nerves produces sweating for some time after amputation.

Hyperhidrosis

In essential hyperhidrosis, the constituents of sweat and sweat gland morphology are normal. The etiology of essential hyperhidrosis is unknown and pharmacologic blockage of sweat gland activity has been unsatisfactory treatment for this condition. Sympathectomy cures the socially embarrassing sweating that usually starts in childhood, but does not become burdensome until adult life. If not treated surgically, hyperhidrosis lasts throughout life, and it is most troublesome when it affects the hands, feet, and axillae. Recently, abnormal vasomotor function has also been noted in some of these patients, and baroreflex activity becomes normal after surgical extirpation of the relevant sympathetic ganglia. Results of biofeedback therapy for essential hyperhidrosis are conflicting and, in cases in which it has been successful, the permanence of reduction in sweating has not been established.

Essential hyperhidrosis must be distinguished from secondary hyperhidrosis which occurs in hypothalamic disorders, due to ingestion of cholinergic agents, thyrotoxicosis or fever. Sweating associated with cold skin occurs with hypoglycemia, the dumping syndrome, withdrawal from alcohol or other drugs, during shock or syncope, and with intense pain. Endocrine abnormalities such as diabetes mellitus or gout have been associated with hyperhidrosis. Patients with familial dysautonomia have hyperhidrosis that affects mainly the limbs, and patients with causalgia have hyperhidrosis confined to the affected extremity.

Sweating abnormalities produced by human nervous system lesions give information about functional pathways in this thermoregulatory activity. Most such studies have involved peripheral nerve disorders associated with complete sympathetic paralysis leading to symptom grouping into syndromes. Horner's syndrome usually occurs after interruption of cervical sympathetic pathways, and pupillary constriction, dilatation of conjunctival vessels, eyelid drooping, anhidrosis, and dilatation of facial vessels ipsilateral to the lesions occur. A partial Horner's syndrome occurs with centrally placed lesions.

Sweating in sympathetically denervated areas of the face during eating has been attributed to facial sweat fibers joining the trigeminal nerve distal to its sensory root for peripheral distribution rather than traversing the paravertebral sympathetic chain and external carotid plexuses to reach the face. These fibers arise in the brainstem and are called accessory sweat secretory fibers. Like other fibers innervating sweat glands, they are cholinergic.

Hyperhidrosis of the face is common. It may be confined to one-half of the face and be associated with tearing and nasal discharge, or sweat may occur only on the cheeks. Emotional or gustatory stimuli provoke this type of sweating. Most exaggerated sweat responses are mediated by accessory sweat fibers except the sweating confined to the cheeks which occurs after injury or parotid gland surgery; this may be related to diffusion or to acetylcholine released by stimulation of parotid secretory nerves.

Anhidrosis is the usual effect of destruction of sympathetic supply to the face. However, in about 35% of patients with sympathetic denervation of the face, accessory fibers (reaching the face through the trigeminal system) become hyperactive and hyperhidrosis occurs, occasionally causing the interesting phenomenon of alternating hyperhidrosis and Horner's syndrome (Ottomo and Heinburger, 1980).

The auriculotemporal syndrome is paradoxic reflex gustatory sweating; it occurs after nerve injury in the face. Sweating and flushing of the skin supplied by the auriculotemporal nerve occur during eating, particularly of spicy or sour foods. Because the auriculotemporal nerve carries sympathetic postganglionic fibers to blood vessels and sweat glands and parasympathetic preganglionic secretomotor fibers to the parotid gland, it may be that reflex sweating during eating is due to cross-excitation between parasympathetic and sympathetic fibers. Successful treatment of this syndrome by division of the ninth cranial nerve has been reported, suggesting that the impulses initiating the abnormal sweating were carried in parasympathetic fibers. The auriculotemporal syndrome has also been attributed to injury of the auriculotemporal nerve by forceps during delivery.

The chorda tympani syndrome is submental gustatory sweating. It occurs after surgical trauma and is attributed to cross-excitation of sympathetic fibers that are in close proximity to parasympathetic secretory fibers to the submaxillary gland.

Diabetic anhidrosis is a condition in which sweating is absent in the lower limbs or trunk of patients with diabetic neuropathy (Goodman, 1966). Patients with this disorder are intolerant to heat, but may experience excessive perspiration on the head, face and neck, or compensatory hyperhidrosis that is particularly profuse on the face at mealtimes (enough to be socially unacceptable). Gustatory sweating in patients with diabetic neuropathy is usually confined to the territory of the superior cervical ganglion. All patients with diabetic anhidrosis or hyperhidrosis of the face have abnormal autonomic function in other systems and organs. Gustatory sweating is attributed to sprouting or cross-innervation of fibers and suggests that in diabetic autonomic neuropathy, despite the persistence of the metabolic abnormality presumably responsible for autonomic disturbances, regeneration of axons is possible (Watkins, 1973).

Hyperhidrosis may be a feature of traumatic peripheral nerve lesions and occasionally occurs in other peripheral neuropathies. It indicates incomplete interruption of peripheral nerve bundles. When it is associated with causalgia, it occurs most commonly in median or sciatic nerve injuries and in those associated with a swollen cyanotic extremely painful limb. Sympathectomy in patients with causalgia relieves the pain, excessive sweating, and other symptoms. The hyperhidrosis of peripheral nerve lesions usually disappears in those with progressive disease and, with advancing disease, the distal extremities eventually become anhidrotic. In some patients with a cervical rib, segmental hyperhidrosis of the ipsilateral limb occurs; it responds to surgical resection of the rib. Non-thermal hyperhidrosis also occurs in involved skin segments of occasional patients with mononeuropathies or mononeuritis multiplex and often manifests as strips of sweating when patients are emotionally stressed, suggesting heightened susceptibility of partially denervated sweat glands to circulating stress hormones or perhaps a sweat gland denervation supersensitivity. This condition occasionally helps diagnose mononeuritis multiplex by pointing to the focal nature of the peripheral nerve involvement.

Excessive sweating of the extremities is the rule in familial dysautonomia in which peripheral nerve dysfunction and morphologic abnormalities also occur. In such patients, the threshold for sweating in response to local heat is much lower than in controls, causing the patient to sweat most of the time. This, together with other evidence, suggests that the hyperhidrosis in familial dysautonomia is due to hyperexcitability of central sudomotor centers.

Sympathectomy causes anhidrosis in appropriate cutaneous segments that is usually permanent, whereas the vasomotor paralysis induced by this surgery may recover after a time. Nevertheless, 'escape areas' of preserved sweating, the result of intermediate ganglia in the rami communicantes, may occur, particularly if the lower limb has been sympathectomized.

Abnormal sweating in patients with collagen disease most often relates to concomitant involvement of peripheral nerves. This occurs in patients with rheumatoid arthritis and polyarteritis nodosa, a well-known cause of peripheral neuropathy.

Anhidrosis corresponding to the territory of small cutaneous sensory branches of peripheral nerves is a feature of some types of leprosy. It is of great diagnostic value

..

Table 4.2 Some tests for the clinical assessment of sweating (from Appenzeller, 1982, courtesy of the Publishers, *The Autonomic Nervous System. An introduction to Basic and Clinical Concepts*, 3rd Edn)

Test	Methods	Normal response	Lesion	Clinical signs or symptoms	Abnormal responses
Body	Heat cradle or two limbs in hot water (43°C) until central temperature 1°C above normal dust body with quinizarin powder purple when wet	Sweating	Central; postganglionic; skin or sweat glands	General or regional hypo- or anhidrosis, heat intolerance	No sweating
Number of functioning sweat glands per unit area	Starch containing paper impregnated with iodine (paper + solid iodine crystals in closed vessel) apply paper to skin; count no. of dark spots	Number of normally active glands varies with area of skin examined	Central; postganglionic; skin or sweat glands	General or regional hypo- or anhidrosis, heat intolerance	Reduced number of dots per unit area
Psycho-galvanic skin reflex	Voltage or current flow change between indifferent area (earlobe) and test skin	Change in voltage or current flow (can be continuously recorded)	Central; postganglionic; skin or sweat glands	General or regional hypo- or anhidrosis, heat intolerance	No change in voltage or current flow
Axon reflex	Faradism; intradermal injection of 5–10 mg acetylcholine solution	Local piloerection; sweating	Sympathetic ganglionic, postglanglionic; skin or sweat glands	General or regional hypo- or anhidrosis, heat intolerance	No piloerection; reduced or absent sweating
Sweat gland function	Pilocarpine iontophoresis	Sweating (can be quantitatively assessed)	Sweat glands (normal function if denervated)	General or regional hypo- or anhidrosis, heat intolerance	No sweating; reduced quantity of sweat
Skin biopsy	Skin punch biopsy	Normal histologic and histochemic appearance of sweat glands and skin	Sweat glands or skin	General or regional hypo- or anhidrosis, heat intolerance, skin lesions	Abnormal sweat composition, morphologic changes

when the small anhidrotic patches on the skin do not follow the cutaneous sensory distribution of major peripheral nerves.

Tests for the clinical assessment of sweating are listed in *Table 4.2*.

NEUROGENIC IMPAIRMENT OF THE CIRCULATION

Afferent or efferent impairment of baroreflexes causes circulatory disturbance. In tabes dorsalis, the Valsalva maneuver is not associated with a normal 'overshoot', but vasodilatation occurs normally in the hands in response to heating the feet, and vasoconstriction following a gasp is preserved. These tests suggest that postural hypotension in tabes dorsalis results from interruption of the afferent side of the baroreflex arc (*see* Table 4.1). Similar reasoning also suggests baroreflex afferent involvement in diabetics with autonomic neuropathy. The point should be made that autonomic neuropathy may not be symptomatic even when cardiovascular reflexes are clearly abnormal when assessed by special tests (*Table 4.1*). Autonomic responses may be abnormal in diabetics during ketoacidosis without clinical autonomic neuropathy. Additionally, parasympathetic function tends to be more widely involved and more commonly abnormal than sympathetic function in patients with diabetes mellitus; progression occurs with time in both parasympathetic and sympathetic deficits.

Animal studies indicate a role for substance P in autonomic function in baro- and chemoreceptor afferent neurotransmission. Substance P occurs in significant amounts in the nucleus of the tractus solitarius, a termination site for baroreceptor reflex afferents. Moreover, removal of the nodose ganglia reduces substance P in parts of the tractus solitarius nucleus, known also to receive vagal afferents. In addition, the aortic arch and carotid sinus tunica adventitia contain considerable amounts of substance P. In animals and man, this neurotransmitter seems necessary for normal baroreceptor function. Postural hypotension, particularly in patients with afferent reflex blockade, may result from atrophy of substance P-containing autonomic structures. Substance P is abnormally low in the CSF of patients with peripheral neuropathy and in some patients with multisystem atrophy (Shy-Drager syndrome) in whom peripheral neuropathy may also be present. The lower CSF levels are attributed to decreased release of substance P from the spinal roots, cord, and dorsal root ganglia because of pathologic involvement of these structures (Nutt *et al.*, 1980).

Baroreflexes are markedly abnormal in hemodialyzed uremic patients and are different from those in patients with primary hypertension. Some uremic patients, however, may have a neurogenic component to their hypertension similar to that found in experimental baroreceptor afferent denervation (Levy *et al.*, 1978). Moreover, in such patients Valsalva's maneuver and the hemodynamic adaptation after amyl nitrite inhalation show severe vasomotor failure, particularly in those with clinical and electrical evidence of peripheral neuropathy.

Reflex vasoconstriction is impaired in patients with chronic hypoxemia because of failure of sympathetic function. However, vasoconstrictor responses in such patients improve promptly when the hypoxemia is temporarily corrected. The abnormal sympathetic function is probably based on both central and peripheral disturbances; patients with chronic hypoxemia may develop peripheral neuropathy. Impaired autonomic neurotramission rather than structural autonomic pathology probably accounts for the vasomotor abnormalities. In an experiment when healthy males inhaled carbon monoxide, vasoconstrictor responses were also impaired even when arterial oxygen tension was normal (Heistad and Wheeler, 1972).

The orthostatic hypotension of primary amyloidosis may suggest the correct diagnosis of this type of peripheral neuropathy prior to nerve biopsy. Abnormal sweating also occurs. These disturbances are attributed to invasion of somatic and autonomic peripheral nerves by the disease process. Clinical and pathologic studies of patients with both primary and secondary amyloidosis show that structural involvement of the autonomic nervous system does not necessarily produce autonomic dysfunction. However, when autonomic structures are severely involved, as they often are in secondary amyloidosis, autonomic disturbances are usually disabling (Nordborg *et al.*, 1973). In dominantly inherited amyloidosis (Andrade, 1952), postural hypotension and widespread sweating abnormalities are common. Similar vasomotor disturbances also occur in alcoholic, porphyric, and several other neuropathies. Abnormal vascular reflexes in patients with Charcot-Marie-Tooth disease have been confirmed repeatedly, and the finding of giant nerve bundles in bowel myenteric plexuses of these patients supports the notion that the autonomic nervous system is involved (Brooks, 1980). Charcot and Marie (1886) noted the bluish or reddish discoloration and mottling of the feet and legs in their patients with this disease, recognizing vasomotor abnormalities commonly found in such individuals.

Features of diabetic autonomic neuropathy, apart from the vasomotor abnormalities, include gastrointestinal symptoms which resemble those found after surgical vagotomy, and the term 'autovagotomy' has been used to describe this condition. In these patients, vagal stimulation or hypoglycemia may not produce gastric acid secretion, but acid secretion still occurs in response to administration of humoral agents such as pentagastrin. Pancreatic polypeptide secretion in response to insulin hypoglycemia is decreased in juvenile diabetics with autonomic neuropathy when compared with those without clinical neuropathy. A significant correlation exists between the duration of diabetes and the response to insulin-induced hypoglycemia. Abnormal responses are attributed to a vagal neuropathy since pancreatic polypeptide release depends normally upon intact vagal innervation of the pancreas.

DYSAUTONOMIA IN MITRAL VALVE PROLAPSE

The recognition of mitral valve prolapse has prompted its frequent diagnosis in recent years. The fundamental anatomic clinical and physiologic aspects of the condition have been fully described and many patients with this condition experience symptoms suggestive of abnormal autonomic function. In addition, a large number also have migraine. Autonomic dysfunction in mitral valve prolapse includes inappropriate changes in heart rate during general anesthesia, excessive bradycardia, and increased tendency to ventricular fibrillation during coronary angiography, widely oscillating heart rates when the patient stands, and exaggerated and prolonged bradycardia during recovery after Valsalva's maneuver. Greater respiratory variations in pulse intervals, prominent during postural changes, occur (Coghlan *et al.*, 1979). These responses suggest that autonomic activity is not blunted or absent, but is rather hypersensitive to autonomic stimulation; these findings are not dissimilar to those in patients with variant angina. In both conditions, an increased incidence of migraine suggests that autonomic disability is a feature of these cardiovascular disorders.

FAMILIAL DYSAUTONOMIA (RILEY-DAY SYNDROME)

This congenital condition is characterized by diminished lacrimation, hyperhidrosis, blotching of the skin, which may be transient, abnormal swallowing reflexes, impaired vestibular reflexes, labile blood pressure, disturbed temperature control, emotional instability associated with episodes of severe vomiting, poor coordination, relative insensitivity to pain and diminished deep tendon reflexes; all suggest peripheral nervous system involvement which has indeed been documented morphologically. Most cases occur in Jewish children, and extensive reviews of the subject have been published (Riley, 1957; McKusick *et al.*, 1967; Aguayo *et al.*, 1971; Pearson *et al.*, 1974).

Clinical-pathologic correlation is now possible for some of the symptoms. Impaired taste results from reduced numbers of, or defective, lingual taste buds. If sural nerve changes are representative of those in the rest of the peripheral nervous system, postural hypotension, altered catecholamine excretion, adrenergic denervation supersensitivity, skin blotching and impaired thermoregulation can be accounted for. Unmyelinated C fiber loss in peripheral nerves is consistent with impaired pain and temperature perception, and absent corneal and axonal reflexes. Because large myelinated fibers are rare, the tendon stretch reflexes dependent on muscle spindle afferents subserved by these fibers are also impaired or abolished. The pathogenesis of familial dysautonomia is not known. It has been suggested that nerve growth factor is involved and that developmental arrest of neuronal migration from the neural crest explains the absence of unmyelinated and large myelinated fibers, including muscle spindle afferents.

Other inherited diseases can produce the clinical manifestations of familial dysautonomia. If the diagnosis is to be made in acutely ill infants, this possibility should be kept in mind. Hyperammonemia due to propionyl-coenzyme-A carboxylase deficiency is an example of a metabolic abnormality that can produce phenocopies of familial dysautonomia (Harris *et al.*, 1980). The diagnosis of familial dysautonomia in infants depends on abnormal responses to intracutaneous histamine and methacholine (absence of flare component of triple response of Lewis that depends on intact small myelinated pain afferents) and abnormal urinary catecholamine excretion. In the infants with hyperammonemia, however, appropriate dietary manipulation results in reversal of the clinical symptoms.

LESCH-NYHAN SYNDROME

The Lesch-Nyhan syndrome, a disorder of purine metabolism, is characterized by hyperuricemia and excessive uric acid production. It is X-linked and manifests profound neurologic dysfunction including spasticity, choreoathetosis, self-mutilation and mental retardation. There is an almost total absence of the enzyme hypoxanthine-guanine-phosphoribosyl transferase (HGPRT). The pathogenesis of behavioral and neurologic disturbances in patients with HGPRT deficiency is not known. Because of self-mutilating behavior induced in animals by caffeine or amphetamine administration, it has been suggested that this part of the Lesch-Nyhan syndrome results from altered function in central nervous system pathways affected by these agents. A study of patients with the HGPRT deficiency and self-mutilating behavior shows a unique pattern of adrenergic dysfunction. Plasma dopamine beta-hydroxylase, an enzyme which catalyzes norepinephrine formation from dopamine, is elevated. This enzyme is released simultaneously into the synaptic cleft with norepinephrine. Circulating dopamine beta-hydroxylase is a quantitative index of peripheral adrenergic function. Though this enzyme was elevated in patients with Lesch-Nyhan syndrome, none of them had autonomic manifestations of excessive adrenergic activity such as hypertension, tachycardia or midriasis. But clinical evaluation of adrenergic responsiveness such as the cold pressor test showed that the normally expected rise in blood pressure (due to vasoconstriction) was absent in those with the HGPRT deficiency syndrome who also exhibited self-mutilation. The mechanism of this failure of vasoconstriction is not known. Any implied relationship of high plasma dopamine beta-hydroxylase activity remains conjectural. The experimentally induced self-mutilation of animals by caffeine injection may link this behavioral abnormality to the endorphin system since caffeine is a potent stimulator of plasma, but not CSF beta-endorphin release.

MISCELLANEOUS DISORDERS ASSOCIATED WITH AUTONOMIC FAILURE

Severe autonomic failure with peripheral sensory neuropathy and incomplete recovery, to be distinguished from acute pandysautonomia, has drawn attention to a number of peripheral nerve disorders with predominant and severely disabling autonomic failure. In one such case, incomplete recovery occurred after 13 months. The patient had high CSF protein at one stage of the disease, and the course was complicated by almost global sensory loss and corneal ulceration. Sural nerve biopsy showed degeneration of both myelinated and unmyelinated fibers. The condition was attributed to an acute ganglionopathy of unknown cause, toxin and viral etiologies having been excluded (Colan *et al.*, 1980).

In Fabry's disease, the glycolipid, ceramide trihexoside, is stored within the nervous system, including the autonomic neurons, and a dying-back neuropathy occurs. Autonomic dysfunction has also been demonstrated in this disease (Cable *et al.*, 1980). Examination of these patients showed impaired sweating, abnormal skin corrugation induced by warm water immersion of the hands and feet, and an abnormal flare component of the triple response of Lewis. The pupils responded abnormally to pilocarpine, and saliva and tear production were reduced. Cardiovascular responses, including decreased reflex increases in plasma norepinephrine, were abnormal in most of the patients. Sympathetic and parasympathetic functions were impaired, and this was attributed to involvement of small fibers in peripheral nerves.

Patients with multiple mucosal neuromas have dysautonomia and abnormal triple responses of Lewis after intradermal histamine injection. This syndrome is characterized by painless greyish yellow tumors on the conjunctivae, tongue, oral cavity, pharynx and larynx. These are usually arranged symmetrically about the midline and a typical site is along the anterior dorsum of the tongue. Such patients also have a Marfanoid habitus, thick everted lips, and multiple endocrine tumors, such as medullary thyroid carcinoma and pheochromocytomas. Funnel chest, myelinated fibers in the cornea, skin pigmentation, hypertrophic nerves, abnormalities of Auerbach's and Meissner's plexuses and a myopathy have also been reported. Certain clinical features may appear in early childhood, but endocrine tumors are not apparent until later life. Autonomic dysfunction includes impaired lacrimation, parasympathetic denervation supersensitivity of the pupil with intact sympathetic responses, orthostatic hypotension with an intact overshoot in response to Valsalva's maneuver, normal responses to vagal stimulation (eyeball pressure and carotid sinus massage), impaired pilomotor activity, absent reflex vasodilatation with preservation of reflex vasoconstriction in hand blood vessels in response to temperature changes, abnormal glucose levels after intravenous insulin, and dermographia. Sweat, salivary, and lacrimal gland functions are normal. The sural nerve shows degeneration and regeneration of unmyelinated fibers similar to the findings in patients with acute pandysautonomia (Horstink *et al.*, 1974).

Autonomic dysfunction occurs in acute botulism. A minor variant of this condition due to intoxication with botulism B and predominant effects upon cholinergic autonomic function has also been described (Jenzer *et al.*, 1975). In this condition, benign, but protracted, symptoms of paresis of accommodation, salivary and lacrimal secretion, constipation, pupillary abnormalities and disturbances of micturition, all due to peripheral cholinergic dysfunction, occur. Orthostatic hypotension and apathetic behavior, not usually attributed to the toxin, are also present. Symptoms may last from 30–80 days with or without otherwise normal neurologic function. Electromyography shows normal neuromuscular transmission. Specific treatment is not available, but most patients eventually recover. It is important to distinguish this condition from acute pandysautonomia, which is different etiologically and morphologically by study of peripheral nerves.

THE TRIPLE RESPONSE OF LEWIS

This response is elicited when the skin is injured by a variety of agents and consists of local blood vessel dilatation, blistering or wheal formation locally, and a surrounding bright red flare due to spreading dilatation of small blood vessels. The flare component is absent in denervated skin, but can be elicited for a few days after peripheral nerve section until the nerve degenerates. Thereafter, only the wheal and central red area without the spreading flare occurs. Transection of dorsal roots does not affect the flare, but it is abolished 7 or more days after dorsal root ganglionectomy, evidence that integrity of afferent fibers arising in dorsal root ganglion cells is essential for the flare response. While the inflammatory reaction is not abolished by peripheral denervation, it is modified in denervated skin as evidenced by the absence of the flare component of the triple response of Lewis. In subjects with intact peripheral nerves it has been shown that the central nervous system modulates the extent of the flare, and thus, in turn, influences the response of the skin to injury. The flare component of the triple response is not, strictly speaking, mediated by the autonomic nervous system since it depends on small myelinated pain afferent fibers that originate from cell bodies in the posterior root ganglia. Though the neurogenic component of the triple response is anatomically outside the autonomic nervous system, it is often included in tests of autonomic function and is abnormal in patients with familial dysautonomia.

THE NERVOUS SYSTEM AND MYOEDEMA

Muscle contraction after percussion is normally associated with an electrical discharge. However, myoedema (mounding) in response to muscle percussion is not associated with a recordable electrical discharge. Moreover, myoedema is fatiguable; it is undoubtedly a physiologic phenomenon and has been recognized in patients with wasting disorders; it is also frequently found in those with peripheral nerve disease. Myoedema has been attributed to an inherent, muscular excitability related predominantly to the contents of the muscle fiber rather than to depolarization of the muscle membrane (Denny-Brown and Pennybacker, 1938). Though this is an intrinsic muscle phenomenon, it is modulated by central and peripheral nervous system lesions. It also occurs in endocrine disorders such as myxedema and is particularly prominent in those with myxedema neuropathy (Appenzeller, 1975).

TROPHIC PHENOMENA IN PERIPHERAL NERVOUS SYSTEM LESIONS

Peripheral nerve lesions are commonly associated with trophic disorders. The characteristic denervation atrophy of muscles is attributed to lack of trophic influence of motor fibers. The trophic skin changes are usually most marked in hands and feet, particularly when pain is a feature of nerve lesions or the affected parts are subjected to continuous trauma or excessive heat or cold that may not be appreciated because of accompanying sensory loss. Characteristically, the skin is tight and smooth. Later it becomes shiny and transparent, and the subcutaneous tissue is atrophic. Pigmentation is common in chronically denervated areas and an eczema-like change may occur that remains sharply localized to denervated dermatomes. Minor mechanical or thermal trauma leads to indolent ulcers, particularly in fingers and toes, that may be painful even in the presence of extensive sensory loss. Eventually, fibrosis of subcutaneous tissue occurs in partial nerve injuries particularly, and the overlying skin is elevated by contraction of fibrous tissue into heavy folds. Fingers may become clubbed and the fingernails transversely striped, thickened, ridged, brittle and often claw-like in areas of severe sensory loss. Nail growth, however, is not retarded except when the limb blood supply is insufficient. The hair is often thin and disappears from denervated areas of limbs but, on occasion, hypertrichosis occurs, particularly on the forearms. The most marked trophic changes occur in traumatic nerve lesions and chronic sensory neuropathy, but trophic ulcerations of the feet are common in neglected patients with diabetic neuropathy and marked sensory loss.

The trophic phenomena relate to connections between nerves and their target tissue. The maintenance of target cell integrity is exemplified by the close dependence of muscles on their nerve supply and the regulation of certain target cell properties by the innervating neurons that adapt the target to an intended task which can be changed by changing the innervation (the regulation of fast–slow, white–red muscle fibers' properties). Evidence now shows that cholinergic blockade of neuromuscular transmission produces the same effect as denervation. Therefore, the neuromuscular cholinergic transmission is, at least, necessary for trophic neuromuscular interaction, which also depends on axoplasmic flow and adequate muscle activity. Stimulation experiments show that use alone, in the absence of innervation, can almost, if not entirely, maintain muscle integrity.

A wide scope of neurotrophic interactions exist which maintain connections and cause regeneration of certain nervous and other body tissues. This has led to the suggestion that the term 'neurotrophic relations' be restricted to functional manifestations necessary for long-term maintenance and regulation of structures by their innervation, but which are independent of nerve impulses. Since a number of different components are involved in intercellular relationships, such as cell-to-cell contact in addition to neuron and non-neuronal contact, it cannot be expected that all trophic relations are based on this same mechanism. Though it is clear that acetylcholine plays a very important role in neuromuscular interactions and maintenance of trophic function, its role has, however, not been definitively established for other organs (Drachman, 1974).

THE PUPIL

Human and mammalian pupils react continuously to changes in lighting due to a balance between sympathetic and parasympathetic innervation of the iris. In some peripheral nervous system disorders, sympathetic or parasympathetic iris denervation can be shown by pharmacologic tests. Thus, parasympathetic denervation supersensitivity results in pupillary constriction with the instillation of 2.5% methacholine, which, in the normal pupil, does not cause constriction. The instillation of 1/1000 epinephrine into the conjunctival sac of a normally innervated iris will not cause pupillary dilatation, but will do so only in the presence of sympathetic denervation.

In patients with acute pandysautonomia, parasympathetic and sympathetic denervation supersensitivity can be shown with the above tests. Parasympathetic denervation supersensitivity occurs in 81% of patients with diabetic autonomic neuropathy (Sigsbee *et al.*, 1974), a finding most prevalent in patients who had been diabetic for at least 2 years. Symptomatic autonomic neuropathy occurred in patients with long-standing disease, but this was only a small portion of those patients who showed pupillary parasympathetic denervation supersensitivity.

APPROACH TO PATIENTS WITH SYMPTOMS SUGGESTIVE OF AUTONOMIC DYSFUNCTION

It is important to establish the presence or absence of autonomic dysfunction in patients with peripheral neuropathy for diagnostic and prognostic purposes. Certain peripheral neuropathies have prominent, if not exclusive, autonomic dysfunction (amyloid neuropathy, diabetic neuropathy, and acute pandysautonomia). In other neuropathies, autonomic dysfunction may be symptomless, but may become important and life-threatening (Landry-Guillain-Barré syndrome). Delineation of autonomic deficits (*Table 4.1*) may, therefore, help with diagnosis, prognosis, or to anticipate and avoid serious complications.

Treatment

General principles

The most disabling symptoms of autonomic failure are due to cardiovascular dysfunction. Orthostatic hypotension with decreased perfusion of the brain is the most troublesome. It is of particular importance, however, not to be too concerned about low standing blood pressures if the patients remain asymptomatic. With chronic autonomic failure, patients may tolerate very low standing blood pressures without dizziness or syncope. This is attributed to maintenance of cerebral blood flow by remarkable cerebrovascular autoregulation leading to considerable vasodilatation and preservation of perfusion in the face of low blood pressures. Whatever the correct explanation may be clinically, patients with autonomic failure have great tolerance to low blood pressures without developing symptoms of cerebral ischemia. Because of defective baroreflexes, orthostatic hypotension may be associated with paradoxic recumbent hypertension which may complicate the treatment of the postural fall in blood pressure.

While the loss of baroreflex function is of primary importance in the immediate response of the blood pressure to standing, the control of blood volume regulated by low pressure receptors in the kidney through the release of antidiuretic hormone and the renin–angiotensin–aldosterone system is important in the long-term adjustment of patients with autonomic failure to postural hypotension.

There are two principles of treatment of postural hypotension. One involves the reduction of the volume which is available for blood pooling on standing, and the second is to increase the volume of blood available for pooling. Drugs which decrease the capacity for blood to pool below the heart, however, have a tendency to increase the occurrence of recumbent hypertension, and those that increase available blood volume may overload the circulation, causing cardiac failure and edema.

Any measure which temporarily restores the patient to his feet irrespective of the actual standing blood pressure will enhance homeostatic mechanisms which are triggered by standing. For example, an increase in extracellular fluid volume will occur and improved myogenic tone of blood vessels can be expected. Thus, a continued symptomatic improvement in postural hypotension may be erroneously attributed to specific treatment where, under controlled conditions, it may be possible to withdraw a dangerous drug and replace it by mechanical supports of the circulation.

In principle, it is advisable to use combination therapy since most patients with autonomic failure have defects at various levels of the baroreflex pathways. Drugs with central or ganglionic and postganglionic effects may have synergistic effects and require lower doses. Other drugs, which increase norepinephrine release, can be combined with those which reduce its re-uptake or which increase receptor sensitivity. In general, however, it is best to attempt therapy by mechanical methods before complicating matters with the administration of powerful pharmacologic agents.

It is possible to increase blood volume by a head-up position at night. This method of treatment, recently tried by Bannister *et al.* (1969), gives evidence of an increase in body weight overnight, presumably due to increases in extracellular fluid volume. Many patients require nothing more than persistent head-up tilting while asleep. Studies have shown that this position prevents the increased sodium and water loss during the night which may explain the retention of fluid and peripheral edema observed in normal subjects who are confined to a head-up position in crowded aircraft on trans-Atlantic flights.

The head-up position also promotes renin release because of reduced renal arterial pressure. Consequently, angiotensin II formation and aldosterone stimulation occur and this, in turn, increases blood volume.

Drugs

Fludrocortisone is commonly used; it has many pharmacologic effects. The initial dose is 0.1 mg per day. The drug increases effective vasoconstriction because it augments the action of norepinephrine release by normal sympathetic efferent activity; it does not usually aggravate recumbent hypertension. Fludrocortisone increases the sensitivity of vascular receptors to pressors and it may increase fluid content of blood vessel walls, therefore decreasing their distensibility. Because patients with postural hypotension are sensitive to sodium intake it is necessary to support all methods of treatment with a high sodium intake provided this is not contraindicated for other reasons.

Simple external supports to reduce the volume for blood pooling in the legs and abdomen are useful, but because they are cumbersome they are not usually accepted for long.

Pressor drugs, which cause improvement in postural hypotension, include phenylephrine, which has a direct sympathomimetic action and, less effectively, ephedrine, an indirect sympathomimetic drug. These drugs have a tendency to aggravate recumbent hypertension. Midodrine (Schirger *et al.*, 1981) has been used. The constrictor effects of this drug are attributed to its alpha-agonist activity on both arterioles and veins.

Monoamine oxidase inhibitors and tyramine have also been used (Diamond *et al.*, 1970). The effects of tyramine are attributed to release and re-uptake of norepinephrine at sympathetic endings. This drug requires an intact sympathetic supply to blood vessels for effectiveness. When tyramine is given with a monoamine oxidase inhibitor in the presence of adrenergic denervation supersensitivity and baroreflex block, severe hypertension can occur. Moreover, careful trials with pure tyramine and monoamine oxidase inhibitors have shown erratic blood pressure responses and aggravation of recumbent hypertension (Bannister, 1983).

Dihydroergotamine has been advocated because of its direct vasoconstrictor effect on smooth muscles of capacitance vessels (veins). It acts as a direct alpha-agonist and increases central blood volume but, in autonomic failure, it causes constriction of resistance vessels as well. After intravenous injection, dihydroergotamine, though highly effective in abolishing postural hypotension, causes severe recumbent hypertension. The oral dose, which may be needed for control of postural hypotension, may be 30–35 mg daily. It is more effective given intramuscularly in smaller doses during the day to avoid recumbent hypertension at night.

The considerations which led to the recommendation of indomethacin for postural hypotension are based on its antiprostaglandin activity. Prostaglandins are potent vasodilators, and the decreased levels of prostaglandins after indomethacin therapy are helpful in autonomic failure. Indomethacin has a number of other effects, however. It increases sensitivity to infused norepinephrine and angiotensin II and its effectiveness is now attributed to these actions rather than to prostaglandin synthesis inhibition.

Propranolol, a beta-blocker, is used in treatment of postural hypotension because beta-agonist-induced vasodilatation might contribute to symptomatic orthostatic hypotension. Beneficial effects have been reported in patients with progressive autonomic failure using doses of 40–240 mg per day, but these patients were also taking fludrocortisone and added salt to their diet. It may, however, be useful in patients with postural hypotension due to tachycardia leading to a falling cardiac output and, eventually, syncope.

Other drugs used with varying success are pindolol, given to patients with diabetic autonomic neuropathy in whom there was a demonstrated denervation supersensitivity to norepinephrine (Frewin *et al.*, 1980). Some patients have an improved cardiac output but unchanged vascular resistance while taking this drug. However, subsequent reports have not been enthusiastic and pindolol, like metoclopramide, a dopamine agonist, has now been abandoned. Clonidine, a partial alpha-receptor agonist, acts centrally and peripherally, causes hypotension normally, and is used in the treatment of hypertension. It causes an inhibition of sympathetic tone by its primary action on the nucleus of the tractus solitarius. Recently, a report in four patients with autonomic failure showed that an oral dose of 0.4 mg twice daily caused long-term improvement in those with low plasma norepinephrine levels and denervation supersensitivity but no further systematic studies in patients with peripheral autonomic failure have been reported.

Treatment of bladder dysfunction (*see* pp. 69–72)

Thermoregulatory activity

Because many patients with peripheral autonomic failure have abnormal sweating and vasomotor responses, heat tolerance may be severely impaired. Proper advice for regulation of microclimate (clothing) and exposure to heat should be given to avoid serious complications resulting from excessive heatloads or hypothermia (Appenzeller, 1982).

CONCLUSIONS

The effects of treatment of postural hypotension and of autonomic peripheral failure in general have been disappointing. In those conditions in which the deficits are transient, all efforts should be made to control the patient's internal and external environment mechanically at first or with the aid of drugs which mimic normal modulatory activity of the autonomic nervous system. Conditions in which recovery is not expected also need treatment, but the long-term effects and, particularly, side effects of therapy should be carefully balanced with the expected benefits. In general, it is better to tolerate minor disability than cause serious complications due to therapy.

References

Aguayo, A. J., Nair, C. P. V. and Bray, G. M. (1971) Peripheral nerve abnormalities in the Riley-Day syndrome. *Archives of Neurology*, **24**, 106–116

Andrade, C. (1952) A peculiar form of peripheral neuropathy: familial atypical generalized amyloidosis with special involvement of peripheral nerves. *Brain*, **75**, 408–427

Appenzeller, O. (1975) Catecholamine fluorescence of perivascular nerve plexuses in neuromuscular disorders. *Neurology*, **25**, 346

Appenzeller, O. (1982) *The Autonomic Nervous System. An Introduction to Basic and Clinical Concepts*, 3rd Edn. Amsterdam: Elsevier Biomedical Press

Appenzeller, O. and Kornfeld, M. (1973) Acute pandysautonomia clinical and morphologic study. *Archives of Neurology*, **29**, 334–339

Appenzeller, O. and Marshall, J. (1963) Vasomotor disturbances in Landry-Guillain-Barré syndrome. *Archives of Neurology*, **9**, 368–372

Bannister, R., Ardill, L. and Fentem, P. (1969) An assessment of various methods of treatment of idiopathic orthostatic hypotension. *Quarterly Journal of Medicine*, **38**, 377–395

Bannister, R. (Ed.) (1983) *Autonomic Failure*. A textbook of clinical disorders of the autonomic nervous system. Oxford: Oxford University Press

British Medical Journal (1980) Function of the transplanted heart. **2**, 529

Brooks, A. P. (1980) Abnormal vascular reflexes in Charcot-Marie-Tooth disease. *Journal of Neurology, Neurosurgery and Psychiatry*, **43**, 348–350

Cable, W. J. L., Kolodny, E. H. *et al.* (1980) Fabry disease: a clinical demonstration of impaired autonomic function. *Neurology*, **30**, 1352

Charcot, J. M. and Marie, P. (1886) Sur une form particulière d'atrophie musculaire progressive souvent familiale debutant par les pieds et les jambes et atteignant plus tard les mains. *Revue Medicin*, **6**, 97–138

Coghlan, H. C., Phares, P. *et al.* (1979) Dysautonomia in mitral valve prolapse. *American Journal of Medicine*, **67**, 236–244

Colan, R. V., Carter Snead, O. *et al.* (1980) Acute autonomic and sensory neuropathy. *Annals of Neurology*, **8**, 441–444

de Burgh Daly, M. and Angell-James, J. E. (1979) The 'diving response' and its possible clinical implications. *International Medicine*, **1**, 12–19

Denny-Brown, D. and Pennybacker, J. B. (1938) Fibrillation and fasciculations in voluntary muscle. *Brain*, **61**, 311

Diamond, M. A., Murray, R. H. and Schmid, P. G. (1970) Idiopathic postural hypotension; physiologic observations and report of a new mode of therapy. *Journal of Clinical Investigation*, **49**, 1341–1348

Drachman, D. B. (1974) The role of acetylcholine as a neurotrophic transmitter. *Annals of the New York Academy of Sciences*, **228**, 160–176

Duchen, L. W., Anjorin, A., Watkins, P. J. and Mackay, J. D. (1980) Pathology of autonomic neuropathy in diabetes mellitus. *Annals of Internal Medicine*, **92**, 301–303

Ellenberg, M. (1980a) Development of urinary bladder dysfunction in diabetes mellitus. *Annals of Internal Medicine*, **92**, 321–323

Ellenberg, M. (1980b) Sexual function in diabetic patients. *Annals of Internal Medicine*, **92**, 331–333

Frewin, D. B., Leonello, P. P., Pentall, R. K., Hughes, L. and Harding, P. E. (1980) Pindolol in orthostatic hypotension; possibly therapy? *Medical Journal of Australia*, **1**, 128

Furness, J. B. and Costa, M. (1981) Types of nerves in the enteric nervous system. *Neuroscience*, **5**, 1–20

Goodman, J. I. (1966) Diabetic anhidrosis. *American Journal of Medicine*, **41**, 831–835

Harris, D. J., Yang, B. I. Y., *et al.* (1980) Dysautonomia in an infant with secondary hyperammonemia due to propionyl-coenzyme-A carboxylase deficiency. *Pediatrics*, **65**, 107–110

Heistad, D. D. and Wheeler, R. C. (1972) Effect of carbon monoxide on reflex vasoconstriction in man. *Journal of Applied Physiology*, **32**, 7–11

Horstink, M. W. I. M., Gabreels, F. J. M., Joosten, E. M. G. *et al.* (1974) Multiple mucosal neuromas, dysautonomia and abnormal intradermal histamine reaction. *Clinical Neurology and Neurosurgery*, **3/4**, 212–224

Jenzer, G., Mumenthaler, M., Ludin, H. P. and Robert, F. (1975) Autonomic dysfunction in botulism B: a clinical report. *Neurology*, **25**, 150–153

Karacan, I. (1980) Diagnosis of erectile impotence in diabetes mellitus. An objective and specific method. *Annals of Internal Medicine*, **92**, 334–337

Levy, S. B., Lilley, J. J. *et al.* (1978) Baroreflex function in uremic and hypertensive man. *American Journal of the Medical Sciences*, **276**, 57–66

Low, P. A., Walsh, J. C., Huang, C. Y. and McLeod, J. G. (1975a) The sympathetic nervous system in diabetic neuropathy. A clinical and pathological study. *Brain*, **98**, 341–356

Low, P. A., Walsh, J. C., Huang, C. Y. and McLeod, J. G. (1975b) The sympathetic nervous system in alcoholic neuropathy. A clinical and pathological study. *Brain*, **98**, 357–364

Mastri, A. R. (1980) Neuropathology of diabetic neurogenic bladder. *Annals of Internal Medicine*, **92**, 316–318

McKusick, V. A., Norum, R. A., Farkas, H. J., Brunt, P. S. and Mahloudii, M. (1967) The Riley-Day syndrome – observations on genetics and survivorship. *Israel Journal of Medical Sciences*, **3**, 372–379

Nordborg, C., Kristensson, K., Olsson, Y. and Sourander, P. (1973) Involvement of the autonomous nervous system in primary and secondary amyloidosis. *Acta Neurologica Scandinavica*, **49**, 31–38

Nutt, J. G., Mroz, E. A., Leeman, S. E., Williams, A. C., Engel, W. K. and Chase, T. N. (1980) Substance P in human cerebrospinal fluid: reductions in peripheral neuropathy and autonomic dysfunction. *Neurology*, **30**, 1280–1285

Ottomo, M. and Heimburger, R. F. (1980) Alternating Horner's syndrome and hyperhidrosis due to dural adhesions following cervical spinal cord injury. *Journal of Neurosurgery*, **53**, 97–100

Pearson, J., Axelrod, R. and Dancis, J. (1974) Current concepts of dysautonomia: neuropathological defects. *Annals of the New York Academy of Sciences*, **228**, 288–300

Riley, C. M. (1957) Familial dysautonomia. *Advances in Pediatrics*, **9**, 157–190

Schirger, A., Sheps, S. G., Thomas, J. E. and Fealey, R. D. (1981) Midodrine – a new agent in the management of idiopathic orthostatic hypotension and Shy-Drager syndrome. *Proceedings of the Staff Meeting, Mayo Clinic*, **56**, 429–433

Sigsbee, B., Torkelson, B., Kadis, G., Wright, J. W. and Reeves, A. G. (1974) Parasympathetic denervation of the iris in diabetes mellitus. *Journal of Neurology, Neurosurgery and Psychiatry*, **37**, 1031–1035

Takagi, K. and Sakurai, T. (1950) A sweat reflex due to pressure on the body surface. *Japanese Journal of Physiology*, **1**, 22–28

Watkins, P. J. (1973) Facial sweating after food: a new sign of diabetic autonomic neuropathy. *British Medical Journal*, **1**, 583–587

Watkins, P. J. and Mackay, J. D. (1980) Cardiac denervation in diabetic neuropathy. *Annals of Internal Medicine*, **92**, 304–307

Ziegler, M. G. (1980) Postural hypotension. *Annual Review of Medicine*, **31**, 239–245

5
Neuropathies in systemic diseases: hidden and overt

James G. McLeod and John D. Pollard

An analysis of 205 cases of undiagnosed peripheral neuropathy referred to the Mayo Clinic demonstrated that a definitive diagnosis could be made in all but 24% (Dyck *et al.*, 1981). Acquired neuropathies represented 13% of the group and included those due to systemic disorders such as myxoedema, carcinoma, multiple myeloma, and monoclonal paraproteinaemia. In our own study, in which the sural nerve biopsies of 519 patients with peripheral neuropathy were analyzed, it was found that acquired neuropathies represented 225 (43%) of the cases and only 67 (13%) of the patients studied remained undiagnosed. Both these series underestimate the proportion of cases in the general population in whom peripheral neuropathy is related to metabolic and other systemic diseases because in most instances the diagnosis is made without referral to a specialized neurological centre. Clearly, it is important to investigate thoroughly all patients with peripheral neuropathy of uncertain cause since in the acquired neuropathies treatment is often effective.

GENERAL CONSIDERATIONS

There is a clear distinction between peripheral neuropathy which is clinically significant, and often a presenting feature of the underlying condition, and that which is asymptomatic and can be detected only by careful neurological examination and electrophysiological studies. In those malignant conditions where systematic electrophysiological studies have been performed on a large number of patients, for example carcinoma, lymphoma and multiple myeloma, the incidence of clinical neuropathy is about 5%, but electrophysiological abnormalities are detected in 30–50% of patients. These findings suggest that although some involvement of the peripheral nerves is common, the degree of the pathological changes varies greatly and only those patients in whom they are severe will have clinical symptoms. In some conditions, such as chronic liver disease, polycythaemia vera, hypothyroidism, acromegaly and chronic obstructive pulmonary disease, peripheral neuropathy is rarely of clinical importance.

DIAGNOSIS AND MANAGEMENT

The clinical features and pathology of the different types of neuropathy due to systemic disease are summarized in *Table 5.1*.

The mode of clinical presentation may suggest the underlying cause of the neuropathy. An *acute onset* is most commonly due to the Guillain-Barré syndrome, but can also be due to toxic causes and may follow injection of foreign proteins by

Table 5.1 Peripheral neuropathy associated with systemic diseases

Systemic disease	Predominant type of neuropathy	Onset and course	Pathology
Metabolic disorders			
Uraemia	Sensory (sensorimotor)	Chronic (acute)	AD ± SD
Porphyria	Motor	Acute	AD
Hypoglycaemia	Motor	Chronic	AD
Endocrine disorders			
Hypothyroidism	Sensory	Chronic	AD
Acromegaly	Sensory	Chronic	AD
Malignancies and reticuloses			
Carcinoma	Sensory, sensorimotor	Subacute or chronic (acute)	AD (SD in acute sensorimotor and relapsing type)
Lymphoma	Sensorimotor	Acute, subacute or chronic	AD, SD (acute relapsing)
Chronic lymphatic leukaemia	Sensorimotor	Acute (subacute)	AD
Polycythaemia vera	Sensory	Chronic	AD
Deficiency states			
Vitamin B_{12}	Sensory	Chronic	AD
Thiamine	Sensorimotor	Chronic	AD
Folic acid	Sensory	Chronic	AD
Vitamin E	Sensory	Chronic	AD
Paraproteinaemias and dysproteinaemias			
Multiple myeloma	Sensorimotor (motor or sensory)	Chronic	AD
Cryoglobulinaemia	Sensorimotor	Chronic	AD
Macroglobulinaemia	Sensorimotor	Subacute or chronic (acute)	AD, SD
Monoclonal gammopathy			
IgA	Sensorimotor, motor	Chronic	AD
IgG	Sensorimotor	Chronic	AD ± SD
IgM	Sensorimotor	Chronic	SD
Miscellaneous			
Chronic liver disease	Sensory (sensorimotor)	Chronic	SD
Primary biliary cirrhosis	Sensory	Chronic	AD
Viral hepatitis	Sensory or sensorimotor	Acute	SD
Adult coeliac disease	Sensorimotor	Chronic	AD
Chronic obstructive pulmonary disease	Sensory (sensorimotor)	Chronic	AD
Sarcoidosis	Sensorimotor, sensory or motor	Acute or chronic	AD

AD = axonal degeneration; SD = segmental demyelination. Words in parentheses indicate less common types vaccinations and inoculations. The systemic diseases associated with an acute onset of neuropathy are listed in *Table 5.2*; diabetic neuropathy may also occasionally have an acute onset. Where the *onset is gradual* and the course is *chronic*, there are many more possible causes (*Table 5.1*). Most of the neuropathies associated with

Table 5.2 Causes of peripheral neuropathy with acute onset

Carcinoma
Chronic lymphatic leukaemia
Lymphoma
Macroglobulinaemia
Porphyria
Sarcoidosis
Uraemia
Viral hepatitis

systemic diseases are *predominantly sensory* and some are painful (*Table 5.3*). *Predominantly motor* neuropathies are associated with porphyria, hypoglycaemia due to insulinoma and sometimes the osteosclerotic type of multiple myeloma. The peripheral neuropathy in systemic disease is usually symmetrical and only in sarcoidosis, polyarteritis nodosa, and less commonly cryoglobulinaemia, may it present as a mononeuritis multiplex. *Predominantly upper limb involvement* may be seen in porphyria, multiple myeloma and hypoglycaemia due to insulinoma. *Autonomic dysfunction* is characteristically associated with porphyria and primary amyloidosis. In the latter condition there is usually a disproportionate loss of pain and temperature sense.

Table 5.3 Painful sensory neuropathies

Amyloidosis
Carcinoma
Cryoglobulinaemia
Hypothyroidism
Insulinoma
Macroglobulinaemia
Multiple myeloma
Thiamine deficiency and alcohol
Uraemia

A full physical examination should always be performed with a careful search for evidence of carcinoma, lymphoma, and paraproteinaemia; it should include palpation for enlarged lymph nodes, liver and spleen and examination of breasts, testes, rectum and vagina. The physician should be alert to the different clinical manifestations of systemic disease, which may provide a clue to the underlying cause of the neuropathy (*Table 5.4*).

Table 5.4 Clinical features associated with peripheral neuropathy due to systemic diseases

Anaemia and bleeding diatheses
    Chronic liver disease
    Cryoglobulinaemia
    Leukaemia
    Lymphoma
    Macroglobulinaemia
    Malabsorption syndromes
    Multiple myeloma
    Uraemia
	Jaundice
	    Chronic liver disease including primary
	        biliary cirrhosis
	    Viral hepatitis

Autonomic dysfunction
    Porphyria
    Primary amyloidosis
	Lymphadenopathy
	    Carcinoma
	    Lymphoma
	    Macroglobulinaemia
	    Sarcoidosis

Constipation
    Amyloid
    Hypothyroidism
    Porphyria
	Mental changes
	    Carcinoma (especially pure sensory
	        neuropathy)
	    Liver disease
	    Porphyria
	    Thiamine deficiency, alcohol
	    Vitamin B_{12} deficiency

Diarrhoea
    Amyloid
    Malabsorption syndromes
	Raynaud's phenomenon
	    Cryoglobulinaemia
	    Macroglobulinaemia
	    IgM paraproteinaemia

Hepatosplenomegaly
    Alcohol
    Amyloidosis
    Chronic liver disease
    Chronic lymphatic and myeloid leukaemia
    Lymphomas
    Macroglobulinaemia
    Polycythaemia vera (usually only splenomegaly)
    Sarcoidosis
    Viral hepatitis
	Renal failure
	    Amyloid
	    Multiple myeloma
	    Uraemia
	
	Tremor and ataxia
	    IgM paraproteinaemia
	
	Uveitis
	    Sarcoidosis

LABORATORY INVESTIGATIONS

Investigations which should be performed on all patients include urinalysis, full blood count, erythrocyte sedimentation rate, fasting blood glucose, serum electrolytes, serum creatinine, serum proteins and plasma electrophoresis, liver function tests and chest radiographs.

Other investigations may be indicated when specific disorders are suspected. They include urinary porphyrins and heavy metals, cryoglobulins, radiological skeletal survey and bone scan, faecal fats and other tests for malabsorption, thyroid function studies, serum B12 and folate levels, urinary Bence-Jones protein, bone marrow biopsy, radiological and endoscopic investigation of the upper and lower gastrointestinal tract. Biopsy of enlarged lymph nodes and liver may be indicated as may be rectal and renal biopsy for amyloidosis.

Electrophysiological studies

Nerve conduction studies should be performed to affirm the neuropathic nature of symptoms. Marked slowing of conduction, suggestive of demyelination, may be seen in diabetes and some cases of neuropathy secondary to carcinoma and lymphoma. Delayed conduction at sites of entrapment, especially the carpal tunnel, is seen commonly in diabetes, acromegaly and hypothyroidism. More details of the clinical uses of electrodiagnosis may be found in *Chapter 1*.

Sural nerve biopsy

When all other investigations have been performed, sural nerve biopsy is indicated in some patients to establish a diagnosis. Specific diagnostic abnormalities are seen in sarcoidosis, primary amyloid disease, primary biliary cirrhosis and primary hyperoxaluria. Characteristic abnormalities, although not necessarily diagnostic, are seen in hypothyroidism, acromegaly and in IgM paraproteinaemia and macroglobulinaemia.

TREATMENT

Acute neuropathies

Spirometry should be performed every 2–4 hours in the initial stages. Intubation, artificial ventilation and sometimes tracheostomy may be necessary. Careful nursing is very important and particular attention should be paid to skin, bladder, bowels, mouth, pharynx and trachea. Lung and urinary tract infections require prompt treatment. Intravenous or intragastric feeding may be necessary. Splints to prevent foot and wrist drop may be necessary and physiotherapy should begin immediately. Treatment of the underlying condition should be commenced. More detail may be found in *Chapter 2*.

Chronic neuropathies

Specific treatment for the underlying cause should be given if possible. Physiotherapy is an important part of treatment. In severe cases splints, calipers and other walking aids will be necessary and occasionally surgical corrective procedures will be required. A programme of rehabilitation should be commenced.

Some of the systemic disorders associated with peripheral neuropathy will now be considered in more detail.

METABOLIC DISORDERS

Uraemia

Peripheral neuropathy as a complication of chronic renal failure was not recognized until about 20 years ago (Asbury, Victor and Adams, 1963). It was noted primarily in patients undergoing haemodialysis and occurs in about two-thirds of those requiring this form of treatment (Dyck *et al.*, 1975). With the earlier recognition and treatment of chronic renal failure and more effective means of dialysis, the condition is now less common. The peripheral neuropathy is not related to the cause of chronic renal failure but rather to its duration and severity.

Clinical features

Males are more commonly affected (Asbury, 1975a). The onset is usually gradual and the clinical features are those of a sensory neuropathy with symptoms of dysaesthesiae (painful tingling feet, sensations of swelling of the fingers and toes, band-like constrictions around the feet and occasional burning sensations), restless legs and muscle cramps. There is a symmetrical, predominantly distal, involvement with the feet being more commonly affected than the hands (Nielsen, 1974a; Asbury, 1975a). On examination it is common to find mild distal wasting in the feet (especially the extensor digitorum brevis muscles), absent ankle jerks, impaired vibration sense and two-point discrimination. Occasionally the onset is acute or subacute, progressing to marked muscle wasting and paralysis (*see* Asbury, Victor and Adams, 1963, case 4). The CSF protein is usually not elevated although in some cases it reaches levels of about 1.0 g/l (Asbury, 1975a).

Effect of dialysis and transplantation

The peripheral neuropathy usually remains stable or improves with dialysis; if not, increasing the frequency and duration of dialysis may result in improvement although this is not a universal finding (Asbury, 1975a). Rapid improvement, even in patients with long-standing neuropathy, usually follows successful renal transplantation (Bolton, Baltzan and Baltzan, 1971; Ibrahim *et al.*, 1974).

Clinical neurophysiology

There is electrophysiological evidence of peripheral neuropathy in patients with chronic renal failure even when they have no signs or symptoms (Preswick and Jeremy, 1964). In patients with chronic renal failure and clinical neuropathy, there is uniformly impaired nerve conduction in upper and lower extremities. The degree of slowing of conduction correlates closely with the creatinine clearance and is not independently related to serum creatinine or blood urea levels. There is no correlation between the slowing of conduction and the clinical signs of neuropathy (Nielsen, 1973a and b). Regular haemodialysis has very little consistent effect on the impaired conduction velocities in patients with uraemic neuropathy, in spite of their clinical improvement (Nielsen, 1974b). Following renal transplantation there is a rapid improvement in nerve conduction during the first few days (Ibrahim *et al.*, 1974; Oh *et al.*, 1978). There is then a second phase of slow improvement which may last for several months although normal values may never be attained (Nielsen, 1974c; Bolton, 1976).

Pathology

There is little doubt that the major pathological features of uraemic neuropathy are those of axonal degeneration affecting the distal nerve trunks more severely than proximal segments (Asbury, Victor and Adams, 1963; Thomas *et al.*, 1971; Dyck *et al.*, 1971). Some workers have emphasized the presence of segmental demyelination in sural nerve biopsies; however these changes are mainly secondary to axonal damage (Dyck *et al.*, 1971; Asbury, 1975a).

Pathogenesis

The pathogenesis of the peripheral neuropathy is almost certainly multifactorial (Asbury, 1975a). No specific toxic factors have been isolated; neither creatinine nor urea have been directly implicated. It has been suggested that substances of molecular weight 500–5000 may be involved (Babb *et al.*, 1971). Increased levels of myoinositol (de Jesus, Clements and Winegrad, 1974) or parathyroid hormone (Avram, Feinfeld and Huatuco, 1978) and accumulation of inhibitors of sodium transport mechanisms (Nielsen, 1978) may be factors but hypermagnesaemia and vitamin deficiencies do not appear to be important (Asbury, 1975a).

Primary hyperoxaluria

Several patients have been reported with primary hyperoxaluria who develop rapidly progressive motor or sensory neuropathies in spite of adequate haemodialysis. In addition to the presence of axonal degeneration and segmental demyelination in peripheral nerves, oxalate crystals have been observed in the nerve fibres (Hall *et al.*, 1976).

Porphyria

Peripheral neuropathy accompanies the hepatic porphyrias (acute intermittent porphyria, variegate porphyria and the rare hereditary coproporphyria) which are dominantly inherited.

It usually has an acute onset and may be preceded or accompanied by autonomic manifestations of tachycardia, hypertension and postural hypotension. Abdominal pain, constipation, vomiting and mental changes frequently herald the attacks which may have been precipitated by barbiturates. The neuropathy is predominantly motor but pain in the limbs and back may precede the weakness. The upper limbs may be more severely affected than the lower and proximal muscles may be affected more than distal muscles. Facial and ocular palsies may be present. These clinical findings may help to distinguish the peripheral neuropathy of porphyria from that due to other causes (Ridley, 1975).

Electromyography reveals signs of denervation and nerve conduction studies may be normal or show only mild slowing of conduction compatible with the underlying pathology of axonal degeneration (Cavanagh and Mellick, 1965; Wochnik-Dyjas, Niewiadomska and Kostrzewska, 1978).

Hypoglycaemia due to insulinoma

An association of peripheral neuropathy with hypoglycaemia caused by insulinoma has been described (Jaspan *et al.*, 1982). The characteristic findings are those of a predominantly or entirely motor peripheral neuropathy which is distal and symmetrical. Upper limb involvement is more frequent and more severe than that of the lower limbs. The weakness is associated with prominent wasting in involved muscles but fasciculations are infrequently observed. Painful paraesthesiae are common but there are usually no objective signs of sensory disturbance. Following removal of the insulinoma, weakness improves but wasting persists or improves only slightly. Sensory symptoms resolve completely. The peripheral neuropathy occurs more commonly in males and during a period when hypoglycaemic episodes are occurring frequently and are manifested by disturbances in cerebral function. The recurrent hypoglycaemia seems to be a major factor in the aetiology of the condition.

Hyperlipaemic neuropathy

Peripheral neuropathy has been described in association with hyperlipidaemia, hyperuricaemia and hypertension (Nausieda, 1977). However, the association remains unproven.

ENDOCRINE DISORDERS

Hypothyroid polyneuropathy

Carpal tunnel syndrome is a well recognized complication of hypothyroidism but a generalized peripheral neuropathy predominantly of a sensory type may also occur. Symptoms of pain and paraesthesiae are frequent (Crevasse and Logue, 1959; Nickel *et al.*, 1961). The sensory symptoms may be present for many years before the diagnosis of hypothyroidism is made. Electrophysiological studies demonstrate moderate slowing of motor conduction and impaired sensory conduction and pathological studies on the peripheral nerve show loss of myelinated fibres, predominantly due to axonal degeneration, abnormalities of mitochondria and prominent glycogen deposition within Schwann cells (Pollard *et al.*, 1982). Thyroid function should be examined in all patients presenting with a sensory neuropathy. An association between thyrotoxicosis and a severe sensorimotor neuropathy remains unproven (Feibel and Campa, 1976).

Acromegaly

Carpal tunnel syndrome is known to be associated with acromegaly, the incidence having been reported to be as high as 35% (O'Duffy, Randall and MacCarty, 1973). Generalized peripheral neuropathy is not so well recognized but in one series, 5 of 11 (45%) patients had clinical symptoms and signs of peripheral neuropathy and 8 of 11 (73%) had electrophysiological evidence of widespread nerve damage. The peripheral neuropathy, which is independent of associated diabetes, is predominantly sensory in type, the patients usually complaining of paraesthesiae of hands and feet; on physical examination there is depression or absence of reflexes and distal sensory impairment. Occasionally, severe distal muscle wasting may be present (Low *et al.*, 1974). The CSF protein is usually not significantly elevated. Pathologically there is enlargement of the fascicles, increase in endoneural and subperineural tissue and a reduction in the density of myelinated fibres (Low *et al.*, 1974). Some improvement may follow treatment.

MALIGNANCIES AND RETICULOSES

Carcinoma

The incidence of clinical peripheral neuropathy in patients with carcinoma (most commonly the lung but also the stomach, breast, colon, rectum and other organs) is of the order of 5%, although some workers have reported a higher figure (Teräväinen and Larsen, 1977). The incidence is as high as 50% if electrophysio-logical and pathological studies are employed in investigation (McLeod, 1975). There is some evidence, at least in oat cell carcinoma of the lung, that the high incidence is related to loss of body weight in the later stages of the illness (Hawley *et al.*, 1980). The incidence seems to depend on the pathological type and site of the tumour, the stage and duration of the illness, the diligence with which it is sought, the techniques of investigation and the criteria for diagnosis (*see* McLeod, 1975; Henson and Urich, 1982).

Clinical features

Two main clinical types are recognized, a sensory neuropathy and a sensorimotor neuropathy.

(1) Sensory neuropathy. Paraesthesiae, dysaesthesiae, aching pains in the limbs, and gait disturbances due to sensory ataxia are the main features. Muscle wasting and weakness are inconspicuous. Reflexes are depressed or absent and there is loss of all sensory modalities in the extremities with occasional involvement of trunk and face. Severe impairment of position and vibration sense with pseudoathetosis is common and sometimes memory loss and

dementia due to an associated encephalomyelitis may be present. The symptoms may precede the signs of malignancy by anything up to 3.5 years. Less commonly the sensory neuropathy develops after the diagnosis of carcinoma is made. The onset is usually subacute but may rarely be acute. Females are affected more commonly. The site of malignancy is usually in the lung and there is a particular association of sensory neuropathy with oat cell carcinoma. However, it should be noted that Hawley *et al.* (1980) found no sensory neuropathy in a series of 71 patients with oat cell carcinoma.

(2) Sensorimotor neuropathy. Sensorimotor neuropathy is more common than the pure sensory type. The primary site of the malignancy is most commonly the lung but may also be in the stomach, breast, colon, rectum, pancreas, uterus, cervix, kidney, thyroid, prostate and testes. The clinical presentation may be acute like the Guillain-Barré syndrome but is more commonly subacute or chronic. In this latter type it is a predominantly distal, mixed motor and sensory neuropathy with occasionally an associated trigeminal neuropathy. The neuropathy may precede the diagnosis of the carcinoma by up to 5 years. On the other hand, it may be mild and distal, occurring late in the disease. The lower limbs are affected to a greater degree than the upper limbs. A relapsing and remitting neuropathy, presumably of the demyelinating type, may also be associated with malignancy; it is not common in carcinoma of the lung, but there may be an association with seminoma of the testis. There is often a high CSF protein (McLeod, 1975).

Electrophysiological studies

In sensory neuropathy sensory action potentials are absent and motor conduction velocities are normal or only mildly slowed. In subacute and chronic types of sensorimotor neuropathy terminal motor latencies may be increased, motor conduction velocities are normal or mildly slowed, consistent with the underlying pathology of axonal degeneration, and sensory conduction may be impaired. In some patients with acute or subacute neuropathies, and in some with the relapsing and remitting types, motor conduction velocities may be markedly slowed, suggesting that the underlying pathology is segmental demyelination.

Pathology

In the pure sensory neuropathy there is degeneration of the dorsal root ganglion cells, dorsal root fibres, posterior columns and sensory fibres in the peripheral nerve (Denny-Brown, 1948). In sensorimotor neuropathy the pathological findings are those of axonal degeneration with loss of myelinated fibres in the peripheral nerve (*Figure 5.1*). The pathogenesis of the paraneoplastic neuropathies is unknown.

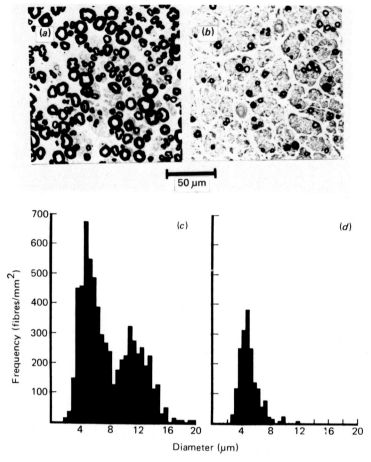

Figure 5.1 Sensorimotor neuropathy associated with carcinoma. Photomicrographs of sural nerves from a control subject (*a*) and a patient with carcinomatous neuropathy (*b*), with corresponding histograms of myelinated fibre distribution (*c, d*). There is a marked loss of myelinated fibres of all diameters.

LYMPHOMAS AND OTHER RETICULOSES

Lymphoma

The incidence of clinical peripheral neuropathy in patients with lymphoma is about 8% but with the aid of electrophysiological techniques it may be demonstrated in about 35% of patients (Walsh, 1971a).

Clinical features

As in carcinomatous neuropathy, two main clinical types are recognized: a sensory neuropathy and a sensorimotor neuropathy.

(1) Sensory neuropathy. Pure sensory neuropathy is considerably less common in lymphoma than it is in carcinoma (McLeod and Walsh, 1975a). The clinical features of paraesthesiae, dysaesthesiae, pain and sensory ataxia are similar to those seen in carcinoma.

(2) Sensorimotor neuropathy. Acute polyneuropathy, of the Guillain-Barré type, is more common in association with lymphomas particularly Hodgkin's disease than with other malignant tumours, probably as a result of the underlying disturbances of immune function in patients with disease of the lymphoreticular system (Lisak *et al.*, 1977). Relapsing and remitting neuropathies also occur more commonly with lymphomas than carcinoma and in both the acute and chronic relapsing neuropathies segmental demyelination is the underlying pathological change. However, chronic neuropathy in which axonal degeneration is the underlying pathology is the most common type of peripheral neuropathy associated with lymphomas (Walsh, 1971a; McLeod and Walsh, 1975a). Malignant infiltration of nerve roots and peripheral nerves occurs more commonly in the lymphomas than in carcinoma.

Leukaemia

Peripheral neuropathy in leukaemia is most commonly the result of infiltration, haemorrhage, and infarction in the peripheral nerves (McLeod and Walsh, 1975a; Henson and Urich, 1982). Paraneoplastic peripheral neuropathy is rare in acute leukaemia and in erythraemic myelosis (Di Guglielmo's disease). It is more common, however, in chronic lymphatic leukaemia in which there may be an associated acute polyneuritis of the Guillain-Barré type or a chronic sensorimotor neuropathy. Peripheral neuropathy is an unusual complication of chronic myeloid leukaemia (McLeod and Walsh, 1975a; Henson and Urich, 1982).

Polycythaemia vera

Neurological manifestations of polycythaemia vera (primary polycythaemia) include headaches, vertigo, strokes, visual symptoms, tinnitus, paraesthesiae and pains in the limbs. Although paraesthesiae of the extremities are common symptoms, peripheral neuropathy is a rare complication of the disease. In a recent study of 26 patients, 11 had sensory symptoms of paraesthesiae, burning sensations or pains in the limbs. Of these, three had clinical signs consistent with a mild peripheral neuropathy, the characteristic clinical findings of which were normal power in all muscle groups but depression of deep tendon reflexes and an impaired perception of all sensory modalities in the distal extremities. Electrophysiological studies revealed impairment of conduction in 7 of the 26 patients, and when the nerve conduction studies of the whole group of patients were compared with those in controls, there was a significant impairment of sensory conduction and mild slowing of motor conduction. Sural nerve biopsies performed on three patients demonstrated features consistent with mild chronic axonal degeneration. It was concluded from the study that there was an association between polycythaemia vera and peripheral neuropathy of a predominantly sensory type (Yiannikas, McLeod and Walsh, 1983).

LIVER DISEASE

Peripheral neuropathy has been associated with: (1) chronic liver disease of different types, and (2) viral hepatitis.

(1) Chronic liver disease

(a) Alcoholic and cryptogenic cirrhosis

A number of workers have reported an association between chronic liver disease, usually alcoholic or cryptogenic cirrhosis, and a mild, frequently asymptomatic, predominantly sensory neuropathy which is unrelated to alcoholism or diabetes (Dayan and Williams, 1967; Seneviratne and Peiris, 1970; Knill-Jones et al., 1972; Kardel and Nielsen, 1974; Chari et al., 1977). The prevalence of this type of neuropathy is variously reported. Kardel and Nielsen (1974) found clinical evidence of neuropathy (absent reflexes and impaired vibration sense) in 23 of 34 (68%) patients with severe chronic hepatic failure but there was clinical and electrophysiological evidence of peripheral nerve dysfunction in 31 of 34 (91%). Chari et al. (1977) found clinical evidence of peripheral neuropathy in 63.3% of patients with hepatic cirrhosis and pathological evidence of demyelination in 80%. Knill-Jones et al. (1972) found mild peripheral neuropathy in 14 of 70 (20%) patients with chronic liver disease due to alcoholic and cryptogenic cirrhosis, haemochromatosis, and active chronic hepatitis; 13 of these had clinical evidence of neuropathy and one additional patient had abnormal nerve conduction studies only. Seneviratne and Peiris (1970) found abnormal nerve conduction studies in 34 of 50 (68%) patients with chronic liver disease but clinical peripheral neuropathy was present in only four of 50 (8%).

The pathological changes in the sural nerve have been most commonly reported to be those of segmental demyelination (Dayan and Williams, 1967; Knill-Jones et al., 1972; Chari et al., 1977) although Kardel and Nielsen (1974) argued that there was a metabolic dysfunction of axonal membranes. It is certainly possible that the changes of segmental demyelination may be secondary to axonal degeneration (Asbury, 1975b).

In summary, a demyelinating neuropathy, usually asymptomatic and of little clinical importance, occurs in chronic liver disease. In all reports, the chronic liver disease has been of mixed aetiologies and it is therefore difficult to determine the cause of the neuropathy. It is not necessarily related to diabetes or alcoholism. In some of the cases it was associated with increased serum IgA and IgM, oesophageal varices and a past history of hepatic encephalopathy (Knill-Jones et al., 1972).

(b) Primary biliary cirrhosis

Thomas and Walker (1965) described a mild sensory neuropathy in three female patients with primary biliary cirrhosis. In two sural nerve biopsies there were myelinated fibre loss and xanthomatous infiltration of the fascicles; the peripheral neuropathy was attributed to the lipid infiltration. Charron, Peyronnard and Marchand (1980) reported the case of a woman, aged 29, with primary biliary cirrhosis who presented with an asymmetrical sensory neuropathy at a time when her liver disease was minimal. Xanthomas were not present in the skin. There was normal motor conduction velocity but impaired sensory conduction. Sural nerve biopsy revealed the pathological changes of chronic axonal degeneration of a dying-back type, but there was no lipid infiltration of the nerve, a finding which indicated that other mechanisms may have been involved in the pathogenesis of the neuropathy.

(c) Infantile obstructive cholangiopathy

A progressive neurological syndrome has been reported in six children with long-standing chronic obstructive liver disease. Three patients came to autopsy; all were found to have biliary cirrhosis and in two there was extrahepatic biliary fibrosis. The neurological syndrome consisted of gaze paresis and nystagmus, ataxia of gait, areflexia and impaired position and vibration sense. Neuropathological findings were loss of large myelinated fibres and axonal degeneration in the peripheral nerves, loss of dorsal root ganglion cells, posterior column degeneration, and swollen dystrophic axons (spheroids) and astrocytosis in the gracile and cuneate nuclei, posterior columns and Clarke's column. The disorder was attributed to vitamin E deficiency (Rosenblum *et al.*, 1981).

(2) Viral hepatitis

Acute polyneuritis of the Guillain-Barré type is sometimes a complication of type A and type B viral hepatitis as it is in other virus infections (Lescher, 1944; Byrne Taylor, 1945; Lovell, 1945; Davison *et al.*, 1972; Asbury, 1975b). Usually it occurs after the onset of jaundice (Boudouresques *et al.*, 1970; Asbury, 1975b) but may occasionally precede it (Lescher, 1944). Chari *et al.* (1977) reported mild clinical neuropathy mainly of a sensory type in two of 12 patients with infectious hepatitis; the pathological findings on sural nerve biopsy were those of segmental demyelination.

Davison *et al.* (1972) found slowing of nerve conduction velocities, followed by recovery, during episodes of severe type B hepatitis in 11 patients undergoing intermittent haemodialysis for chronic renal failure. They attributed the occurrence of neuropathy to the viral infection. Farivar *et al.* (1976) described a severe sensorimotor neuropathy that developed over a period of 4–5 weeks and persisted for over 12 months in a patient with HBsAg-positive chronic active hepatitis and cryoproteinaemia; they considered that cryoprotein deposition in small blood vessels may have been reponsible for the neuropathy. We have also seen patients with acute polyneuritis complicating both type A and type B hepatitis.

GASTROINTESTINAL DISEASE

The subject of peripheral neuropathy and other neurological disorders associated with gastrointestinal disease was thoroughly reviewed by Pallis and Lewis (1974).

Peripheral neuropathy of a predominantly sensory type is a common manifestation of *pernicious anaemia*. The symptoms are those of numbness and tingling in the extremities and there are signs of distal sensory loss with diminished position and vibration sense and depressed reflexes. Electrophysiological studies have demonstrated peripheral nerve involvement in 65% of patients with untreated pernicious anaemia (Cox-Klazinga and Endtz, 1980). They reveal impaired sensory conduction and mild slowing of motor conduction (Gilliatt, Goodman and Willison, 1961; Mayer, 1965; Cox-Klazinga and Endtz, 1980; Fine and Hallett, 1980). Subacute combined degeneration may be associated with the peripheral neuropathy; extensor plantar responses in the presence of absent reflexes and loss of sensation should always alert the clinician to the possibility of vitamin B_{12} deficiency. Improvement in symptoms follows treatment. Thiamine deficiency may also contribute to the neuropathy (Hornabrook and Marks, 1960; Cox-Klazinga and Endtz, 1980). The underlying pathology appears to be that of axonal degeneration (McLeod, Walsh and Little, 1969).

Peripheral neuropathy of a predominantly sensory type may also result from vitamin B_{12} deficiency due to malabsorption following total gastrectomy, carcinoma of the stomach, partial gastrectomy, small bowel resection, tropical sprue, regional ileitis, coeliac disease, Whipple's disease, scleroderma (systemic sclerosis), blind loops, strictures, jejunal and ileal diverticulosis, and stagnant loops due to gastrocolic and other fistulae. Cooke *et al.* (1963) studied neuropathy in patients with jejunal diverticulosis and it was not uncommonly the presenting feature of the condition with symptoms of paraesthesiae. In some patients there were possibly nutritional factors other than the B_{12} deficiency relevant to the aetiology of the neuropathy.

Thiamine deficiency, causing peripheral neuropathy, and even Wernicke's encephalopathy, may also be a complication of malabsorption or of persistent vomiting. The pathological changes in the peripheral nerves are those of axonal degeneration with secondary segmental demyelination (Ohnishi *et al.*, 1980). 'Burning feet' may be a complication of riboflavin, pyridoxine or pantothenic acid deficiency, although the precise mechanism of the symptoms has not been adequately demonstrated (Pallis and Lewis, 1974).

Folate deficiency may result from malnutrition, malabsorption, or drugs, e.g. phenytoin. There are a number of documented cases of patients with predominantly sensory neuropathy attributed to folic acid deficiency in whom clinical and electrophysiological improvement occurred following folic acid administration (Fehling *et al.*, 1974; Botez *et al.*, 1978; Botez, Peyronnard and

Charron, 1979; Shorvon and Reynolds, 1979; Martinez-Figueroa *et al.*, 1980). The pathological features in the peripheral nerve are those of axonal degeneration (Bischoff, Lutschg and Meier, 1975).

Tropical sprue may present with paraesthesiae due to peripheral neuropathy (Pallis and Lewis, 1974). Iyer *et al.* (1973) reported clinical and electrophysiological studies in patients with tropical sprue and found that peripheral neuropathy was relatively common. It was associated with a megaloblastic bone marrow but not with low folate levels.

Cooke and Smith (1966) described clinical and pathological findings in 16 patients with *adult coeliac disease* who developed neurological complications including peripheral neuropathy, myelopathy and cerebellar degeneration. The neuropathy appeared to be of the axonal or dying-back type (Cooke, Johnson and Woolf, 1966). The cause remains unknown but does not seem to be due to vitamin B_{12} or folate deficiency.

Vitamin E deficiency may also occasionally be responsible for peripheral neuropathy in chronic intestinal malabsorption. Cerebellar ataxia may be associated with a predominantly sensory neuropathy (Harding *et al.*, 1982). It seems likely that vitamin E deficiency causes a central-peripheral distal axonopathy (Harding *et al.*, 1982). The patients described by Rosenblum *et al.* (1981) also had low vitamin E levels.

Peripheral neuropathy which improved following treatment of the infection has been described in two patients with giardiasis (Bassett, Danta and Cook, 1978).

CHRONIC OBSTRUCTIVE PULMONARY DISEASE

A mild sensorimotor, usually asymptomatic, neuropathy has been demonstrated clinically and electrophysiologically in some patients with chronic obstructive pulmonary disease (Appenzeller, Parks and MacGee, 1968; Faden, Mendoza and Flynn, 1981). In one study the patients had muscle wasting and in some cases improvement followed treatment of the pulmonary disease and associated malnutrition; it seems likely that nutritional and metabolic disturbances were mainly responsible for the peripheral neuropathy (Appenzeller, Parks and MacGee, 1968). In the other study, in which the patients had only mild sensory neuropathy and no evidence of muscle wasting, an association with tobacco smoking was described and a toxic aetiology suggested (Faden, Mendoza and Flynn, 1981). Further studies on this type of neuropathy are required but at the present time it seems to be of little clinical importance and so far has not been described as a presenting or dominant clinical feature of any patients with chronic obstructive pulmonary disease.

SARCOIDOSIS

Peripheral neuropathy may occur as an isolated manifestation of sarcoidosis or as part of the more generalized systemic manifestations of the disease. Females are affected more commonly (Matthews, 1975).

Facial nerve palsy is the most common neurological manifestation of the condition. The peripheral nervous system is most commonly affected by an asymmetrical involvement of nerve trunks (mononeuritis multiplex). Characteristically, there is sensory loss over large areas on the trunk which may be associated with dysaesthesiae or pain (Matthews, 1975). Symmetrical polyneuropathy is less common; it may have an acute onset, indistinguishable from the Guillain-Barré syndrome, or a slower evolution with a more chronic course. It may be predominantly sensory, predominantly motor, or mixed sensorimotor in type. In the acute form and in mononeuritis multiplex there are often systemic manifestations of sarcoidosis but in the chronic forms there may be little associated evidence of the disease. The association of cranial nerve palsies with a chronic neuropathy should alert the clinician to the possibility of sarcoidosis.

Nerve conduction studies may be normal or show only mild degrees of slowing of conduction (Matthews, 1975; Oh, 1980). There have been few pathological studies of the peripheral nervous system. Granulomas may be found in the epineurium or endoneurium of the peripheral nerves and in some cases granulomas have been seen to surround and invade the walls of arterioles (Oh, 1980; Nemni *et al.*, 1981; Vital *et al.*, 1982a). The diagnosis can often be made clinically when there are associated features of hilar lymphadenopathy, uveitis, parotitis and erythema nodosum. Sarcoid granulomas may be seen on muscle and sural nerve biopsy. The cerebrospinal fluid examination is usually unhelpful in sarcoid neuropathy but there may be a slight increase in cells and an elevated total protein (Matthews, 1975). The natural history of sarcoid neuropathy is uncertain although the prognosis is better than in central nervous system sarcoidosis. It is therefore difficult to be confident of the value of steroid therapy although it is usually given.

PARAPROTEINAEMIAS AND DYSPROTEINAEMIAS

Multiple myeloma

There is clinical evidence of peripheral neuropathy in about 13% of patients with multiple myeloma, but the incidence is as high as 39% when electrophysiological studies are carried out on all patients with the condition (Walsh, 1971b). The symptoms of peripheral neuropathy may precede the diagnosis of multiple myeloma by several months or a year, or may be late manifestations of the established disease (McLeod and Walsh, 1975b; Kelly *et al.*, 1981a). The onset of the neuropathy is usually gradual but may be subacute. In most cases it is symmetrical and of mixed sensorimotor type but pure sensory and pure motor types also occur. Although symptoms most commonly begin in the lower limbs, in some reported cases the clinical manifestations have been predominantly in the upper limbs. The neuropathy is usually progressive and may advance to almost complete quadriplegia but remissions have been reported in some instances. Bone pain and radicular pain due to root compression are characteristic of myelomatous neuropathy. Peripheral neuropathy has been reported in association with solitary myeloma in a number of cases (McLeod and Walsh, 1975b; Read and Warlow, 1978; Kelly *et al.*, 1981a).

There is a particularly high incidence (about 50%) of peripheral neuropathy in the osteosclerotic type of myeloma (Morley and Schwieger, 1967; Kelly *et al.*, 1981a). The neuropathy is predominantly motor and is usually the presenting feature. Rarely a syndrome of hypogonadism, hypertrichosis, skin pigmentation and hypothyroidism is linked with osteosclerotic myeloma and peripheral neuropathy (Iwashita *et al.*, 1977). See also Chapter 12 for a thorough review by Ohnishi of this problem in Japan.

The CSF protein may be normal but is sometimes raised to levels of 2 g/l or more, particularly in patients with osteosclerotic myeloma. The gammaglobulin fractions are mainly increased. There is usually no increase in the number of lymphocytes in the CSF. Nerve conduction studies are usually impaired but there is rarely gross slowing of conduction and the electrophysiological findings are consistent with the underlying pathology of predominantly axonal degeneration. Segmental demyelination may sometimes occur but is usually secondary to the axonal changes. Amyloid deposits may sometimes be seen in the peripheral nerves, in the endoneurium and around blood vessels, but they are likely to be only an epiphenomenon and not a causative factor in the development of peripheral neuropathy (McLeod and Walsh, 1975b). Plasma cells have been noted to infiltrate the endoneurium (Vital *et al.*, 1982b).

The pathogenesis of peripheral neuropathy in multiple myeloma remains uncertain. It is not normally due to amyloid or myelomatous infiltration of nerves or roots. A hyperviscosity syndrome causing ischaemia has been suggested but seems unlikely. Toxic or metabolic disturbances may also be factors. The most plausible explanation is that there is an abnormal immunoglobulin which reacts with specific antigens in the peripheral nervous system. The finding of IgA binding to the myelin in a nerve biopsy of one patient lends support to this hypothesis (Rousseau *et al.*, 1978). Moreover, Besinger *et al.* (1981) produced neuropathy in mice by passive transfer of immunoglobulin from patients with neuropathy and multiple myeloma.

The peripheral neuropathy usually progresses in spite of treatment of the underlying myeloma, although in some cases with single lesions improvement has followed radiation therapy (McLeod and Walsh, 1975b; Read and Warlow, 1978; Kelly *et al.*, 1981a).

Macroglobulinaemia

Macroglobulinaemia is a disease mainly affecting the elderly and characterized by fatigue, weakness, weight loss, anaemia, bleeding from mucous membranes, visual disturbances, lymphadenopathy and hepatosplenomegaly. There is a proliferation of lymphocytoid cells, with infiltration of the bone marrow, lymph nodes and other tissues. The erythrocyte sedimentation rate is usually high. A dense narrow band in the beta–gamma region is seen on paper electrophoresis and a markedly increased IgM fraction on immunoelectrophoresis of the plasma. Less frequently, macroglobulinaemia occurs in association with chronic lymphatic leukaemia, lymphosarcoma, carcinoma, cirrhosis of the liver, connective tissue disorders, haemolytic anaemia of the cold antibody type and other diseases, but in these conditions levels of IgM are not so markedly elevated.

It has been estimated that about 25% of patients with macroglobulinaemia have neurological complications (Logothetis, Silverstein and Coe, 1960).

Where peripheral neuropathy is associated in elderly people with malaise, fatigue, weakness, anaemia, lymphadenopathy, hepatosplenomegaly, and a bleeding diathesis, macroglobulinaemia is a likely cause. The symptoms of peripheral neuropathy may antedate the other symptoms but, in most cases, the neuropathy develops after the systemic manifestations. Sensory symptoms consisting of paraesthesiae, pain and muscle cramps are usually prominent and are accompanied by objective evidence of distal sensory loss. Muscle wasting also occurs and may be severe in upper and lower extremities. In some patients fasciculations have been observed. Foot drop and steppage gait are common and occasionally motor weakness may proceed to almost total paralysis of limbs. Cranial nerves may also be affected and deafness has been described by several authors.

The neuropathy most commonly commences insidiously but, in rare instances, may have an acute onset with a Guillain-Barré type of picture. Initially it may be asymmetrical but in later stages usually has the distribution of a symmetrical sensorimotor neuropathy. A cauda equina syndrome has been reported. The condition is progressive, and remissions with treatment are most unusual. The CSF protein may be normal but is usually elevated and the globulin fraction may be increased. An increase in cells is very unusual.

Electrophysiological studies demonstrate impairment of sensory conduction and normal or mild slowing of motor conduction in most cases (McLeod and Walsh, 1975b; Iwashita *et al.*, 1974). Gross slowing of conduction has also been reported (Julien *et al.*, 1978).

Pathologically, the peripheral nerves are infiltrated by mononuclear cells, mainly lymphocytes, with an occasional plasma cell (McLeod and Walsh, 1975b; Julien *et al.*, 1978, Vital *et al.*, 1982b). Degeneration of myelinated fibres occurs and both axonal degeneration and segmental demyelination have been observed. Myelin may appear uncompacted with widening of the intraperiod line (Propp *et al.*, 1975; Julien *et al.*, 1978). Amyloid deposits have been found in some cases. An amorphous hyaline-like PAS-positive substance has been demonstrated in the perineurium, endoneurium and the blood vessel walls which contains IgM (Iwashita *et al.*, 1974). IgM deposits have also been found on the myelin sheath (Propp *et al.*, 1975; Julien *et al.*, 1978; Iwashita *et al.*, 1974; Vital *et al.*, 1982b).

The pathogenesis of the polyneuropathy in Waldenström's macroglobulinaemia still remains uncertain but the reaction of immunoglobulins against myelin and possibly other nerve antigens may be an important factor. Dellagi *et al.* (1979) found shared idiotypic determinants in five of 16 patients with macroglobulinaemia and neuropathy and one case of IgG paraproteinaemia and polyneuropathy; the finding suggests that certain neural antigens may be involved more frequently than others. Moreover, the shared determinants were located in the Fab fragment of the immunoglobulin, a finding which provides some evidence that the monoclonal immunoglobulin of these patients may mediate the nerve injury via their antibody activity. Other possible mechanisms include cellular infiltration, amyloid deposits and hyperviscosity causing ischaemia.

Cryoglobulinaemia

Cryoglobulinaemia is a disorder characterized by the presence in the serum of a protein (cryoglobulin) that precipitates on cooling and redissolves on warming to 37°C. Cryoglobulins are usually IgG or IgM although mixed cryoglobulins of both fractions have been reported. Cryoglobulinaemia may occur as a primary condition without any apparent underlying process (essential cryoglobulinaemias). More commonly it may be secondary to a large number of other diseases which include the monoclonal gammopathies, such as myeloma, macroglobulinaemia, and lymphomas in which the M component has cryoproperties and also the polyclonal gammopathies such as connective tissue disorders, chronic infections and mesothelioma.

The usual clinical manifestations of cryoglobulinaemia are those related to cold sensitivity such as Raynaud's phenomenon and sometimes even gangrene of the extremities; bleeding diatheses, including purpura, ecchymoses, bleeding from the mouth, nose or gastrointestinal tract and retinal haemorrhage; arthralgia; weakness; malaise; and ulceration of the skin.

The incidence of clinical neuropathy in cryoglobulinaemia, essential and secondary, is about 7% (Logothetis *et al.*, 1968).

Characteristically, the patients present with Raynaud's phenomenon, purpuric skin eruptions and ulceration of the lower limbs. After a variable period of time, from 1–8 years, they develop symptoms of neuropathy which are often precipitated by cold weather, the most prominent of which are pain in the limbs and paraesthesiae. Wasting and weakness of distal muscles may also occur. The neuropathy is commonly asymmetrical at least initially, and it may present as a mononeuritis multiplex. Gradual progression occurs.

Peripheral neuropathy may also occur in cryoglobulinaemia secondary to malignant lymphoma, polyarteritis, and multiple myeloma (McLeod and Walsh, 1975b; Vallat *et al.*, 1980).

Nerve conduction studies reveal impairment of sensory conduction and mild slowing of motor conduction in those cases where they have been performed (McLeod and Walsh, 1975b).

Pathological changes in the peripheral nerve are those of predominantly axonal degeneration. Lymphocyte and plasma cell infiltration has been observed around blood vessels which may show evidence of vasculitis (Cream *et al.*, 1974; Chad *et al.*, 1982; Konishi *et al.*, 1982). Vasculitis and inflammatory cell infiltration may extend into the perineurium. In a case of cryoglobulinaemic neuropathy complicating multiple myeloma, closely packed tubular structures whose ultrastructure was identical to cryoprecipitate extracted from serum, were seen in the endoneurial space, walls of vasa nervorum and within the lumen of some blood vessels (Vallat *et al.*, 1980). The pathogenetic mechanism is uncertain but possibly vasculitis and cryoprotein precipitation may interfere with local microcirculation leading to ischaemic injury of the peripheral nerve. Immune-mediated demyelination, increased blood viscosity, thrombosis and haemorrhage have also been postulated.

The treatment of the neuropathy is that of the underlying condition by the administration of cytotoxic drugs, corticosteroids, and sometimes plasma exchange. There is little evidence that the treatment influences the course of peripheral neuropathy.

Neuropathy associated with benign monoclonal gammopathy

Benign monoclonal gammopathy is the name applied to conditions in which a monoclonal paraprotein is present without any other evidence of a malignant B cell disorder. The incidence of this finding increases with age, and is found in 19% of people over 90 years of age (Kohn, 1976). An association between benign monoclonal gammopathy and peripheral neuropathy is well recognized and has been reported in 10% of patients with peripheral neuropathy of unknown cause (Kelly *et al.*, 1981b). IgG, IgM and IgA paraproteinaemias have been found in these cases.

IgG paraproteinaemia

Most of the cases of IgG paraproteinaemia described have been chronic progressive sensorimotor polyneuropathies (Dalakas and Engel, 1981) although three cases described by Read, Vanhegan and Matthews (1978) remitted spontaneously and the case of Contamin *et al.* (1976) followed a relapsing and remitting course. In a small number only of these cases low nerve conduction velocities have been reported (Dalakas and Engel, 1981). Immunofluorescent studies have shown binding of IgG or light chain fragments to myelin sheaths in some cases (Chazot *et al.*, 1976; Sewell *et al.*, 1981; Dalakas and Engel, 1981). Both axonal degeneration and demyelination have been reported in sural nerve biopsies (Read, Vanhegan and Matthews, 1978).

IgA paraproteinaemia

IgA is the least common paraprotein found (Chazot *et al.*, 1976; Kahn, Riches and Kohn, 1980; Bosch *et al.*, 1982). Few cases have been described in detail but two patients presented with features of anterior horn cell degeneration (Chazot *et al.*, 1976; Bosch *et al.*, 1982).

IgM paraproteinaemia

Greater homogeneity exists among patients with IgM than with other classes of paraproteinaemia. Smith *et al.* (1983) have described the clinical features as those of a chronic sensorimotor polyneuropathy presenting insidiously in the sixth or seventh decades with paraesthesiae and then numbness in the feet, followed by similar symptoms in the hands. In their series of 12 cases, nine were male, all had tremor or ataxia and in five there was a history of Raynaud's phenomenon. The tremor was evident in the fingers and hands when arms were outstretched and it was increased by action. Ataxia in the legs was common. These movement disorders have previously been described in patients with neuropathy and IgM paraproteinaemia (Fitting *et al.*, 1979; Bajada, Mastaglia and Fisher, 1980; Spencer and Moench, 1980).

Immunology

IgM antibodies binding to surviving myelin sheaths have been reported in sural nerve biopsy specimens (*Figure 5.2*; Chazot *et al.*, 1976; Fitting *et al.*, 1979; Swash *et al.*, 1979; Dalakas and Engel, 1981; Smith *et al.*, 1983). Latov *et al.* (1981a) demonstrated that the serum IgM fraction in four cases displayed antimyelin activity (as detected by a complement fixation assay) and that the antigen in peripheral nerve against which these antibodies appear to be directed is a protein of approximately 100 000 daltons. This protein is also present in the central nervous

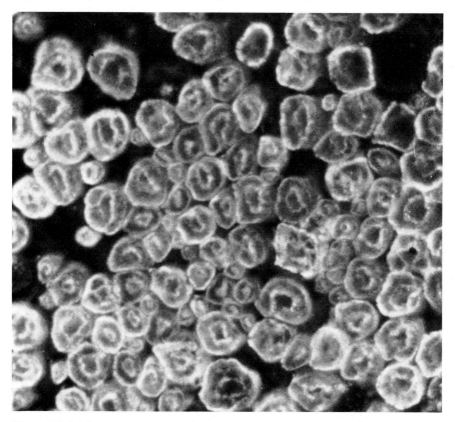

Figure 5.2 IgM κ paraproteinemia and neuropathy. Indirect immunofluorescence on normal sural nerve treated with 1:10 serum and immunostained with fluorescein labelled anti IgM. (Frozen section, acetone fixation ×480)

system and current evidence suggests that it is myelin-associated-glycoprotein (MAG) (Latov *et al.*, 1981b; Braun, Frail and Latov, 1982). In the cases described by Smith *et al.* (1983) monoclonal IgM was attached to peripheral nerve myelin in all of eight biopsied cases and the heavy-chain class and the light-chain type were identical to those of the circulating paraprotein. In 11 of 12 cases the light chain type was κ, and the heavy chain class μ. Non-specific binding to myelin via the IgM Fc region was excluded by demonstrating affinity of Fab μ and F(ab)$_2$ μ fragments for myelin. Latov *et al.* (1981a) and Smith *et al.* (1983) have demonstrated considerable species restriction in the antigen antibody binding, the antibody not recognizing mouse, rat or rabbit myelin. Bosch *et al.* (1982) injected serum from three patients with paraproteinaemic neuropathy into rat sciatic nerve but were unable to produce disease; similar studies in appropriate species and passive transfer experiments have yet to be reported.

Cerebrospinal fluid

CSF protein values have been raised in many cases (Thrush, 1970; Latov *et al.*, 1980; Dalakas and Engel, 1981). A monoclonal immunoglobulin peak has been detected in the CSF on agar gel electrophoresis (Dalakas and Engel, 1981).

Electrophysiology

Motor conduction velocities have been slowed to less than 50% of the lower limit of normal in most cases of IgM paraproteinaemic neuropathy (Swash *et al.*, 1979; Fitting *et al.*, 1979; Dalakas and Engel, 1981; Smith *et al.*, 1983).

Histopathology

Consistent histological changes have been found on examination of sural nerve biopsies (Swash *et al.*, 1979; Latov *et al.*, 1980; Smith *et al.*, 1983). All eight cases biopsied by Smith *et al.* (1983) showed a chronic demyelinating neuropathy with extensive axonal loss. Myelinated fibres of all sizes were involved and hypertrophic changes were seen in half the cases. A considerable number of reports have drawn attention to the presence of uncompacted myelin related to widening of the intraperiod line (*Figure 5.3*) in IgM paraproteinaemia (Sluga, 1974; Smith *et al.*, 1983) and in other dysglobulinaemias (Propp *et al.*, 1975; Julien *et al.*, 1978; Nardelli *et al.*, 1981; Ohnishi and Hirano, 1981). Pertinent to these changes is the location of MAG within the intraperiod line, i.e. on the outer surface of the Schwann-cell plasma membrane. It is consistent with the proposed immunological mechanism that unmyelinated fibres are spared (Swash *et al.*, 1979; Latov *et al.*, 1980; Smith *et al.*, 1983).

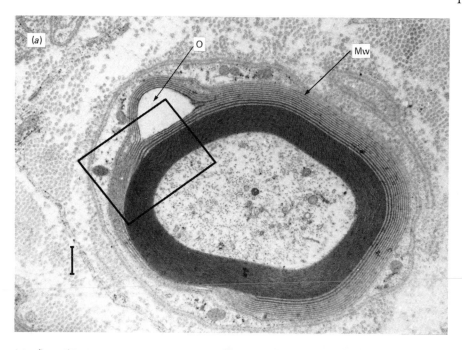

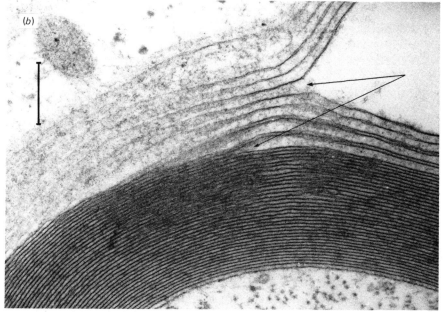

Figure 5.3 (*a*) Electronmicrograph (sural nerve) of a patient with IgM κ paraprotein and neuropathy, showing a myelinated fibre. The outer myelin lamellae (Mw) are widened to about twice the normal periodicity. Intramyelinic oedema (O) has accumulated within the widened lamellae. Bar = 0.5 μm. (*b*) A higher magnification of area outlined in (*a*). Arrows point to the separation of myelin lamellae by opening of intraperiod line. Myelin associated glycoprotein (MAG) is located within intraperiod line. Bar = 0.25 μm

Treatment

No controlled therapeutic trials in monoclonal gammopathy have been published. Several authors have reported improvement in some patients following the use of plasma exchange and immunosuppressive therapy (Latov *et al.*, 1980; Abrams *et al.*, 1982) but a consistent relationship between outcome and reduction of the monoclonal immunoglobulin has not been found (Dalakas and Engel, 1981; Bosch *et al.*, 1982).

Intensive therapy aimed to lower antibody levels (plasma exchange and immunosuppressive therapy) will be justified only if it can be shown that the antibody has not only an affinity for a myelin component (MAG) but actually causes the demyelination.

PRIMARY AMYLOIDOSIS

There is clinical evidence of peripheral neuropathy in 14–15% of patients with primary amyloidosis (Cohen and Benson, 1975; Kyle and Bayrd, 1975) and it may also be present when amyloidosis is associated with dysproteinaemias such as multiple myeloma and macroglobulinaemia.

The clinical manifestations of primary amyloidosis depend upon which organ systems are involved. Gastrointestinal symptoms of diarrhoea, constipation, nausea, abdominal pain and weight loss are common. Renal involvement is present in about 80% of patients with primary amyloid and results in proteinuria, nephrotic syndrome and chronic renal failure. Heart failure due to cardiac infiltration occurs in about 30% of patients. Purpura, macroglossia and hepatomegaly are characteristic findings on physical examination.

When the peripheral nervous system is involved, sensory symptoms of numbness and pain in the extremities are the usual presenting features; carpal tunnel syndrome is commonly associated (Kelly *et al.*, 1979). Because of loss of pain and temperature sense, some patients experience painless burns on the hands and feet; they also later complain of weakness. Autonomic dysfunction is frequently present and patients complain of symptoms of postural hypotension (light headedness, dizziness and syncope), impotence and bladder disturbances.

On neurological examination there is distal wasting and weakness with hyporeflexia or areflexia, but the sensory signs are predominant. There is frequently dissociated sensory loss, with pain and temperature sense being disproportionately affected (Dyck and Lambert, 1969; Kelly *et al.*, 1979). Most patients have postural hypotension and impairment of sweating.

On electrophysiological examination normal or mildly impaired motor conduction velocities and absent or reduced sensory action potentials are found. Sural nerve biopsy characteristically reveals a severe loss of myelinated fibres especially those of small diameter and of unmyelinated fibres (*Figures 5.4* and *5.5*). Axonal degeneration is seen in teased nerve fibres (Thomas and King, 1974). Amyloid deposits are seen around capillaries in the endoneurium, epineurium and perineurium. The CSF protein levels are frequently elevated and there is

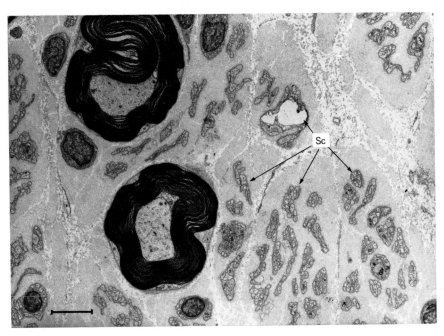

Figure 5.4 Electronmicrograph of sural nerve from a patient with amyloid disease. Large myelinated fibres are present but there is a gross loss of unmyelinated fibres, with empty Schwann-cell subunits (Sc). Bar = 2 μm

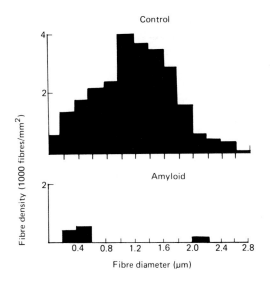

Figure 5.5 Unmyelinated fibre diameter distribution in the sural nerve of a control subject, and that of the patient with amyloid disease shown in *Figure 5.4*. Very few unmyelinated fibres remain

occasionally a pleocytosis (Kelly *et al.*, 1979). The neuropathy is relentlessly progressive and unaffected by medical treatment (Kelly *et al.*, 1979).

In amyloidosis associated with multiple myeloma, plasma cells constitute more than 15% of the nucleated cells in the bone marrow. IgG or IgA monoclonal protein is frequently present in the plasma and monoclonal light chains are found in the urine. Anaemia is usually more severe in myeloma than in primary amyloidosis and lytic bone lesions occur in multiple myeloma but not in primary amyloidosis (Kelly *et al.*, 1979).

References

Abrams, G. M., Latov, N., Hays, A. P., Sherman, W. and Zimmerman, E. A. (1982) Immunocytochemical studies of human peripheral nerve with serum from patients with polyneuropathy and paraproteinaemia. *Neurology (NY)*, **32**, 821–826

Appenzeller, O., Parks, R. D. and MacGee, J. (1968) Peripheral neuropathy in chronic disease of the respiratory tract. *American Journal of Medicine*, **44**, 873–880

Asbury, A. K. (1975a) Uremic neuropathy. In *Peripheral Neuropathy*, edited by P. J. Dyck, P. K. Thomas and E. H. Lambert, pp. 982–992. Philadelphia: W. B. Saunders

Asbury, A. K. (1975b) Hepatic neuropathy. In *Peripheral Neuropathy*, edited by P. J. Dyck, P. K. Thomas and E. H. Lambert, pp. 993–998. Philadelphia: W. B. Saunders

Asbury, A. K., Victor, M. and Adams, R. D. (1963) Uremic polyneuropathy. *Archives of Neurology*, **8**, 413–428

Avram, M. M., Feinfeld, D. A. and Huatuco, A. H. (1978) Search for the uremic toxin. Decreased motor-nerve conduction velocity and elevated parathyroid hormone in uremia. *New England Journal of Medicine*, **298**, 1000–1003

Babb, A. L., Popovich, R. P., Christopher, T. G. and Scribner, B. H. (1971) The genesis of the square meter-hour hypothesis. *Transactions of the American Society of Artificial Internal Organs*, **17**, 81–91

Bajada, S., Mastaglia, F. L. and Fisher, A. (1980) Amyloid neuropathy and tremor in Waldenström's macroglobulinaemia. *Archives of Neurology*, **37**, 240–242

Bassett, M. L., Danta, G. and Cook, T. A. (1978) Giardiasis and peripheral neuropathy. *British Medical Journal*, **2**, 19

Besinger, U. A., Toyka, K. V., Anzil, A. P., Fateh-Moghadem, A., Neumeier, D., Rauscher, R. and Heininger, K. (1981) Myeloma neuropathy: passive transfer from man to mouse. *Science*, **213**, 1027–1030

Bischoff, A., Lutschg, J. and Meier, C. (1975) Polyneuropathie bei vitamin-B$_{12}$ und Folsauremangel. *Munchen Med. Wochenschrift*, **117**, 1593–1598

Bolton, C. F. (1976) Electrophysiologic changes in uremic neuropathy after successful renal transplantation. *Neurology (NY)*, **26**, 152–161

Bolton, C. F., Baltzan, M. A. and Baltzan, R. B. (1971) Effects of renal transplantation on uremic neuropathy. A clinical and electrophysiologic study. *New England Journal of Medicine*, **284**, 1170–1175

Bosch, E. P., Ansbacker, C. E., Goeken, J. A. and Cancilla, P. A. (1982) Peripheral neuropathy associated with monoclonal gammopathy. Studies of intraneural injections of monoclonal immunoglobulin sera. *Journal of Neuropathology and Experimental Neurology*, **41**, 446–459

Botez, M. I., Peyronnard, J.-M., Bachevalier, J. and Charron, L. (1978) Polyneuropathy and folate deficiency. *Archives of Neurology*, **35**, 581–584

Botez, M. I., Peyronnard, J.-M. and Charron, L. (1979) Polyneuropathies responsive to folic-acid therapy. In *Folic Acid in Neuropathy*, edited by M. I. Botez and E. H. Reynolds, pp. 401–412. New York: Raven Press

Boudouresques, J., Khalil, R., Vigouroux, R. A., Daniel, F. and Gosset, A. (1970) Infectious diseases of nerves. In *Handbook of Clinical Neurology*, Volume 7, edited by P. J. Vinken and G. W. Bruyn, pp. 486–000. Amsterdam: North Holland Publishing Company

Braun, P. E., Frail, D. E. and Latov, N. (1982) Myelin-associated glycoprotein is the antigen for a monoclonal IgM in polyneuropathy. *Journal of Neurochemistry*, **39**, 1261–1265

Byrne, E. A. J. and Taylor, G. F. (1945) An outbreak of jaundice with signs in the nervous system. *British Medical Journal*, **1**, 477–478

Cavanagh, J. B. and Mellick, R. S. (1965) The nature of peripheral nerve lesions associated with acute intermittent porphyria. *Journal of Neurology, Neurosurgery and Psychiatry*, **28**, 320–327

Chad, D., Pariser, K., Bradley, W. G., Adelman, L. S. and Pinn, V. W. (1982) The pathogenesis of cryoglobulinemic neuropathy. *Neurology (NY)*, **32**, 725–729

Chari, V. B., Katiyar, B. C., Rastogi, B. L. and Bhattacharya, S. K. (1977) Neuropathy in hepatic disorders. A clinical electrophysiological and histopathological appraisal. *Journal of the Neurological Sciences*, **31**, 93–111

Charron, L., Peyronnard, J.-M. and Marchand, L. (1980) Sensory neuropathy associated with primary biliary cirrhosis. Histologic and morphometric studies. *Archives of Neurology*, **37**, 84–87

Chazot, G., Berger, B., Carrier, H. *et al.* (1976) Manifestations neurologiques des gammopathies monoclonales. Formes neurologiques pures – étude en immunofluorescence. *Revue Neurologique (Paris)*, **132**, 195–212

Cohen, A. S. and Benson, M. D. (1975) Amyloid neuropathy. In *Peripheral Neuropathy*, edited by P. J. Dyck, P. K. Thomas and E. H. Lambert, pp. 1082–1084. Philadelphia: W. B. Saunders

Contamin, F., Singer, B., Mignot, R., Ecoffet, M. and Kazatchkine, M. (1976) Polyneuropathie à rechutes évoluant depuis 19 ans, associée à une gammapathie monoclonale IgG benigne. Effet favorable de la corticotherapie. *Revue Neurologique (Paris)*, **132**, 741–762

Cooke, W. T., Cox, E. V., Fone, D. J., Meynell, M. J. and Gaddi, R. (1963) The clinical and metabolic significance of jejunal diverticula. *Gut*, **4**, 115–137

Cooke, W. T., Johnson, A. G. and Woolf, A. L. (1966) Vital staining and electron microscopy of the intramuscular nerve endings in the neuropathy of adult coeliac disease. *Brain*, **89**, 663–682

Cooke, W. T. and Smith, W. T. (1966) Neurological disorders associated with adult coeliac disease. *Brain*, **89**, 683–722

Cox-Klazinga, M. and Endtz, L. J. (1980) Peripheral nerve involvement in pernicious anaemia. *Journal of the Neurological Sciences*, **45**, 367–371

Cream, J. J., Hern, J. E. C., Hughes, R. A. C. and MacKenzie, I. C. K. (1974) Mixed or immune complex cryoglobulinaemia and neuropathy. *Journal of Neurology, Neurosurgery and Psychiatry*, **37**, 82–87

Crevasse, L. E. and Logue, R. B. (1959) Peripheral neuropathy in myxoedema. *Annals of Internal Medicine*, **50**, 1433–1437

Dalakas, M. C. and Engel, W. K. (1981) Polyneuropathy with monoclonal gammopathy. Studies of 11 patients. *Annals of Neurology*, **10**, 45–52

Davison, A. M., Williams, I. R., Mawdsley, C. and Robson, J. S. (1972) Neuropathy associated with hepatitis in patients maintained on haemodialysis. *British Medical Journal*, **1**, 409–411

Dayan, A. D. and Williams, R. (1967) Demyelinating peripheral neuropathy and liver disease. *Lancet*, **2**, 133–134

De Jesus, P. V. Jr, Clements, R. S. Jr and Winegrad, A. I. (1974) Hypermyoinositolemic polyneuropathy in rats. A possible mechanism for uremic polyneuropathy. *Journal of the Neurological Sciences*, **21**, 237–249

Dellagi, K., Brouet, J.-C. and Danom, F. (1979) Cross-idiotypic antigens among monoclonal immunologulin M from patients with Waldenström's macroglobulinemia and polyneuropathy. *Journal of Clinical Investigation*, **64**, 1530–1534

Denny-Brown, D. (1948) Primary sensory neuropathy with muscular changes associated with carcinoma. *Journal of Neurology, Neurosurgery and Psychiatry*, **11**, 73–87

Dyck, P. J., Johnson, W. J., Lambert, E. H. and O'Brien, P. C. (1971) Segmental demyelination secondary to axonal degeneration in uremic neuropathy. *Mayo Clinic Proceedings*, **46**, 400–431

Dyck, P. J., Johnson, W. J., Lambert, E. H., Bushek, W. and Pollock, M. (1975) Detection and evaluation of uremic peripheral neuropathy in patients on hemodialysis. *Kidney International*, **7**, Suppl. 2, 201–205

Dyck, P. J. and Lambert, E. H. (1969) Dissociated sensation in amyloidosis. *Archives of Neurology*, **20**, 490–507

Dyck, P. J., Oviatt, K. F. and Lambert E. H. (1981) Intensive evaluation of unclassified neuropathies yields improved diagnosis. *Annals of Neurology*, **10**, 222–226

Faden, A, Mendoza, E. and Flynn, F. (1981) Subclinical neuropathy associated with chronic obstructive pulmonary disease. Possible pathophysiologic role of smoking. *Archives of Neurology*, **38**, 639–642

Farivar, M., Wands, J. R., Benson, G. D., Dienst, J. L. and Isselbacher, K. J. (1976) Cryoprotein complexes and peripheral neuropathy in a patient with chronic active hepatitis. *Gastroenterology*, **71**, 490–493

Fehling, C., Jagerstaff, M., Lindstrand, K. and Elmqvist, D. (1974) Folate deficiency and neurological disease. *Archives of Neurology*, **30**, 263–265

Feibel, J. H. and Campa, J. F. (1976) Thyrotoxic neuropathy (Basedow's paraplegia). *Journal of Neurology, Neurosurgery and Psychiatry*, **39**, 491–497

Fine, E. J. and Hallett, M. (1980) Neurophysiological study of subacute combined degeneration. *Journal of the Neurological Sciences*, **45**, 331–336

Fitting, J.W., Bischoff, A., Regli, F. and De Crousaz, G. (1979) Neuropathy, amyloidosis and monoclonal gammopathy. *Journal of Neurology, Neurosurgery and Psychiatry*, **42**, 193–202

Gilliatt, R. W., Goodman, H. B. and Willison, R. G. (1961) The recording of lateral popliteal nerve action potentials in man. *Journal of Neurology, Neurosurgery and Psychiatry*, **24**, 305–318

Hall, B. M., Walsh, J. C., Horvath, J. S. and Lytton, D. G. (1976) Peripheral neuropathy complicating primary hyperoxaluria. *Journal of the Neurological Sciences*, **29**, 343–349

Harding, A. E., Muller, D. P. R., Thomas, P. K. and Willison, H. J. (1982) Spinocerebellar degeneration secondary to chronic intestinal malabsorption: a vitamin E deficiency syndrome. *Annals of Neurology*, **12**, 419–424

Hawley, R. J., Cohen, M. H., Saini, N. and Armbrustmacher, V. W. (1980) The carcinomatous neuromyopathy of oat cell lung carcinoma. *Annals of Neurology*, **7**, 65–72

Henson, R. A. and Urich, H. (1982) *Cancer and the Nervous System*. Oxford: Blackwell Scientific Publications

Hornabrook, R. W. and Marks, V. (1960) The effect of vitamin B_1 therapy on blood pyruvate levels in subacute combined degeneration of the cord. *Lancet*, **2**, 893–895

Ibrahim, M. M., Barnes, A. D., Crosland, J. M. *et al.* (1974) Effect of renal transplantation on uraemic neuropathy. *Lancet*, **2**, 739–742

Iwashita, H., Argyrakis, A., Lowitzsch, K. and Spaar, F.-W. (1974) Polyneuropathy in Waldenström's macroglobulinaemia. *Journal of the Neurological Sciences*, **21**, 341–354

Iwashita, H., Ohnishi, A., Asada, M., Kawazawa, Y. and Kuriowa, Y. (1977) Polyneuropathy, skin hyperpigmentation, edema, and hypertrichosis in localized osteosclerotic myeloma. *Neurology (NY)*, **27**, 675–681

Iyer, J. V., Taori, G. M., Kapadia, C. R., Mathan, V. I. and Baker, S. J. (1973) Neurological manifestations in tropical sprue: a clinical and electrodiagnostic study. *Neurology (Minneapolis)*, **23**, 959–966

Jaspan, J. B., Wollran, R. Z., Bernstein, L. and Rubenstein, A. H. (1982) Hypoglycaemic peripheral neuropathy in association with insulinoma: implications of glucopenia rather than hyperinsulinism. *Medicine (Baltimore)*, **61**, 33–44

Julien, J., Vital, C., Vallat, J. M., Lagueny, A., Demoniere, C. and Darriet, D. (1978) Polyneuropathy in Waldenström's macroglobulinaemia. Deposition of M-component on myelin sheaths. *Archives of Neurology*, **35**, 423–425

Kahn, S. N., Riches, P. G. and Kohn, J. (1980) Paraproteinaemia in neurologic disease: incidence, associations and classifications of monoclonal immunoglobulins. *Journal of Clinical Pathology*, **33**, 617–621

Kardel, T. and Nielsen, V. K. (1974) Hepatic neuropathy. A clinical and electrophysiological study. *Acta Neurologica Scandinavica*, **50**, 513–526

Kelly, J. J., Kyle, R. A., O'Brien, P. C. and Dyck, P. J. (1979) The natural history of peripheral neuropathy in primary systemic amyloidosis. *Annals of Neurology*, **6**, 1–7

Kelly, J. J. Jr, Kyle, R. A., Miles, J. M., O'Brien, P. C. and Dyck, P. J. (1981a) The spectrum of peripheral neuropathy in myeloma. *Neurology (NY)*, **31**, 24–31

Kelly, J. J., Kyle, R. A., O'Brien, P. C. and Dyck, P. J. (1981b) The prevalence of monoclonal gammopathy in peripheral neuropathy. *Neurology (NY)*, **31**, 1480–1483

Knill-Jones, R. P., Goodwill, C. J., Dayan, A. D. and Williams, R. (1972) Peripheral neuropathy in chronic liver disease: clinical, electrodiagnostic and nerve biopsy findings. *Journal of Neurology, Neurosurgery and Psychiatry*, **35**, 22–30

Kohn, J. (1976) Benign paraproteinaemias. *Journal of Clinical Pathology*, **8**, Suppl. 6, 77–82

Konishi, T., Saida, K., Ohnishi, A. and Nishitani, H. (1982) Perineuritis in mononeuritis multiplex with cryoglobulinemia. *Muscle and Nerve*, **5**, 173–177

Kyle, R. A. and Bayrd, E. D. (1975) Amyloidosis: review of 236 cases. *Medicine (Baltimore)*, **54**, 271–299

Latov, N., Sherman, W. H., Nemni, R. *et al.* (1980) Plasma cell dyscrasia and peripheral neuropathy with a monoclonal antibody to peripheral nerve myelin. *New England Journal of Medicine*, **303**, 618–621

Latov, N., Gross, R. B., Kastelman, J. *et al.* (1981a) Complement-fixing antiperipheral nerve myelin antibodies in patients with inflammatory poly-neuritis and with polyneuropathy and paraproteinaemia. *Neurology (NY)*, **31**, 1530–1534

Latov, N., Braun, P. E., Gross, R. B., Sherman, W. H., Penn, A. S. and Chess, L. (1981b) Plasma cell dyscrasia and peripheral neuropathy. Identification of the myelin antigens that react with human paraproteins. *Proceedings of the National Academy of Sciences USA*, **78**, 7139–7142

Lescher, F. G. (1944) The nervous complications of infective hepatitis. *British Medical Journal*, **1**, 554–556

Lisak, R. P., Mitchell, M., Zweiman, B., Orrechio, E. and Asbury, A. K. (1977) Guillain-Barré syndrome and Hodgkin's disease: three cases with immunological studies. *Annals of Neurology*, **1**, 72–78

Logothetis, J., Silverstein, P. and Coe, J. (1960) Neurologic aspects of Waldenström's macroglobulinemia. *Archives of Neurology (Chicago)*, **5**, 564–573

Logothetis, J., Kennedy, W. R., Ellington, A. and Williams, R. C. (1968) Cryoglobulinemic neuropathy: incidence and clinical characteristics. *Archives of Neurology*, **19**, 389–397

Lovell, C. (1945) Neurological symptoms in infective hepatitis. *British Medical Journal*, **1**, 569

Low, P. A., McLeod, J. G., Turtle, J. R., Donnelly, P. and Wright, R. G. (1974) Peripheral neuropathy in acromegaly. *Brain*, **97**, 139–152

McLeod, J. G. (1975) Carcinomatous neuropathy. In *Peripheral Neuropathy*, edited by P. J. Dyck, P. K. Thomas and E. H. Lambert, pp. 1301–1313. Philadelphia: W. B. Saunders

McLeod, J. G. and Walsh, J. C. (1975a) Peripheral neuropathy associated with lymphomas and other reticuloses. In *Peripheral Neuropathy*, edited by P. J.

Dyck, P. K. Thomas and E. H. Lambert, pp. 1314–1325. Philadelphia: W. B. Saunders

McLeod, J. G. and Walsh, J. C. (1975b) Neuropathies associated with paraproteinemias and dysproteinemias. In *Peripheral Neuropathy*, edited by P. J. Dyck, P. K. Thomas and E. H. Lambert, pp. 1012–1029. Philadelphia: W. B. Saunders

McLeod, J. G., Walsh, J. C. and Little, J. M. (1969) Sural nerve biopsy. *Medical Journal of Australia*, **2,** 1092–1096

Martinez-Figueroa, A., Johnson, R. H., Lambie, D. G. and Shakir, A. A. (1980) The role of folate deficiency in the development of peripheral neuropathy caused by anticonvulsants. *Journal of the Neurological Sciences*, **48,** 315–323

Matthews, W. B. (1975) Sarcoid neuropathy. In *Peripheral Neuropathy*, edited by P. J. Dyck, P. K. Thomas and E. H. Lambert, pp. 1199–1206. Philadelphia: W. B. Saunders

Mayer, R. F. (1965) Peripheral nerve function in vitamin B_{12} deficiency. *Archives of Neurology (Chicago)*, **13,** 355–362

Morley, J. B. and Schwieger, A. C. (1967) The relation between chronic polyneuropathy and osteosclerotic myeloma. *Journal of Neurology, Neurosurgery and Psychiatry*, **30,** 432–442

Nardelli, E., Pizzighella, S., Tridente, G. and Rizzuto, N. (1981) Peripheral neuropathy associated with immunoglobulin disorders. An immunological and ultrastructural study. *Acta Neuropathologica (Berlin)* Suppl. 7, 258–261

Nausieda, P. A. (1977) Hyperlipemic neuropathy. In *Handbook of Clinical Neurology*, edited by P. J. Vinken and G. W. Bruyn, Vol. 29. Metabolic and deficiency diseases of the nervous system. Part III, pp. 429–433. Amsterdam: North-Holland Publishing Company

Nemni, R., Gallassi, G., Cohen, M. *et al.* (1981) Symmetric sarcoid polyneuropathy: analysis of a sural nerve biopsy. *Neurology (NY)*, **31,** 1217–1223

Nickel, S. N., Frame, B., Bebin, J., Tourtelotte, W. W., Parker, J. A. and Hughes, B. R. (1961) Myxoedema neuropathy and myopathy – a clinical and pathological study. *Neurology (Minneapolis)*, **8,** 511–517

Nielsen, V. K. (1973a) The peripheral nerve function of chronic renal failure, V. Sensory and motor conduction velocity. *Acta Medica Scandinavica*, **194,** 445–454

Nielsen, V. K. (1973b) The peripheral nerve function in chronic renal failure, VI. The relationship between sensory and motor nerve conduction and kidney function, azotemia, age, sex, and clinical neuropathy. *Acta Medica Scandinavica*, **194,** 455–462

Nielsen, V. K. (1974a) The peripheral nerve function in chronic renal failure: a survey. *Acta Medica Scandinavica*, Suppl. 573, 10–32

Nielsen, V. K. (1974b) The peripheral nerve function in chronic renal failure, VII. Longitudinal course during terminal renal failure and regular hemodialyses. *Acta Medica Scandinavica*, **195,** 155–162

Nielsen, V. K. (1974c) The peripheral nerve function in chronic renal failure, IX. Recovery after renal transplantation; electrophysiological aspects. *Acta Medica Scandinavica*, **195,** 171–180

Nielsen, V. K. (1978) Pathophysiological aspects of uraemic neuropathy. In *Peripheral Neuropathies*, edited by N. Canal and G. Pozza, pp. 197–210. Amsterdam: Elsevier/North Holland Biomedical Press

O'Duffy, J. D., Randall, R. V. and MacCarty, C. S. (1973) Median neuropathy (carpal tunnel syndrome) in acromegaly. *Annals of Internal Medicine*, **78**, 379–383

Oh, S. J. (1980) Sarcoid polyneuropathy: a histologically proved case. *Annals of Neurology*, **7**, 178–181

Oh, S. J., Clements, R. S. Jr, Lee, Y. W. and Diethelm, A. G. (1978) Rapid improvement in nerve conduction velocity following renal transplantation. *Annals of Neurology*, **4**, 369–373

Ohnishi, I. and Hirano, A. (1981) Uncompacted myelin lamellae in dysglobulin-aemic neuropathy. *Journal of the Neurological Sciences*, **51**, 131–140

Ohnishi, A., Tsuji, S., Igisu, H. *et al.* (1980) Beri-beri neuropathy. Morphometric study of sural nerve. *Journal of the Neurological Sciences*, **45**, 177–190

Pallis, C. A. and Lewis, P. D. (1974) *The Neurology of Gastrointestinal Disease*. London: W. B. Saunders

Pollard, J. D., McLeod, J. G., Angel-Honnibal, T. G. and Verheijden, M. A. (1982) Hypothyroid polyneuropathy. Clinical, electrophysiological and nerve biopsy findings in two cases. *Journal of the Neurological Sciences*, **53**, 461–471

Preswick, G. and Jeremy, D. (1964) Subclinical polyneuropathy in renal insufficiency. *Lancet*, **2**, 731–732

Propp, R. P., Means, E., Deibel, R., Sherer, G. and Barron, K. (1975) Waldeström's macrogobulinemia and neuropathy. Deposition of M-component on myelin sheaths. *Neurology (Minneapolis)*, **25**, 980–988

Read, D. J., Vanhegan, R. I. and Matthews, W. B. (1978) Peripheral neuropathy and benign IgG paraproteinaemia. *Journal of Neurology, Neurosurgery and Psychiatry*, **41**, 215–219

Read, D. and Warlow, C. (1978) Peripheral neuropathy and solitary plasmacytoma. *Journal of Neurology, Neurosurgery and Psychiatry*, **41**, 177–184

Ridley, A. (1975) Porphyric neuropathy. In *Peripheral Neuropathy*, edited by P. J. Dyck, P. K. Thomas and E. H. Lambert, pp. 942–955. Philadelphia: W. B. Saunders

Rosenblum, J. L., Keating, J. P., Prensky, A. L. and Nelson, J. S. (1981) A progressive neurologic syndrome in children with chronic liver disease. *New England Journal of Medicine*, **304**, 503–508

Rousseau, J. J., Franck, G., Grisar, T., Reznik, M., Heynen, G. and Salmon, J. (1978) Osteosclerotic myeloma with polyneuropathy and ectopic secretion of calcitonin. *Cancer*, **14**, 133–140

Seneviratne, K. N. and Peiris, O. A. (1970) Peripheral nerve function in chronic liver disease. *Journal of Neurology, Neurosurgery and Psychiatry*, **33**, 609–614

Sewell, H. F., Mathews, J. B., Gooch, E. *et al.* (1981) Autoantibody to nerve tissue in a patient with a peripheral neuropathy and an IgG paraprotein. *Journal of Clinical Pathology*, **34**, 1163–1166

Shorvon, S. D. and Reynolds, E. H. (1979) Folate deficiency and peripheral neuropathy. In *Folic Acid in Neurology*, edited by M. I. Botez and E. H. Reynolds, pp. 413–421. New York: Raven Press

Sluga, E. (1974) Demyelinsieren des neuropathie-syndrome mit Struktueränderungen der Marklamellen. In *Polyneuropathien. Typen und Differenzietung. Ergebnisse bioptische Untersuchungen. Schriftenreihe Neurologie.* Berlin: Springer Verlag, 51

Smith, I. S., Kahn, S. N., Lacey, B. W. *et al.* (1983) Chronic demyelinating neuropathy associated with benign IgM paraproteinaemia. *Brain*, **106**, 169–196

Spencer, S. S. and Moench, J. C. (1980) Progressive and treatable cerebellar ataxia in macroglobulinaemia. *Neurology (NY)*, **30**, 536–538

Swash, M., Perrin, J. and Schwartz, M. S. (1979) Significance of immunoglobulin deposition in peripheral nerve in neuropathies associated with paraproteinaemias. *Journal of Neurology, Neurosurgery and Psychiatry*, **42**, 179–183

Teräväinen, H. and Larsen, A. (1977) Some features of the neuromuscular complications of pulmonary carcinoma. *Annals of Neurology*, **2**, 495–502

Thomas, P. K. and Walker, J. G. (1965) Xanthomatous neuropathy in primary biliary cirrhosis. *Brain*, **88**, 1079–1088

Thomas, P. K., Hollinrake, K., Lascelles, R. G. *et al.* (1971) The polyneuropathy of chronic renal failure. *Brain*, **94**, 761–780

Thomas, P. K. and King, R. H. M. (1974) Peripheral nerve changes in amyloid neuropathy. *Brain*, **97**, 395–406

Thrush, D. C. (1970) Neuropathy, IgM paraproteinaemia and autoantibodies in hypernephroma. *British Medical Journal*, **4**, 474

Vallat, J. M., Desproges-Gotteron, R., LeBouter, M. J., Loubet, A., Gualde, N. and Treves, R. (1980) Cryoglobulinemic neuropathy: a pathological study. *Annals of Neurology*, **8**, 179–185

Vital, C., Oubertin, J., Ragnault, J. M., Amigues, H., Mouton, L. and Bellance, R. (1982a) Sarcoidosis of the peripheral nerve: a histological and ultrastructural study of two cases. *Acta Neuropathologica (Berlin)*, **58**, 111–114

Vital, C., Vallat, J. M., Deminiere, C., Loubet, A. and Lebouter, M. J. (1982b) Peripheral nerve damage during multiple myeloma and Waldenström's macroglobulinemia. An ultrastructural and immunopathologic study. *Cancer*, **50**, 1491–1497

Walsh, J. C. (1971a) Neuropathy associated with lymphoma. *Journal of Neurology, Neurosurgery and Psychiatry*, **34**, 42–50

Walsh, J. C. (1971b) Neuropathy of multiple myeloma. *Archives of Neurology*, **25**, 404–414

Wochnik-Dyjas, D., Niewiadomska, M. and Kostrzewska, E. (1978) Porphyric polyneuropathy and its pathogenesis in the light of electrophysiological investigations. *Journal of the Neurological Sciences*, **35**, 243–256

Yiannikas, C., McLeod, J. G. and Walsh, J. C. (1983) Peripheral neuropathy associated with polycythemia vera. *Neurology (NY)*, **33**, 139–143

6
Diabetic neuropathy: pathophysiology and management
Mark J. Brown and Douglas A. Greene

INTRODUCTION

Diabetes mellitus is not one disease but a group of disorders expressed by abnormal glucose metabolism. The two forms of primary diabetes, previously called 'juvenile onset, ketosis prone' and 'adult onset, ketosis resistant' are now referred to as insulin dependent (Type I) or non-insulin dependent (Type II), since either may occur at any age. Current knowledge of the etiology of diabetes mellitus and modern approaches to management have been reviewed recently (Albin and Rifkin, 1982; Brown and Asbury, 1983; Defronzo and Ferrannini, 1982; Genuth, 1982).

Table 6.1 Classification of diabetic neuropathies by topography

(1) Distal symmetrical polyneuropathy
    (a) Mixed sensory-motor-autonomic neuropathy
    (b) Predominantly sensory neuropathy
        (i) predominantly large fiber
        (ii) mixed large and small fiber
        (iii) predominantly small fiber
    (c) Predominantly motor neuropathy
    (d) Predominantly autonomic neuropathy

(2) Symmetrical proximal motor neuropathy

(3) Focal and multifocal neuropathies
    (a) Asymmetrical proximal motor neuropathy
    (b) Cranial neuropathy
    (c) Intercostal and other mononeuropathies
    (d) Entrapment neuropathy

Three major neuropathic syndromes occur in diabetes (*Table 6.1*), of which distal symmetrical polyneuropathy is the most common. Proximal motor neuropathy and focal neuropathies are rare in comparison, but the neurologist is more likely to become involved in their management. Although the presence of any one of these syndromes should raise the possibility of underlying diabetes, none is unique to diabetic individuals. To make matters more complex, two or more forms of neuropathy often are encountered in the same diabetic patient.

In this chapter we review the present clinical knowledge of diabetic polyneuropathy and other diabetic neuropathies. In addition we summarize portions of the growing literature on experimental diabetic neuropathy and nerve metabolism. The justification for inclusion of this material in a volume intended for clinicians is that diabetic polyneuropathy has become the best understood human metabolic neuropathy. Approaches used for investigating the biochemical basis of diabetic neuropathy may prove applicable to the study of other axonal neuropathies as well.

DIABETIC POLYNEUROPATHY

Polyneuropathy is unquestionably the most common form of diabetic neuropathy. The prevalence of polyneuropathy in diabetic populations has been estimated at from 0–93% (Bruyn and Garland, 1970; Thomas and Eliasson, 1975). This wide range results from patient selection factors, investigators' criteria for diagnosis of neuropathy, and the sensitivity of detection methods. A balanced view of prevalence comes from the studies of Pirart, who found evidence of neuropathy by clinical examination in about 8% of diabetics at the time of diagnosis, increasing to 50% after 25 years of diabetes (Pirart, 1978).

In most cases diabetic polyneuropathy involves a combination of sensory, motor and autonomic nerve fiber abnormalities. Cutaneous sensibility is reduced in a stocking and glove distribution, often associated with decreased vibratory and proprioceptive perception in the limbs, reduced or absent ankle jerks, mild distal muscle weakness, and autonomic dysfunction. These features may be indistinguishable from those that occur in other acquired polyneuropathies.

Pathology

Diabetic polyneuropathy is best classified as an axonal neuropathy, in that the predominant neuropathic feature is nerve fiber loss (Vital and Vallat, 1980; Brown, Martin and Asbury, 1976; Brown *et al.*, 1979; Greenbaum *et al.*, 1964; Chopra and Hurwitz, 1969; Behse, Buchthal and Carlsen, 1977). A proximal to distal gradient of myelinated fiber abnormalities has been found at autopsy (Chopra and Fannin, 1971) and in an intramuscular twig nerve biopsy study of asymptomatic diabetic patients (Reske-Nielsen, Harmsen and Vorre, 1977). Denervation changes are evident in histologic sections of distal muscles. When examined, the extent of fiber loss has paralleled the degree of clinical dysfunction, and it appears that denervation changes are sufficient to account for the symptoms and signs in diabetic polyneuropathy. Ultrastructural studies of diabetic nerves have not demonstrated distinctive features in affected axons (Brown, Martin and Asbury, 1976; Bischoff, 1973; Vital *et al.*, 1973). This pattern of nerve fiber damage and neurogenic atrophy is shared with most toxic and metabolic neuropathies (Asbury and Johnson, 1978), and is not unique to diabetes.

Thomas and Lascelles (1966) and others (Chopra, Hurwitz and Montgomery, 1969; Dyck *et al.*, 1980; Bishoff, 1973; Behse, Buchthal and Carlsen, 1977) described an increased incidence of segmental demyelination in diabetic nerves. On occasion extensive demyelinative–remyelinative changes lead to frank onion bulb formations (Vital and Vallat, 1980; Ballin and Thomas, 1968). Demyelination in diabetic neuropathy cannot be explained as a secondary response to axonal atrophy (Sugimura and Dyck, 1981), and the occurrence of segmental demyelination suggests a selective Schwann cell disorder that is independent of axonal loss (Thomas and Lascelles, 1966; Chopra, Hurwitz and Montgomery, 1969). While segmental demyelination is prominent in some cases of diabetic polyneuropathy, it may be only a minor neuropathological feature in others (Behse, Buchthal and Carlsen, 1977; Brown, Martin and Asbury, 1976).

Traditional silver-staining techniques have demonstrated a decrease in unmyelinated fiber numbers in somatic and autonomic nerves of diabetics (Martin, 1953), and unmyelinated fiber loss has been confirmed by electron microscopy (Behse, Buchthal and Carlsen, 1977; Bischoff, 1973; Vital *et al.*, 1973). In a morphometric study of two cases with painful neuropathy, increased numbers of very small unmyelinated axons ($0.1–0.2\,\mu$m diameter) suggested axonal regeneration with sprouting in concert with reduced unmyelinated fibers of normal caliber ($0.2–2.0\,\mu$m diameter) (Brown, Martin and Asbury, 1976). This probably reflects concurrent fiber degeneration and regeneration, which also occurs in other axonal polyneuropathies.

The pathology of blood vessels in diabetic peripheral nerves has been examined with interest because the other important late complications of diabetes are microvascular disorders. Endoneurial capillaries are thickened (Fagerberg, 1959; Vital and Vallat, 1980; Behse, Buchthal and Carlsen, 1977), and perineurial basement membranes are widened (Johnson, Brendel and Meezan, 1981). A permeability disorder at the blood-nerve or blood-perineurial barrier in diabetics could lead to endoneurial metabolic derangements, possibly resulting in neuropathy. However, vascular abnormalities and neuropathy could occur independently as a consequence of long-standing diabetes, and their association does not indicate a causal relationship. Small vessel occlusion has been described in diabetic nerves (Timperley *et al.*, 1976; Williams *et al.*, 1980), and Sugimura and Dyck (1982) found focal areas of myelinated fiber loss in proximal nerves of two autopsied patients with polyneuropathy, in a pattern similar to that seen distal to experimental nerve infarcts (Parry and Brown, 1982). This raises the intriguing possibility that proximal occlusion microvascular disease could underlie the diffuse distal polyneuropathy that occurs in diabetes.

Neurophysiology

Nerve conduction abnormalities in diabetics were observed in some of the earliest clinical neurophysiological studies of peripheral neuropathy (Gilliatt and Willison,

1962; Mulder *et al.*, 1961). In asymptomatic patients with established diabetes of short duration motor conduction often is normal (Eng, Hung and August, 1975), but in most cases of symptomatic neuropathy there is mild to moderate slowing of conduction velocities (Mulder *et al.*, 1961; Kimura *et al.*, 1979). This is the degree of impairment that would be expected if larger-diameter motor axons were lost and only the smaller, slower-conducting motor fibers remained. Conduction in leg nerves is slowed before that of arm nerves (Eng, Hung and August, 1975) and, in the same nerves, conduction along distal segments is impaired more than that of proximal segments (Kimura *et al.*, 1979). Although longitudinal studies have not documented progression over time in individual patients, motor conduction abnormalities are most severe in clinically advanced cases. EMG studies are more sensitive to neuropathic changes than conduction velocities (Mulder *et al.*, 1961; Lamontagne and Buchthal, 1970), and have detected denervation abnormalities before the fastest motor velocities became slowed (Hansen and Ballantyne, 1977).

With the introduction of signal averagers, sensory nerve studies have become a standard part of the electrophysiologic assessment of diabetic neuropathy. Reduction of sensory potential amplitudes (Lamontagne and Buchthal, 1970; Noel, 1973) and slowing of spinal somatosensory conduction (Gupta and Dorfman, 1981) are early electrophysiologic signs of diabetic polyneuropathy. In general, sensory potential amplitudes fall in the foot before amplitudes are reduced in the hand, and distal portions of sensory nerves are affected before proximal portions (Noel, 1973). This pattern appears to reflect the early loss of distal myelinated sensory axons. In advanced diabetic neuropathy, as fiber loss progresses, sensory potential responses may be impossible to detect in the legs and difficult to obtain in the arms.

At times, nerve conduction velocities are slowed to a greater degree than would be expected by axonal loss alone. This additional slowing probably reflects the consequences of segmental demyelination. There may be a very small degree of further slowing that has not been explained on a structural basis (Behse, Buchthal and Carlsen, 1977). This poorly understood 'metabolic' phenomenon seems to underlie the small improvement in motor conduction velocity that follows insulin or other treatment in early diabetes (Ward *et al.*, 1971; Gregerson, 1968b; Judzewitsch *et al.*, 1983). These small fluctuations in conduction velocity, which do not have known clinical or pathological correlates, should be considered as independent from the process causing nerve fiber damage until a relationship can be established.

Diabetic patients with or without symptomatic neuropathy are usually resistant to the loss of vibration perception and motor and sensory nerve conduction failure that follows limb ischemia (Horowitz and Ginsberg-Fellner, 1979; Gregerson, 1968a). The basis for this resistance is unknown. However, nerves of patients with other metabolic or neurological disorders are occasionally more resistant to ischemia than normals, suggesting that the persistence of conduction in diabetics results from factors other than elevated blood glucose alone.

Nerve conduction studies can be reliable tools for following large-diameter myelinated fiber function in diabetes, if proper care is given to skin temperature and electrode placement. Routine electrophysiological methods do not measure unmyelinated fiber conduction (Asbury and Brown, 1982), but functional tests of modalities served by these fibers, both somatic and autonomic, are being developed for clinical use. These include quantitative psychophysiological testing of the threshold for appreciating sensory stimuli (Conomy, Barnes and Conomy, 1979; Dyck *et al.*, 1976), measurement of resting heart rate and cardiac responses to the Valsalva maneuver (Appenzeller, 1982) and determination of cutaneous sweat gland density (Kennedy and Sakuta, 1982).

Clinical features

The clinical manifestations of diabetic polyneuropathy can vary considerably among individuals (Martin, 1953; Greenbaum, 1964; Mayne, 1968; Thomas and Eliasson, 1975; Eng, Hung and August, 1975). Onset may be abrupt or insidious; progression may be rapid or slow. The course may appear static, or there can be partial recovery. The neuropathy may be asymptomatic or lead to severe disability. In addition, the spectrum of nerve fiber involvement may follow a number of different patterns. Although mixed polyneuropathy is the most common form, relatively pure subtypes are encountered (*Table 6.1*).

Mixed sensory-motor-autonomic polyneuropathy

This is the most common clinical type of diabetic neuropathy. The symptoms and signs of sensory, motor and autonomic fiber involvement, considered individually below, are present to varying degrees in this group of patients. Sensory disturbances are common in symptomatic patients. Weakness and atrophy may not be striking, but motor nerve conduction and EMG studies are nevertheless abnormal. Autonomic nervous systemic abnormalities range from clinically inapparent to severe.

Sensory polyneuropathy

Both large and small fiber modalities may be involved in this relatively common subtype. Sensory abnormalities range from mild toe numbness to profound anesthesia with neuropathic ulcers and arthropathy. Corneal sensation and hearing may be affected (Schwartz, 1974; Friedman, Schulman and Weiss, 1975). Sensory deficits occur in a symmetrical stocking-glove pattern, a feature that is easily overlooked if the level of hypesthesia reaches more proximally than the groin and shoulders. At that point the presence of a coexisting vertical anterior chest band of hypesthesia will be demonstrable (Sabin, Geschwind and Waxman, 1978), confirming the fiber length-dependent nature of this polyneuropathy.

   In one group of sensory polyneuropathy patients there is a disproportionate loss of large fiber functions, manifested by impaired balance, decreased perception of distal vibration and position stimuli, and loss of ankle jerks. In its most severe form, position sense loss may result in sensory ataxia, the 'pseudotabetic' form of diabetic neuropathy. Further confusion with tabes dorsalis may arise if the pupils are small and sluggishly reactive to light, as occurs in diabetes (Smith *et al.*, 1978). In another group small fiber modalities are most affected. Pain and temperature sensibility are disturbed, with relative preservation of position and vibration perception, and reflexes are normal or nearly so (Brown, Martin and Asbury, 1976). Disabling spontaneous pains, dysesthesias and paresthesias are common associated features. Orthostatic hypotension and sexual dysfunction seem to be especially common in this group, reflecting the coexisting autonomic nervous system involvement.

Several kinds of pains may be associated with diabetic sensory neuropathy. Most patients will have typical neuropathic distal paresthesias (spontaneously occurring uncomfortable sensations) or dysesthesias (contact paresthesias). Occasional individuals with otherwise mild neuropathy have excessive skin hypersensitivity to light touch, reminiscent of reflex sympathetic dystrophy (causalgia). There may be shooting or stabbing pains which are multifocal in location, and arresting in their impact. Some individuals complain of superficial cutaneous burning pain. Most troublesome is the bone-deep, aching, tearing pain that is present throughout the day, although with varying intensity. Cramps in the small muscles of the feet, later ascending to calves or thighs, are similar to those that occur in muscle denervated from other disorders.

The paradoxical coexistence of spontaneous pain and insensitivity to painful stimuli in neuropathic individuals has not been explained fully. Melzack and Wall's 'gate' theory suggests that the selective loss of large-diameter pain-suppressing fibers would result in painful neuropathy, but pain is not a feature of some large fiber neuropathies (Nathan, 1976). It seems more likely that pain results from increased activity of injured small-diameter fibers (Brown, Martin and Asbury, 1976; Dyck, Lambert and O'Brien, 1976). Regenerating nerve fibers in experimental neuromas fire at abnormally low thresholds and with rapid rates (Wall and Gutnick, 1974), and depolarization of damaged or regenerating fibers in humans with neuropathy could contribute to the pain in these patients. The loss or dysfunction of small diameter fibers would account for the associated cutaneous hypesthesia.

Motor polyneuropathy

Chronic motor polyneuropathy is unusual in diabetes and its presence should prompt the search for another etiology. In many apparent cases sensory abnormalities can be found on careful examination. We and others (Thomas, 1982) have followed several young diabetic individuals who developed acute motor neuropathy after a period of ketoacidosis. They presented with quadriparesis, slowed nerve conduction and elevated spinal fluid protein concentration. It seems most likely that these ill patients had the Guillain-Barré syndrome and not a new disorder unique to diabetics.

Motor neuropathy or anterior horn cell loss may occur in psychiatric patients who have been treated with exogenous insulin-induced coma, and patients with hypoglycemia from an insulinoma can develop a neuronopathy which is clinically and electrophysiologically indistinguishable from a predominantly motor polyneuropathy (Mulder, Bastron and Lambert, 1956). Strength and the mild sensory symptoms may improve if hyperinsulinism is relieved (Rosner and Elstad, 1964; Jaspan *et al.*, 1982). Experimentally, acute hypoglycemia in otherwise normal rats may cause neuronopathy and axonal loss (Sidenius and Jakobsen, 1983). Thus the possibility of insulin excess should be considered in a diabetic patient with motor neuropathy and a history of cerebral hypoglycemic episodes. (*See also section on hypoglycemia and neuropathy in Chapter 5.*)

Autonomic neuropathy

Only a small number of diabetic patients have preferential autonomic nervous system involvement. There seems to be a disproportionate number of young Type I diabetics in this group. Abnormalities include gastroparesis, diarrhea, resting tachycardia, orthostatic hypotension, sweating disorders, incomplete bladder emptying, and impotence. Diabetic autonomic neuropathy has been the subject of recent reviews (Hosking, Bennett and Hampton, 1978; Clarke, Ewing and Campbell, 1979; Hilsted, 1982; Feldman and Schiller, 1983; Bradley, 1980) and is discussed in *Chapter 4*. The morphological basis of diabetic autonomic neuropathy appears to be both axonal loss and segmental demyelination (Low *et al.*, 1975; Faerman *et al.*, 1973), but this has not been studied as extensively as in somatic neuropathy. Electrophysiological studies of these patients almost always show some evidence of associated sensory and motor nerve involvement. Conversely, autonomic dysfunction is often present in diabetic individuals without autonomic symptoms (Pfeifer *et al.*, 1982). Diabetics with autonomic neuropathy may have an increased incidence of cardiac arrest and sudden death (Page and Watkins, 1978; Clarke, Ewing and Campbell, 1979).

Role of hyperglycemia in human diabetic polyneuropathy

Most investigators now believe that neuropathy and other long-term complications of diabetes in humans result from the interaction of multiple metabolic, genetic, and other factors, of which the most important is chronic hyperglycemia. A number of observations have led to the conclusion that chronic insulin deficiency and/or hyperglycemia influence the development of diabetic neuropathy (Clements, 1979; Sidenius, 1982). The prevalence of all forms of diabetic neuropathy increases with duration of diabetes in a similar linear rate in both Type I and Type II diabetes (Pirart, 1978). Although the pathogenesis and pathophysiology of these two forms of diabetes are distinct (Roiter and Rimoin, 1981; Kolterman and Olefsky, 1981), they share in common reduced insulin effect and hyperglycemia. Neuropathy is more prevalent in patients whose diabetes is poorly controlled (Pirart, 1978), and clinical neuropathy usually does not appear until after 5–10 years of hyperglycemia. Electrophysiological evidence of subclinical neuropathy correlates with the degree of hyperglycemia in stable Type II diabetics (Graf *et al.*, 1979).

As additional evidence for the pathogenic importance of hyperglycemia, intensive metabolic therapy can improve neurophysiologic abnormalities in diabetics with neuropathy. Motor conduction velocities can increase with treatment (Gregerson, 1968b; Graf *et al.*, 1981; Ward *et al.*, 1971; Boulton *et al.*, 1982) and the resistance of diabetic nerves to ischemic failure can be lessened (Horowitz and Ginsberg-Fellner, 1979; Gregerson, 1968a). Because these rapidly reversible changes may have a different pathogenesis from axonal degeneration or segmental demyelination, the improvement in these tests cannot be taken as being synonymous with reversal of neuropathy.

Convincing evidence for the clinical importance of chronic hyperglycemia in the production diabetic neuropathy is that treatment which maintains relative euglycemia also may effect reversal of neurological symptoms. Neuropathic pains may decrease within a few weeks after institution of insulin therapy (Boulton *et al.*, 1982), and sensory signs and symptoms may diminish over several months (Greene *et al.*, 1981; Greenbaum, 1964; Mayne, 1968; Fry, Hardwick and Scott, 1962). These favorable responses suggest that the past reports of failure of diabetic neuropathy to improve with therapy (Greenbaum, 1964; Fry, Hardwick and Scott, 1962) could reflect the inability of those patients to achieve good control, as defined by present-day standards.

In summary, diabetic polyneuropathy is best thought of as a distal axonal neuropathy with variable manifestations (Thomas, 1982). Severity of the neuropathy is related to duration of hyperglycemia and other as yet unknown factors. The distribution of symptoms and signs is length-dependent, a pattern that would result if diabetic polyneuropathy were a dying-back neuropathy or distal axonopathy (Spencer and Schaumberg, 1976). However, an alternative neurophysiologic mechanism has been proposed that would explain distal symptoms and signs if diabetes produced widespread randomly distributed abnormalities of axonal function (Waxman *et al.*, 1976)

Relationship between metabolic abnormalities and impaired nerve function

The pathogenetically relevant biochemical alterations in diabetic neuropathy have been difficult to study because structurally intact human peripheral nerve in early diabetes has not been accessible for biochemical study, and the regulation of normal peripheral nerve metabolism has been poorly understood. Recent studies employing animal models of human diabetes and *in vitro* tissue preparations derived from animal and human peripheral nerves have led to important advances in studying nerve metabolism in diabetes. A set of biochemically interrelated functionally significant abnormalities in diabetic peripheral nerve has emerged in conjunction with a newly-recognized fabric of peripheral nerve metabolic regulation and integration. The resulting pathogenetic scheme appears to relate metabolic defects to functional abnormalities in diabetic peripheral nerve. The relevance of these experimental observations to human neuropathy derives from the assumption that the metabolic mediators of acute nerve dysfunction have some degree of commonality with the factors responsible for chronic diabetic peripheral neuropathy.

Impaired nerve conduction in experimental diabetes

Experimental animal models of diabetic peripheral nerve disease originated with Eliasson's observation in 1964 that acute alloxan or pancreatic diabetes in the rat resulted in impaired peripheral motor nerve conduction velocity. Although simulating the reversible conduction impairment of newly-diagnosed Type I diabetes, the original model was limited because a histological or biochemical basis for the conduction defect, as well as its unequivocal cause-and-effect relationship with insulin deficiency, could not be established. Since 1974 numerous studies in the streptozotocin and spontaneously-diabetic BB rat have demonstrated that conduction impairment is a consequence of insulin deficiency (Greene, DeJesus and Winegrad, 1975; Jakobsen, 1979; Sima, 1980). Axonal changes may appear in chronic streptozotocin diabetes (Jakobsen, 1976; Brown *et al.*, 1980; Powell *et al.*, 1977; Yagihashi, Kudo and Nishihira, 1979), but conduction slowing may occur acutely in the absence of prominent segmental demyelination or axonal degeneration (Sharma and Thomas, 1974; Jakobsen, 1979).

Although a variety of biochemical peripheral nerve defects have been uncovered in experimental diabetes, thus far only one sequence, that involving altered neural sorbitol and *myo*-inositol metabolism and the sodium-potassium ATPase, is directly implicated in conduction slowing (Greene, DeJesus and Winegrad, 1975; Greene *et al.*, 1982; Mayer and Tomlinson, 1983a; Finegold *et al.*, 1983; Greene and Lattimer, 1983; Greene, 1983). This last conclusion is based on the observed parallel responses of nerve *myo*-inositol content, sodium-potassium ATPase activity and motor nerve conduction velocity to metabolic intervention in acute streptozotocin diabetes.

Impaired axonal transport in experimental diabetes

Acute experimental diabetes produces abnormalities in axonal transport. Virtually all neuronal proteins necessary for axonal function are transported from the cell body where they are synthesized to the peripheral axon by several distinct axonal transport mechanisms. 'Fast axonal transport' ('fast component' or FC) consists of membrane-associated proteins, glycoproteins and lipids which travel peripherally through the axon at rates as high as 400 mm/day. 'Slow axonal transport' consists of 'slow component a' (SCa), carrying the microtubular-neurofilament network at a rate of 0.3–1.0 mm/day, and 'slow component b' (SCb) carrying the actin-containing microfilaments and the associated axoplasmic matrix at 2–4 mm/day. It is generally felt that the biologically relevant units of axonal transport are likely to be cytological structures rather than individual macromolecules (Tytell *et al.*, 1981).

Axonal transport occurs in a series of steps. Cytological structures synthesized in the cell body are 'loaded' via the Golgi apparatus and then transported peripherally at various rates. Upon arriving at the axon terminal, components are 'turned around', reinserted on a retrograde transport system which carries them centripetally to the cell body. Retrograde transport is thought to permit degradation of 'worn-out' organelles, recycling of cell constituents, and the transfer to the cell body of 'trophic' substances which enter via the nerve terminals (Brimijoin, 1982). Neither the mechanism nor the regulation of axonal transport are entirely understood; however, it is generally conceded to be energy-, ATP- and calcium-dependent, and to involve contractile proteins such as actin and myosin, possibly in association with microtubules (Brimijoin, 1982). Axonal transport is disordered in a variety of human and experimental nerve diseases, including human diabetic neuropathy (Brimijoin and Dyck, 1979; Brimijoin, 1982). Patients with diabetic neuropathy not only have a markedly reduced average FC transport rate for the enzyme dopamine-B-hydroxylase, but a reduced concentration of the enzyme as well (Brimijoin and Dyck, 1979). However, reduced apparent FC transport may represent a consequence rather than a cause of diabetic neuropathy (Brimijoin, 1982).

Axonal transport has been studied in animals with acute experimental diabetes, with conflicting results. Decreased FC transport by ligature-accumulation (Schmidt *et al.*, 1975) and radiolabel techniques (McLean and Meiri, 1979) has been reported in motor axons of acutely streptozotocin-diabetic rats. In contrast, Jakobsen and Sidenius (1980) and Bisby (1980) found normal sensory axon FC transport. Whether this inconsistency is attributable to methodological differences, or characteristics of the axon populations studied, is not clear. Jakobsen and Sidenius (1980) also reported a reduction in the anterograde transport of structural proteins in SCa in streptozotocin diabetic rat sciatic nerve, an observation which has been confirmed by others. Thus, various abnormalities in axoplasmic flow have been identified in acute experimental diabetes, but the nature of the defect remains obscure; however, a possible role for abnormal axonal transport has been postulated in the axonal atrophy of acute experimental diabetes and the axonal degeneration in human diabetic neuropathy (Sidenius, 1982). Recent observations implicate nerve *myo*-inositol metabolism in some components of disordered axonal transport in experimental diabetes (Mayer and Tomlinson, 1983).

Nerve carbohydrate and energy metabolism

An understanding of the mechanism(s) by which metabolic perturbations in diabetes alter nerve electrophysiology and motility requires an examination of normal and diabetic nerve carbohydrate and energy metabolism. Recently developed *in vitro* tissue preparations from rodent sciatic nerve have altered our classical view of peripheral nerve metabolic control (Greene *et al.*, 1979; Greene and Winegrad, 1979; Greene and Winegrad, 1981; Greene and Lattimer, 1982; Simmons, Winegrad and Martin, 1982; Gillon and Hawthorne, 1983a; Greene and Lattimer, 1983b). Peripheral nerve, like brain, is sequestered behind a specialized and relatively impermeable diffusion barrier *in vivo*, which severely limits the choice of substrates available for energy production (Bradbury and Crowder, 1976; Olsson, 1975). Brain is exquisitely dependent on glucose oxidation for energy. *In vitro* studies of peripheral nerve energy metabolism demonstrate a similar dependency on exogenous glucose and an independence from insulin control, with regulation primarily by intrinsic energy needs. (Earlier *in vitro* studies, which found an important insulin effect, were confounded by contaminating insulin-sensitive epineurial adipocytes and connective tissue elements (Greene *et al.*, 1979; Greene and Winegrad, 1979; Brown, Pleasure and Asbury, 1976.)) Thus, neither insulin deficiency nor hyperglycemia *per se* should directly or acutely derange glucose-derived oxidative energy production in diabetic peripheral nerve. Hence, the notion that diabetic neuropathy simply represents the failure of an insulin-dependent tissue in an insulin-deficient state is not supported by our present understanding of peripheral nerve metabolism.

Relationship of energy metabolism to sodium-potassium ATPase function and *myo*-inositol

Although insulin and glucose concentrations do not directly or acutely influence overall peripheral nerve glucose metabolism, peripheral nerve energy and substrate metabolism is significantly altered in acute experimental diabetes. *In vitro* resting nerve energy utilization is reduced by 25–30% despite the presence of augmented endogenous tissue substrate stores in the form of free glucose and fructose (Greene and Winegrad, 1981). The reduced energy utilization of diabetic peripheral nerve has been ascribed to an alteration in nerve sodium-potassium ATPase activity. A major fraction of resting peripheral nerve energy utilization occurs via the Mg^{++}-dependent, Na^+- and K^+-stimulated, adenosinetriphosphatase ('sodium-potassium ATPase,' EC 3.6.1.3) (Ritchie, 1967). *In vitro* studies have demonstrated that the reduction in steady-state diabetic nerve resting energy utilization is confined to and quantitatively equals the ouabain-inhibitable respiratory fraction (Greene and Lattimer, 1983b) which, in nerve, is an expression of sodium-potassium ATPase activity (Ritchie, 1967).

In mammalian cells the membrane-bound sodium-potassium ATPase is regulated by a variety of intrinsic intracellular modulators (including cytoplasmic sodium, potassium, magnesium, calcium, ATP, pH), by the characteristics of the plasma membrane into which it is embedded, and by extracellular sodium and potassium concentrations (Trachtenberg, Packey and Sweeney, 1981). Extrinsic modulation may be expressed through phosphorylation-dephosphorylation of either the sodium-potassium ATPase itself, or an associated membrane protein, or by regulation of sodium-potassium ATPase protein turnover (Trachtenberg, Packey and Sweeney, 1981; Lingham and Sen, 1982). The sodium-potassium ATPase defect in diabetic peripheral nerve is not acutely influenced by insulin *in vitro* (Greene and Winegrad, 1981), and is expressed in broken cell nerve homogenates, where the concentration of water-soluble modulators is controlled (Das *et al.*, 1976; Greene and Lattimer, 1983a). Therefore, the sodium-potassium ATPase defect in experimental diabetes is intrinsic to the enzyme-membrane complex. The defect is entirely prevented or reversed by *in vivo* *myo*-inositol supplementation, a manipulation that prevents the characteristic slowing of motor conduction velocity in diabetic rats (Greene and Lattimer, 1983a). Thus, the impairment of diabetic rat sodium-potassium ATPase activity can be explained as a consequence of altered diabetic nerve *myo*-inositol metabolism, which must secondarily alter the structure and/or function of the sodium-potassium ATPase-membrane complex. Since *myo*-inositol is a substrate for the synthesis of membrane phosphatidylinositol, an endogenous regulator of renal microsomal sodium-potassium ATPase (Roelofsen, 1981; Mandersloot, Roelofsen and DeGrier, 1978), it is tempting to speculate that the effect of *myo*-inositol on nerve sodium-potassium ATPase is membrane phosphatidylinositol-mediated. Support for this contention comes from the recent observation of Simmons, Winegrad and Martin (1982) that free *myo*-inositol levels may limit phosphatidylinositol turnover in peripheral nerve.

Normal peripheral nerve maintains a tissue-to-plasma *myo*-inositol concentration gradient of 90–100-fold; this gradient is reduced in both human (Mayhew, Gillon and Hawthorne, 1983) and animal (Greene, DeJesus and Winegrad, 1975; Palmano, Whiting and Hawthorne, 1977) diabetic peripheral nerves. A specific high-affinity sodium-dependent carrier-mediated *myo*-inositol transport system has been identified in peripheral nerve (Greene and Lattimer, 1982) and probably contributes to the establishment and/or maintenance of this gradient. High concentrations of glucose competitively inhibit *myo*-inositol uptake via this transport system (Greene and Lattimer, 1982), providing a potential mechanism by which diabetes could reduce nerve *myo*-inositol content. The low transport capacity and high concentration gradient characteristic of this transport system suggests that factors which influence passive efflux of *myo*-inositol might also greatly affect the tissue-to-plasma *myo*-inositol concentration gradient.

The peripheral nerve *myo*-inositol transport system is driven by the sodium gradient generated by the sodium-potassium ATPase (Greene and Lattimer, 1982). Therefore, the reduced sodium-potassium ATPase activity of diabetic peripheral nerve might secondarily impair sodium-dependent *myo*-inositol uptake. Recent experiments confirm that sodium-dependent *myo*-inositol uptake remains reduced in diabetic peripheral nerve even after tissue glucose concentrations are normalized; this remaining impairment correlates with the sodium-potassium ATPase reduction under various experimental conditions (Greene and Lattimer, 1983b), suggesting that reduced diabetic nerve sodium-potassium ATPase activity further compromises endoneurial sodium-dependent *myo*-inositol uptake. These relationships thus set the stage for a self-reinforcing cyclic metabolic derangement involving *myo*-inositol and the sodium-potassium ATPase in diabetic peripheral nerve.

Since nerve action potential generation and sodium-dependent *myo*-inositol uptake are altered by sodium-potassium ATPase reduction, it is likely that other sodium-gradient dependent processes are also impaired in diabetic nerve. With the exception of Ca^{++}, H^+ and K^+ ions, all known examples of net extrusion or accumulation of any substance against its concentration gradient across an animal cell plasma membrane involve the coupling of that movement to the electro-chemical gradient of sodium created by sodium-potassium ATPase (Kyte, 1981). Therefore, a defect in diabetic peripheral nerve sodium-potassium ATPase activity could lead not only to an acute reduction in nerve action potential generation (Brismar and Sima, 1981), but also to multiple biochemical and physiological abnormalities affecting all substrates and metabolites actively transported across the cell membrane. Resultant long-term metabolic and electrolyte imbalances might culminate in structural alterations in peripheral nerve which contribute to clinical diabetic neuropathy.

Other effects of hyperglycemia on nerve metabolism

Although the major pathways of nerve glucose metabolism are unaffected by high ambient glucose concentrations *in vitro* (Greene and Winegrad, 1981), several potentially important intracellular biochemical alterations are directly attributable to elevated extracellular glucose levels. These include increased polyol pathway activity and nonenyzmatic protein glycosylation.

Increased polyol pathway activity

In vivo tissue glucose concentrations reflect plasma glucose levels (Stewart *et al.*, 1967; Winegrad, Clements and Morrison, 1972). Polyol pathway activity, in turn, is regulated by the intracellular glucose concentration, since the Michaelis constants (K_m) of aldose reductase and sorbitol dehydrogenase for their respective substrates glucose and sorbitol exceed tissue levels by at least an order of magnitude (Winegrad, Clements and Morrison, 1972; Kinoshita, Merola and Dikmak, 1962). Peripheral nerve glucose, sorbitol and fructose levels are raised in experimental diabetes but fall quickly when plasma glucose is lowered with insulin (Stewart *et al.*, 1967), suggesting that sorbitol and fructose turn over rapidly. In the diabetic lens, sorbitol, which is poorly diffusible across cell membranes, accumulates in millimolar concentrations, implying a possible important polyol osmotic contribution in the pathogenesis of the 'sugar cataract' (Gabbay, 1975; Kinoshita, Merola and Dikmak, 1962). Uncritical extrapolation of this osmotic hypothesis to diabetic nerve ignores the micromolar (versus millimolar) sorbitol concentration range in nerve, which is unlikely to be osmotically significant unless sorbitol were highly localized to a minute tissue fraction. Furthermore, increased tissue water and edema is neither a constant nor necessary feature of diabetic nerve conduction impairment (Brown *et al.*, 1980; Greene, 1983).

Although polyol osmotic effects are unlikely to contribute prominently to diabetic peripheral nerve dysfunction, other manifestations of increased polyol pathway activity may be of pathogenetic relevance. Polyol pathway hyperactivity is known to perturb cytoplasmic NAD^+-NADH and $NADP^+$-NADPH couples in erthyrocytes (Travis *et al.*, 1971) and similar effects may occur in peripheral nerve. Recent studies in man and rats demonstrate that specific aldose reductase inhibitors may improve nerve function in diabetes (Yue *et al.*, 1982; Judzewitsch *et al.*, 1983; Mayer and Tomlinson, 1983; Fagius and Jameson, 1981) although the effects in humans are small. Polyol pathway hyperactivity may reduce peripheral nerve *myo*-inositol content (Gillon and Hawthorne, 1983b; Mayer and Tomlinson, 1983;

Finegold *et al.*, 1983), and extrapolation from studies in the lens would imply that the increased polyol pathway activity might enhance nerve *myo*-inositol efflux (Broekhuyse, 1968). Thus, increased peripheral nerve polyol pathway flux contributes to the derangement in diabetic nerve *myo*-inositol metabolism, and may influence diabetic nerve function in part by a *myo*-inositol-mediated mechanism.

Non-enzymatic protein glycosylation

In the late 1940s it was appreciated that glucose could react non-enzymatically with the alpha- and epsilon-amino groups of proteins *in vitro*. The *in vivo* occurrence of this process was demonstrated by the discovery of a naturally existing glycosylated minor hemoglobin component, hemoglobin A_1C (Bunn, Gabbay and Gallop, 1978). The non-enzymatic glycosylation reaction is thought to occur by slow condensation of the aldehyde group of glucose with the NH_2 terminus of the beta-chain of hemoglobin A to a more stable ketoamine form. Once the ketoamine linkage is formed, the reaction is irreversible and the linkage persists throughout the life of the protein molecule.

Patients with diabetes mellitus have significant elevations in erythrocyte hemoglobin A_1C concentration. Elevated hemoglobin A_1C levels were subsequently demonstrated in both the ob/ob and db/db genetically diabetic mouse and in the streptozotocin diabetic rat, implying a metabolic rather than a genetic basis for the hemoglobin A_1C elevation. The rate of hemoglobin A_1C formation is a reflection of the ambient glucose concentration, so that the concentration of hemoglobin A_1C is proportional to the average concentration of glucose in the erythrocyte. Numerous clinical studies have demonstrated that the concentration of hemoglobin A_1C in blood accurately reflects the mean plasma glucose over the preceding several months.

Non-enzymatic glycosylation can occur in a variety of tissue proteins as a result of increased ambient glucose concentration (Day, Thorpe and Baynes, 1979; Pande, Garner and Spector, 1979; Miller, Gravallese and Bunn, 1980; Schnider and Kohn, 1981; Vlassara, Brownlee and Cerami, 1981) and, in some instances, protein function is secondarily altered (Bunn, Gabbay and Gallop, 1978). This process has been implicated in diabetic cataractogenesis (Pande, Garner and Spector, 1979). Peripheral nerve protein glycosylation is increased in acute experimental diabetes (Vlassara, Brownlee and Cerami, 1981). Although the glycosylated proteins have not been identified, and their function remains unknown, these altered proteins could have a possible role in the functional and/or structural alterations in diabetic peripheral nerve. Of interest is the recent discovery that brain tubulin may be non-enzymatically glycosylated *in vitro* and *in vivo*, with dramatic alteration in its self-assembly and solubility characteristics (Williams *et al.*, 1982). Such glycosylation of peripheral nerve tubulin might well have important consequences on both fast and slow axonal transport, and on the physical characteristics of the axon cylinder.

Unifying hypothesis

Hyperglycemia alters nerve metabolism in several ways. Through competitive inhibition of sodium-dependent *myo*-inositol uptake and increased polyol (sorbitol) pathway activity, hyperglycemia reduces nerve *myo*-inositol content, alters nerve phosphoinositide metabolism and impairs sodium-potassium ATPase activity. The impairment of the electrogenic sodium-potassium ATPase secondarily and acutely slows nerve conduction velocity and inhibits other sodium-gradient dependent processes such as *myo*-inositol and amino acid uptake and intracellular water hemostasis. Other membrane defects occur as a consequence of altered inositol phospholipid metabolism, independent of the sodium-potassium ATPase, possibly involving other membrane-bound proteins such as the voltage-dependent sodium channel, or other membrane cationic ATPases. Elevated tissue glucose levels also result in non-enzymatic glycosylation of nerve proteins, potentially impairing their function. These abnormalities become self-reinforcing cyclic defects, with potentially widespread pathophysiological implications, leading to chronically slowed nerve conduction, impaired axonal transport, altered intermediary metabolism and, eventually, structural damage to diabetic peripheral nerve fibers.

Therapy of diabetic polyneuropathy

The first step in the treatment of diabetic polyneuropathy is to establish the diagnosis with reasonable certainty. This may be difficult at times because both diabetes mellitus and axonal neuropathies are common and may occur independently in some individuals. In most cases the course, clinical setting, and anatomic pattern of neuropathy will not suggest another condition. Because almost all cases of symptomatic diabetic neuropathy appear after many years of diabetes, another cause must be sought if the diagnosis of diabetes is not firmly established or if blood glucose has been elevated for only a short time. Nerve conduction studies are helpful to identify superimposed compression neuropathies which occur with increased frequency in diabetics and may confuse the clinical picture. Spinal fluid examination and sensory nerve biopsy are seldom useful except for research purposes. The workup of an undiagnosed polyneuropathy is discussed in *Chapter 1*.

Because of the accumulating evidence that severity of diabetic neuropathy correlates with the magnitude and duration of hyperglycemia, one should strive to obtain the most normal level of blood glucose control possible for each patient. Rigor of control depends largely on the patient's intelligence and motivation. At present the most widely advocated means of obtaining 'good' control is by monitoring finger stick blood sugar levels at home, using glucose oxidase strips and a portable colorimeter (e.g. Dextrometer), and adjusting insulin dosage accordingly. This method has supplanted urine glucose testing, which often gives a poor reflection of blood sugar levels. Hemoglobin A_1C levels can serve as a cumulative record of prior blood glucose elevation for long-term monitoring. In the future, islet cell transplantation may become the ultimate therapy for diabetes. In animal experiments both allograft and xenograft islet cells have survived and ameliorated hyperglycemia in previously diabetic hosts (Lacy, Davie and Finke, 1981).

Vitamin supplementation has no demonstrable value in the treatment of diabetic neuropathy except for individuals with poor nutrition. Clinical trials of *myo*-inositol (Greene *et al.*, 1981; Clements *et al.*, 1979) and aldose reductase inhibitors (Judzewitsch *et al.*, 1983) have been carried out, and more are under way. As yet the results are inconclusive, and since both inositol and aldose reductase inhibitors may be associated with unpleasant side effects neither should be considered for routine clinical use at this time.

Patients with diabetic polyneuropathy are most likely to be referred to a neurologist if they experience pain or prominent sensory symptoms. Unfortunately, none of the forms of diabetic neuropathic pain respond predictably to therapy. The most important step in reducing pain may be to increase the opportunity for nerve regeneration by improving the degree of blood glucose control. Thus, most patients with symptomatic diabetic neuropathy will require insulin therapy. Occasional patients will have a transient increase in pain intensity after restoration of blood glucose levels toward normal, but there is no evidence that this represents a worsening of the neuropathy. In fact, it may indicate that sensibility is returning.

The treatment of pain in diabetic neuropathy is often disappointing. We and others have observed that pain subsides after a number of months (Mayne, 1968), although not all investigators agree on this point (Boulton *et al.*, 1982). If deep burning pain occurs at the end of the day after elevating the feet, elastic stockings may reduce its severity. Simple analgesics should be tried but their effectiveness with neuropathic pain is limited. About half of patients with shooting, stabbing pains will respond to either phenytoin (Dilantin) or carbamazepine (Tegretol), given in doses sufficient to achieve therapeutic anticonvulsant levels. In contrast, anticonvulsants do not seem to be of value for deep, constant, aching pains. Amitriptyline (Elavil) 50–150 mg orally at bedtime, often brings partial relief of aching pains. The beneficial effect may be apparent in only a few days, before the onset of its antidepressant effect, but the potent analgesic and antidepressant effects of amitriptyline are difficult to distinguish (Spiegel, Kalb and Pasternak, 1983). The full dose should be reached very slowly, not only to avoid early lethargy, but also to watch for anticholinergic side effects such as urinary retention and impotence which may be especially likely in a diabetic with neuropathy. The addition of fluphenazine (Prolixin) (1 mg three times a day) may be useful, but the risk of inducing tardive dyskinesias must be considered before using phenothiazines for a potentially reversible condition.

Skin care is of particular importance to diabetics or other patients with cutaneous sensory loss. Arthropathy is another complication of insensitive extremities. Dysfunction of pain or proprioceptive fibers results in unsensed trauma with subluxation, degeneration of joint surfaces, bony resorption and Charcot joints (Lippmann, Perotto and Farrar, 1976; Sinha, Munichoodappa and Kozack, 1972). Unlike the more familiar Charcot joints seen in syphilis, diabetic neurogenic arthropathy tends to involve the distal articular surfaces of the small joints in the feet. Unusual foot deformities or the appearance of calluses in new areas should suggest this disorder, indicate the need for X-rays, and prompt referral to a knowledgeable orthopedic surgeon or physiatrist.

Strength will be normal or nearly so in the majority of patients with symmetrical diabetic polyneuropathy, although those referred to a neurologist are more likely to have severe neuropathy and a greater degree of muscle weakness. Simple ankle braces and other mechnical measures should be considered as with any neuromuscular disorder. If weakness is asymmetrical or in the distribution of a major nerve trunk, a search for superimposed compression neuropathy should be carried out. The therapy of neurogenic autonomic dysfunction is discussed in *Chapter 4*. Disordered gastrointestinal motility, orthostatic hypotension and sexual dysfunction are managed in diabetes as in other autonomic neuropathies.

DIABETIC SYMMETRICAL PROXIMAL MOTOR NEUROPATHY

Diabetic symmetrical proximal motor neuropathy is an uncommon disorder. It presents as slowly progressive weakness of hip and thigh muscles, sometimes associated with aching thigh pain. The length of the progressive phase may be weeks or months. This figure is difficult to obtain because published reports include phases of early recovery as part of the duration of disability. Proximal sensory loss is unusual, although most patients will have evidence of distal sensory loss as part of an associated sensory-motor polyneuropathy (Greenbaum, 1964; Williams and Mayer, 1976; Chokroverty *et al.*, 1977; Noel, 1973; Locke, Lawrence and Legg, 1963). Careful muscle testing may show minor asymmetries in the degree of iliopsoas, quadriceps, and other muscle involvement, and anterior compartment leg muscles may be involved. The pattern may suggest a myopathic disorder, especially when shoulder girdle muscles are affected (Locke, Lawrence and Legg, 1963). Electromyography and biopsy of affected muscles has shown convincing evidence of denervation and subsequent re-innervation (Casey and Harrison, 1972; Hamilton, Dobson and Marshall, 1968; Locke, Lawrence and Legg, 1963; Williams and Mayer, 1976; Gilliatt and Willison, 1962) and there is no modern evidence of primary myopathy in these patients.

The nature of diabetic symmetrical proximal motor neuropathy remains obscure (Asbury, 1977). Clinical and EMG findings could be explained by dysfunction of anterior horn cells, motor roots, the lumbosacral plexus, or intramuscular nerve twigs (Chokroverty *et al.*, 1977). Garland's original view (Garland, 1955) that the lesion is in the anterior spinal cord remains plausible and is supported by the occurrence of extensor toe signs and elevated spinal fluid protein in some cases. However, selective lumbar anterior horn cell loss has not been demonstrated at autopsy. The overlap with polyneuropathy has led to the suggestion that the two disorders are in fact one (Gregerson, 1969), but this view is not widely accepted.

Both diffuse metabolic and vascular abnormalities have been suggested as the basis of this disorder. Metabolic factors do seem to have a role because weakness sometimes appears after a period of weight loss or poor diabetic control (Hamilton, Dobson and Marshall, 1968). Satisfactory functional recovery occurs in most cases (Garland, 1955; Casey and Harrison, 1972), often shortly after institution of insulin therapy (Hamilton, Dobson and Marshall, 1968).

DIABETIC FOCAL AND MULTIFOCAL NEUROPATHIES

Asymmetrical proximal motor neuropathy

Acute mononeuropathy multiplex affecting the femoral nerve or lumbar plexus occasionally develops in older diabetics, often during periods of poor control (Goodman, 1954; Raff and Asbury, 1968; Calverley and Mulder, 1960). The progressive phase is short, over a few hours or days. Clinically, anterior thigh and knee pain is prominent and weakness is most apparent in the iliopsoas and quadriceps muscles, with loss of the ipsilateral knee jerk. Detailed examination may show that obturator-innervated and other muscles are affected, and the disorder may coexist with distal sensory-motor polyneuropathy (Calverley and Mulder, 1960). If the progressive phase is longer and the contralateral leg is affected, the syndrome may be clinically indistinguishable from symmetrical proximal motor neuropathy.

It is our impression that there is an initial period of rapid recovery and a later interval, lasting many months, when improvement proceeds more slowly. This biphasic course suggests that weakness results from two components, conduction block and axonal destruction. In one case of asymmetrical proximal motor neuropathy examined in detail at autopsy, there were multifocal infarctive lesions in the distribution of the lumbar plexus and proximal obturator and femoral nerve trunks (Raff, Sangalang and Asbury, 1968), strongly supporting the presumed ischemic basis of this acute disorder.

Cranial neuropathy

Ocular mononeuropathies are sufficiently common in diabetes that their occurrence in isolation should suggest the diagnosis. Oculomotor neuropathy is most often encountered, manifested by painful ophthalmoplegia of sudden onset, with pupillary sparing in a setting of established or previously unrecognized diabetes. The basis of this mononeuropathy appears to be centrofascicular ischemia of the oculomotor nerve (Asbury *et al.*, 1970). The preservation of circumferentially located parasympathetic fibers explains the pupillary sparing that is usually found in this syndrome. Acute trochlear, abducens, and facial nerve palsies are thought to occur with increased frequency in diabetes, and presumably have the same acute ischemic basis. Prognosis for recovery is good. If the neuropathy does not improve within 3–6 months, or if more than one nerve is affected, another etiology should be sought.

Intercostal and other mononeuropathies

Ellenberg (1978) called attention to the occurrence of acute thoracic sensory mononeuropathies or radiculopathies in individuals with diabetic polyneuropathy.

This disorder can mimic the pain of acute cardiac or intra-abdominal medical emergencies (Longstreth and Newcomer, 1977). The unilateral nature, acute onset and good resolution suggest a vascular basis, and distinguish this entity from the symmetrical anterior chest sensory loss which occurs with advanced polyneuropathy (Waxman, 1982). Other rare isolated mononeuropathies occur in diabetic individuals, but their low incidence makes it difficult to determine whether they are more common in diabetes.

Entrapment neuropathy

Single and multiple entrapment mononeuropathies, either clinically evident or demonstrable only electrophysiologically, are frequently associated with diabetic polyneuropathy (Mulder *et al.*, 1961; Gilliatt and Willison, 1962). In one unpublished series of 38 patients, we found clinical or electrophysiological evidence of entrapment neuropathy in 40% of all individuals examined. Diabetic mononeuropathies occur at the common sites of nerve compression, including the wrist and palm (median nerve); the elbow (ulnar nerve); and the fibular head (peroneal nerve). These entrapment neuropathies may respond favorably to the same conservative or surgical measures that are effective in patients without polyneuropathy.

Acknowledgements

We thank Kathy McDevitt for typing the manuscript and gratefully acknowledge research support from the Muscular Dystrophy Association, the Kroc Foundation, the Juvenile Diabetes Foundation, the Harry Soffer Memorial Research Fund, and NIH Grants NS08075 and RO1-AM2982.

References

Albin, J. and Rifkin, H. (1982) Etiologies of diabetes mellitus. *Medical Clinics of North America*, **66**, 1209–1226

Appenzeller, O. (1982) *The Autonomic Nervous System. An Introduction to Basic and Clinical Concepts*. Amsterdam: Elsevier Biomedical Press

Asbury, A. K. (1977) Proximal diabetic neuropathy. *Annals of Neurology*, **2**, 179–180

Asbury, A. K., Aldredge, H., Hershberg, R. and Fisher, C. M. (1970) Oculomotor palsy in diabetes mellitus: a clinicopathological study. *Brain*, **93**, 555–566

Asbury, A. K. and Brown, M. J. (1982) Clinical and pathological studies of diabetic neuropathies. In *Diabetic Neuropathy*, edited by Y. Goto, A. Horiuchi and K. Kogure. Amsterdam: Excerpta Medica

Asbury, A. K. and Johnson, P. C. (1978) *Pathology of Peripheral Nerve*. Philadelphia: W. B. Saunders

Ballin, R. H. M. and Thomas, P. K. (1968) Hypertrophic changes in diabetic neuropathy. *Acta Neuropathologica*, **11**, 93–102

Behse, F., Buchthal, F. and Carlsen, F. (1977) Nerve biopsy and conduction studies in diabetic neuropathy. *Journal of Neurology, Neurosurgery and Psychiatry*, **40**, 1072–1082

Bisby, M. A. (1980) Axonal transport of labelled protein and regeneration rate in nerves of streptozotocin diabetic rats. *Experimental Neurology*, **69**, 74–84

Bishoff, A. (1973) Ultrastructural pathology of peripheral nervous system in early diabetes. In *Vascular and Neurologic Changes in Early Diabetes*, edited by R. A. Camerini-Davalos and H. S. Cole, pp. 441–449. New York: Academic Press

Boulton, A. J. M., Drury, J., Clarke, B. and Ward, J. D. (1982) Continuous subcutaneous insulin infusion in the management of painful diabetic neuropathy. *Diabetes Care*, **5**, 386–390

Bradbury, M. W. B. and Crowder, J. (1976) Compartments and barriers in the sciatic nerve of the rabbit. *Brain Research*, **103**, 515–526

Bradley, W. E. (Ed.) (1980) Aspects of diabetic autonomic neuropathy. *Annals of Internal Medicine*, **92** (Part 2), 289–342

Brimijoin, W. S. (1982) Abnormalities of axonal transport. Are they a cause of peripheral nerve disease? *Mayo Clinic Proceedings*, **57**, 707–714

Brimijoin, W. S. and Dyck, P. J. (1979) Axonal transport of dopamine-B-hydroxylase and acetyl-cholinesterase in human peripheral neuropathy. *Experimental Neurology*, **66**, 467–478

Brismar, T. and Sima, A. A. F. (1981) Changes in nodal function in nerve fibers of the spontaneously diabetic BB-Wistar rat: potential clamp analysis. *Acta Physiologica Scandinavica*, **113**, 499–506

Broekhuyse, R. M. (1968) Changes in *myo*-inositol permeability in the lens due to cataractous conditions. *Biochemistry and Biophysical Acta*, **163**, 269–272

Brown, M. J. and Asbury, A. K. (1984) Diabetic neuropathy. *Annals of Neurology* (in press)

Brown, M. J., Iwamori, M., Kishimoto, Y., Rapoport, B., Moser, H. W. and Asbury, A. K. (1979) Nerve lipid abnormalities in human diabetic neuropathy: a correlative study. *Annals of Neurology*, **5**, 245–252

Brown, M. J., Martin, J. R. and Asbury, A. K. (1976) Painful diabetic neuropathy. A morphometric study. *Archives of Neurology*, **33**, 164–171

Brown, M. J., Pleasure, D. E. and Asbury, A. K. (1976) Microdissection of peripheral nerve: collagen and lipid distribution with morphological correlations. *Journal of Neurological Science*, **29**, 361–369

Brown, M. J., Sumner, A. J., Greene, D. A., Diamond, S. M. and Asbury, A. K. (1980) Distal neuropathy in experimental diabetes mellitus. *Annals of Neurology*, **8**, 168–178

Bruyn, G. W. and Garland, H. (1970) Neuropathies of endocrine origin. In *Handbook of Clinical Neurology*, Volume 1, edited by P. J. Vinken and G. W. Bruyn, pp. 29–71. Amsterdam: North-Holland

Bunn, H. F., Gabbay, K. H. and Gallop, P. M. (1978) The glycosylation of hemoglobin: relevance to diabetes mellitus. *Science*, **200**, 21–27

Calverley, J. R. and Mulder, D. W. (1960) Femoral neuropathy. *Neurology*, **10**, 963–967

Casey, E. G. and Harrison, M. J. G. (1972) Diabetic amyotrophy: a follow-up study. *British Medical Journal*, **1**, 656–659

Chokroverty, S., Reyes, M. G., Rubino, F. A. and Tonaki, H. (1977) The syndrome of diabetic amyotrophy. *Annals of Neurology*, **2**, 181–194

Chopra, J. S. and Fannin, T. (1971) Pathology of diabetic neuropathy. *Journal of Pathology*, **104**, 175–184

Chopra, J. S. and Hurwitz, L. J. (1969) Sural nerve myelinated fiber density and size in diabetics. *Journal of Neurology, Neurosurgery and Psychiatry*, **32**, 149–154

Chopra, J. S., Hurwitz, L. J. and Montgomery, D. A. D. (1969) The pathogenesis of sural nerve changes in diabetes mellitus. *Brain*, **92**, 391–418

Clarke, B. F., Ewing, D. J. and Campbell, I. W. (1979) Diabetic autonomic neuropathy. *Diabetologia*, **17**, 195–212

Clements, R. S. Jr (1979) Diabetic neuropathy – new concepts of its etiology. *Diabetes*, **28**, 604–611

Clements, R. S. Jr, Vourganti, B., Kuba, T., Oh, S. J. and Darnell, B. (1979) Dietary myoinositol intake and peripheral nerve function in diabetic nerve. *Metabolism*, **28**, 477–483

Conomy, J. P., Barnes, K. L. and Conomy, J. M. (1979) Cutaneous sensory function in diabetes mellitus. *Journal of Neurology, Neurosurgery and Psychiatry*, **42**, 656–661

Das, P. K., Bray, G. M., Aguayo, A. J. and Rasminsky, M. (1976) Diminished ouabain-sensitive, sodium-potassium ATPase activity in sciatic nerves of rats with streptozotocin-induced diabetes. *Experimental Neurology*, **53**, 285–288

Day, J. F., Thorpe, S. R. and Baynes, J. W. (1979) Non-enzymatically glycosylated albumin. *In vitro* preparation and isolation from normal human serum. *Journal of Biological Chemistry*, **254**, 595–597

DeFronzo, R. A. and Ferrannini, E. (1982) The pathogenesis of non-insulin-dependent diabetes. An update. *Medicine*, **61**, 125–140

Dyck, P. J., Lambert, E. H. and O'Brien, P. C. (1976) Pain in peripheral neuropathy related to rate and kind of fiber degeneration. *Neurology*, **26**, 446–471

Dyck, P. J., O'Brien, P. C., Bushek, W., Oviatt, K. F., Schilling, K. and Stevens, J. C. (1976) Clinical vs. quantitative evaluation of cutaneous sensation. *Archives of Neurology*, **33**, 651–655

Dyck, P. J., Sherman, W. R., Hallcher, L. M. *et al.* (1980) Human diabetic endoneurial sorbitol, fructose, and *myo*-inositol related to sural nerve morphometry. *Annals of Neurology*, **8**, 590–596

Eliasson, S. G. (1964) Nerve conduction changes in experimental diabetes. *Journal of Clinical Investigation*, **43**, 2353–2358

Ellenberg, M. (1978) Diabetic truncal mononeuropathy – a new clinical syndrome. *Diabetes Care*, **1**, 10–13

Eng, G. D., Hung, N. and August, G. P. (1975) Nerve conduction velocity determination in juvenile diabetes. *Modern Problems of Pediatrics*, **12**, 213–219

Faerman, I., Glocer, L., Celener, D. *et al.* (1973) Autonomic nervous system and diabetes. Histological and histochemical study of the autonomic nerve fibers of the urinary bladder in diabetic patients. *Diabetes*, **22**, 225–237

Fagerberg, S. E. (1959) Diabetic neuropathy, a clinical and histological study on the significance of vascular affections. *Acta Medica Scandinavica*, **164** (Suppl. 345), 1–97

Fagius, J. and Jameson, S. (1981) Effects of aldose reductase inhibitor treatment in diabetic polyneuropathy – a clinical and neurophysiological study. *Journal of Neurology, Neurosurgery and Psychiatry*, **44**, 991–1001

Feldman, M. and Schiller, L. R. (1983) Disorders of gastrointestinal motility associated with diabetes mellitus. *Annals of Internal Medicine*, **98**, 378–384

Finegold, D., Lattimer, S. A., Nolle, S., Bernstein, M. and Greene, D. A. (1983) Polyol pathway activity and *myo*-inositol metabolism: a suggested relationship in the pathogenesis of diabetic neuropathy. *Diabetes* (in press)

Friedman, S. A., Schulman, R. H. and Weiss, S. (1975) Hearing and diabetic neuropathy. *Archives of Internal Medicine*, **135**, 573–576

Fry, I. K., Hardwick, C. and Scott, G. W. (1962) Diabetic neuropathy: a survey and follow-up of 66 cases. *Guy's Hospital Report*, **111**, 113–129

Gabbay, K. H. (1975) Hyperglycemia, polyol metabolism and complications of diabetes mellitus. *Annual Review of Medicine*, **36**, 521–536

Garland, H. T. (1955) Diabetic amyotrophy. *British Journal of Medicine*, **2**, 1287–1290

Genuth, S. (1982) Classification and diagnoses of diabetes mellitus. *Medical Clinics of North America*, **66**, 1191–1207

Gilliatt, R. W. and Willison, R. G. (1962) Peripheral nerve conduction in diabetic neuropathy. *Journal of Neurology, Neurosurgery and Psychiatry*, **25**, 11–18

Gillon, K. R. W. and Hawthorne, J. N. (1983a) Transport of *myo*-inositol into endoneurial preparations of sciatic nerve from normal and streptozotocin-diabetic rats. *Biochemical Journal*, **210**, 775–781

Gillon, K. R. W. and Hawthorne, J. N. (1983b) Sorbitol, inositol and nerve conduction in diabetes. *Life Sciences*, **32**, 1943–1947

Goodman, J. I. (1954) Femoral neuropathy in relation to diabetes mellitus. Report of 17 cases. *Diabetes*, **3**, 266–273

Graf, R. J., Halter, J. B., Halar, E. and Porte, D. (1979) Nerve conduction abnormalities in untreated maturity-onset diabetes: relation to levels of fasting plasma glucose and glycosylated hemoglobin. *Annals of Internal Medicine*, **90**, 298–303

Graf, R. J., Halter, J. B., Pfeifer, M. A., Halar, E., Brozovich, F. and Porte, D. F. Jr (1981) Glycemic control and nerve conduction abnormalities in non-insulin-dependent diabetic subjects. *Annals of Internal Medicine*, **94**, 307–311

Greenbaum, D. (1964) Observations on the homogeneous nature and pathogenesis of diabetic neuropathy. *Brain*, **87**, 215–232

Greenbaum, D., Richardson, P. C., Salmon, M. V. and Urich, H. (1964) Pathological observations on six cases of diabetic neuropathy. *Brain*, **87**, 201–214

Greene, D. A. (1983) Metabolic abnormalities in diabetic peripheral nerve: relation to impaired function. *Metabolism*, **32**(Suppl. 1) 118–123

Greene, D. A., Brown, M. J., Braunstein, S. N., Schwartz, S. S., Asbury, A. K. and Winegrad, A. I. (1981) Comparison of clinical course and sequential electrophysiological tests in diabetics with symptomatic polyneuropathy and its implications for clinical trials. *Diabetes*, **30**, 139–147

Greene, D. A., DeJesus, P. V. and Winegrad, A. I. (1975) Effects of insulin and dietary myoinositol on impaired peripheral motor nerve conduction velocity in adult streptozotocin diabetes. *Journal of Clinical Investigation*, **55**, 1326–1336

Greene, D. A. and Lattimer, S. A. (1982) Sodium- and energy-dependent uptake of *myo*-inositol by rabbit peripheral nerve. Competitive inhibition by glucose and lack of an insulin effect. *Journal of Clinical Investigation*, **70**, 1009–1018

Greene, D. A. and Lattimer, S. A. (1983a) Na/K ATPase defect in diabetic rat peripheral nerve: correction by *myo*-inositol administration. *Journal of Clinical Investigation*, **72**, 1058–1063

Greene, D. A. and Lattimer, S. A. (1983b) A self-reinforcing metabolic defect in diabetic peripheral nerve involving *myo*-inositol and the sodium-potassium ATPase. *Clinical Research*, **31**, 501A (Abstract)

Greene, D. A., Lewis, R. A., Lattimer, S. A. and Brown, M. J. (1982) Selective effects of myo-inositol administration on sciatic and tibial motor nerve conduction parameters in the streptozotocin-diabetic rat. *Diabetes*, **31**, 573–578

Greene, D. A. and Winegrad, A. I. (1979) *In vitro* studies of the substrates for energy production and the effects of insulin on glucose utilization in the neural components of peripheral nerve. *Diabetes*, **28**, 878–887

Greene, D. A. and Winegrad, A. I. (1981) Effects of acute experimental diabetes on composite energy metabolism in peripheral nerve axons and Schwann cells. *Diabetes*, **30**, 967–974

Greene, D. A., Winegrad, A. I., Carpentier, J.-L., Brown, M. J., Fukuma, M. and Orci, L. (1979) Rabbit sciatic nerve fascicle and 'endoneurial' preparations for *in vitro* studies of peripheral nerve glucose metabolism. *Journal of Neurochemistry*, **33**, 1007–1018

Gregerson, G. (1968a) A study of the peripheral nerves in diabetic subjects during ischemia. *Journal of Neurology, Neurosurgery and Psychiatry*, **31**, 175–181

Gregerson, G. (1968b) Variations in motor conduction velocity produced by acute changes of the metabolic state in diabetic patients. *Diabetologia*, **4**, 273–277

Gregerson, G. (1969) Diabetic amyotrophy – a well defined syndrome? *Acta Medica Scandinavica*, **185**, 303–310

Gupta, P. R. and Dorfman, L. J. (1981) Spinal somatosensory conduction in diabetes. *Neurology*, **31**, 841–845

Hamilton, C. R., Dobson, H. L. and Marshall, J. (1968) Diabetic amyotrophy: clinical and electronmicroscopic studies of six patients. *American Journal of Medical Sciences*, **256**, 81–90

Hansen, S. and Ballantyne, J. P. (1977) Axonal dysfunction in the neuropathy of diabetes mellitus: a quantitative electrophysiological study. *Journal of Neurology, Neurosurgery and Psychiatry*, **40**, 555–564

Hilsted, J. (1982) Pathophysiology in diabetic autonomic neuropathy: cardiovascular, hormonal and metabolic studies. *Diabetes*, **31**, 730–737

Horowitz, S. H. and Ginsberg-Fellner, F. (1979) Ischemia and sensory nerve conduction in diabetes mellitus. *Neurology*, **29**, 695–704

Hosking, D. J., Bennett, T. and Hampton, J. R. (1978) Diabetic autonomic neuropathy. *Diabetes*, **27**, 1043–1054

Jakobsen, J. (1976) Axonal dwindling in early experimental diabetes. I. A study of cross sectioned nerves. *Diabetologia*, **12**, 539–546

Jakobsen, J. (1979) Early and preventable changes of peripheral nerve structure and function in insulin-deficient diabetic rats. *Journal of Neurology, Neurosurgery and Psychiatry*, **42**, 509–518

Jakobsen, J. and Sidenius, P. (1980) Transport of structural proteins in streptozotocin diabetic rats. *Journal of Clinical Investigation*, **66**, 292–297

Jaspan, J. B., Wollman, R. L., Bernstein, L. and Rubenstein, A. H. (1982) Hypoglycemic peripheral neuropathy in association with insulinoma: implication of glucopenia rather than hyperinsulinism. *Medicine*, **61**, 33–44

Johnson, P. C., Brendel, K. and Meezan, E. (1981) Human diabetic perineurial cell basement membrane thickening. *Laboratory Investigation*, **44**, 265–270

Judzewitsch, R. G., Jaspan, J. B., Polonsky, K. S. *et al.* (1983) Aldose reductase inhibition improves nerve conduction velocity in diabetic patients. *New England Journal of Medicine*, **308**, 119–125

Kennedy, W. R. and Sakuta, M. (1982) Sweat gland dysfunction in diabetic neuropathy. *Annals of Neurology*, **12**, 106

Kimura, J., Yamada, T. and Stevland, N. P. (1979) Distal slowing of motor nerve conduction velocity in diabetic polyneuropathy. *Journal of Neurological Science*, **42**, 291–302

Kinoshita, J. H., Merola, L. O. and Dikmak, E. (1962) The accumulation of dulcitol and water in rabbit lens incubated with galactose. *Biochemical and Biophysical Acta*, **62**, 176–178

Kolterman, O. G. and Olefsky, J. M. (1981) Insulin receptor in diabetes mellitus and obesity. In *Etiology and Pathogenesis of Insulin-Dependent Diabetes Mellitus*, edited by J. M. Martin, R. M. Ehrlich and R. J. Holland, pp. 99–125. New York: Raven Press

Kyte, J. (1981) Molecular considerations relevant to the mechanism of active transport. *Nature*, **16**, 201–204

Lacy, P. E., Davie, J. M. and Finke, E. H. (1981) Transplantation of insulin-producing tissue. *Medicine*, **70**, 589–594

Lamontagne, A. and Buchthal, F. (1970) Electrophysiological studies in diabetic neuropathy. *Journal of Neurology, Neurosurgery and Psychiatry*, **33**, 442–452

Lingham, R. B. and Sen, A. K. (1982) Regulation of rat brain $(Na^+ + K^+)$-ATPase activity by cyclic AMP. *Biochemical and Biophysical Acta*, **688**, 475–485

Lippmann, H. I., Perotto, A. and Farrar, R. (1976) The neuropathic foot of the diabetic. *Bulletin of the New York Academy of Medicine*, **52**, 1159–1178

Locke, S., Lawrence, D. G. and Legg, M. A. (1963) Diabetic amyotrophy. *American Journal of Medicine*, **34**, 775–785

Longstreth, G. F. and Newcomer, A. D. (1977) Abdominal pain caused by diabetic radiculopathy. *Annals of Internal Medicine*, **86**, 166–168

Low, P. A., Walsh, J. C., Huang, C. Y. and McLeod, J. G. (1975) The sympathetic nervous system in diabetic neuropathy – a clinical and pathological study. *Brain*, **98**, 341–356

Mandersloot, J. G., Roelofsen, B. and DeGrier, J. (1978) Phosphatidylinositol as the endogenous activator of the $(Na^+ + K^+)$-ATPase in microsomes of rabbit kidney. *Biochemical and Biophysical Acta*, **508**, 478–485

Martin, M. M. (1953) Diabetic neuropathy: a clinical study of 150 cases. *Brain*, **76**, 594–624

Mayer, J. H. and Tomlinson, D. R. (1983) The influence of aldose reductase inhibition and nerve *myo*-inositol on axonal transport and nerve conduction velocity in rats with experimental diabetes. *Journal of Physiology (London)*, **340**, 25P–26P

Mayhew, J. A., Gillon, K. R. W. and Hawthorne, J. N. (1983) Free and lipid inositol, sorbitol and sugars in sciatic nerve obtained post-mortem from diabetic patients and control subjects. *Diabetologia*, **24**, 13–15

Mayne, N. (1968) The short-term prognosis in diabetic neuropathy. *Diabetes*, **17**, 270–273

McLean, W. G. and Meiri, K. F. (1979) Rapid axonal transport of protein in rat sciatic motor nerves during early experimental diabetes. *Journal of Physiology*, **301**, 43P–44P

Miller, J. A., Gravallese, E. and Bunn, H. B. (1980) Non-enzymatic glucosylation of erythrocyte membrane proteins. *Journal of Clinical Investigation*, **65**, 896–901

Mulder, D. W., Bastron, J. A. and Lambert, E. H. (1956) Hyperinsulin neuropathy. *Neurology*, **6**, 627–635

Mulder, D. W., Lambert, E. H., Bastron, J. A. and Sprague, R. G. (1961) The neuropathies associated with diabetes. A clinical and electromyographic study of 103 unselected diabetic patients. *Neurology*, **11**, 275–284

Nathan, P. W. (1976) The gate-control theory of pain – a critical review. *Brain*, **99**, 123–158

Noel, P. (1973) Sensory nerve conduction in the upper limbs at various stages of diabetic neuropathy. *Journal of Neurology, Neurosurgery and Psychiatry*, **36**, 786–796

Olsson, Y. (1975) Vascular permeability in the peripheral nervous system. In *Peripheral Neuropathy, Volume I*, edited by P. J. Dyck, P. K. Thomas and E. M. Lambert, pp. 190–200. Philadelphia: W. B. Saunders

Page, M. McB. and Watkins, P. J. (1978) Cardiorespiratory arrest and diabetic autonomic neuropathy. *Lancet*, **1**, 14–16

Palmano, K. P., Whiting, P. H. and Hawthorne, J. N. (1977) Free and lipid *myo*-inositol in tissues from rats with acute and less severe streptozotocin-induced diabetes. *Biochemical Journal*, **167**, 229–235

Pande, A., Garner, W. H. and Spector, A. (1979) Glycosylation of human lens protein and cataractogenesis. *Biochemical and Biophysical Research Communications*, **89**, 1260–1266

Parry, G. J. and Brown, M. J. (1982) Selective fiber vulnerability in acute ischemic neuropathy. *Annals of Neurology*, **11**, 147–154

Pfeifer, M. A., Cook, D., Brodsky, J. *et al.* (1982) Quantitative evaluation of cardiac parasympathetic activity in normal and diabetic man. *Diabetes*, **31**, 339–345

Pirart, J. (1978) Diabetes mellitus and its degenerative complications, a prospective study of 4400 patients observed between 1947 and 1973. *Diabetes Care*, **1**, 168–188 and 252–263

Powell, H., Knox, D., Lee, S. *et al.* (1977) Alloxan diabetic neuropathy: electron microscopic studies. *Neurology*, **27**, 60–66

Raff, M. C. and Asbury, A. K. (1968) Ischemic mononeuropathy and mononeuropathy multiplex in diabetes mellitus. *New England Journal of Medicine*, **279**, 17–22

Raff, M. C., Sangalang, V. and Asbury, A. K. (1968) Ischemic mononeuropathy multiplex associated with diabetes mellitus. *Archives of Neurology*, **18**, 487–499

Reske-Nielsen, E., Harmsen, A. and Vorre, P. (1977) Ultrastructure of muscle biopsies in recent, short-term and long-term juvenile diabetes. *Acta Neurologica Scandinavica*, **55**, 345–362

Ritchie, J. M. (1967) The oxygen consumption of mammalian non-myelinated nerve fibers at rest and during activity. *Journal of Physiology*, **188**, 309–329

Roelofsen, B. (1981) The (non)specificity in the lipid requirement of the calcium- and (sodium plus potassium)-transporting adenosine triphosphatase. *Life Sciences*, **29**, 2235–2247

Roiter, J. I. and Rimoin, D. L. (1981) Genetics of insulin-dependent diabetes. In *Etiology and Pathogenesis of Insulin-Dependent Diabetes Mellitus*, edited by J. M. Martin, R. M. Ehrlich and R. J. Holland, pp. 37–59. New York: Raven Press

Rosner, L. and Elstad, R. (1964) The neuropathy of hypoglycemia. *Neurology*, **14**, 1–6

Sabin, T. D., Geschwind, N. and Waxman, S. G. (1978) Patterns of clinical deficits in peripheral nerve disease. In *Physiology and Pathobiology of Axons*, edited by S. G. Waxman, pp. 431–438. New York: Raven Press

Schmidt, R. E., Matschinsky, F. M., Godfrey, D. A., Williams, A. D. and McDougal, D. B. Jr (1975) Fast and slow axoplasmic flow in sciatic nerve of diabetic rats. *Diabetes*, **24**, 1081–1085

Schnider, S. L. and Kohn, R. R. (1981) Glucosylation of human collagen in aging and diabetes mellitus. *Journal of Clinical Investigation*, **66**, 1179–1181

Schwartz, D. E. (1974) Corneal sensitivity in diabetics. *Archives of Ophthalmology*, **91**, 174–178

Sharma, A. K. and Thomas, P. K. (1974) Peripheral nerve structure and function in experimental diabetes. *Journal of Neurological Science*, **23**, 1–15

Sidenius, P. (1982) The axonopathy of diabetic neuropathy. *Diabetes*, **31**, 356–363

Sidenius, P. and Jakobsen, J. (1983) Peripheral neuropathy in rats induced by insulin treatment. *Diabetes*, **22**, 383–386

Sima, A. A. F. (1980) Peripheral neuropathy in the spontaneously diabetic BB-Wistar-rat. An ultrastructural study. *Acta Neuropathologica*, **51**, 223–227

Simmons, D. A., Winegrad, A. I. and Martin, D. B. (1982) Significance of tissue *myo*-inositol concentrations in metabolic regulation in nerve. *Science*, **217**, 848–851

Sinha, S., Munichoodappa, C. S. and Kozack, G. P. (1972) Neuroarthropathy (Charcot joints) in diabetes mellitus. Clinical study of 101 cases. *Medicine*, **51**, 191–210

Smith, S. E., Smith, S. A., Brown, P. M., Fox, C. and Sonksen, P. H. (1978) Pupillary signs in diabetic autonomic neuropathy. *British Medical Journal*, **2**, 924–927

Spencer, P. S. and Schaumburg, H. H. (1976) Central-peripheral distal axonopathy: the pathology of dying-back polyneuropathies. *Progress in Neuropathology*, **3**, 253–295

Spiegel, K., Kalb, R. and Pasternak, G. W. (1983) Analgesic activity of tricyclic antidepressants. *Annals of Neurology*, **13**, 462–465

Stewart, M. A., Sherman, W. R., Kurien, M. M., Moonsammy, G. I. and Wisgerhof, M. (1967) Polyol accumulations in nervous tissue of rats with experimental diabetes and galactosaemia. *Journal of Neurochemistry*, **14**, 1057–1066

Sugimura, K. and Dyck, P. J. (1981) Sural nerve myelin thickness and axis cylinder caliber in human diabetes. *Neurology*, **31**, 1087–1091

Sugimura, K. and Dyck, P. J. (1982) Multifocal fiber loss in proximal sciatic nerve in symmetrical distal diabetic neuropathy. *Journal of Neurological Science*, **53**, 501–509

Thomas, P. K. (1982) Diabetic neuropathy. In *Complications of Diabetes*, edited by H. Keen and J. Jarrett. London: Edward Arnold

Thomas, P. K. and Eliasson, S. G. (1975) Diabetic neuropathy. In *Peripheral Neuropathy*, edited by P. J. Dyck, P. K. Thomas and E. H. Lambert. Philadelphia: W. B. Saunders

Thomas, P. K. and Lascelles, R. G. (1966) The pathology of diabetic neuropathy. *Quarterly Journal of Medicine*, **35**, 489–509

Timperley, W. R., Ward, J. D., Preston, F. E., Duckworth, T. and O'Malley, B. C. (1976) Clinical and histological studies in diabetic neuropathy. A reassessment of vascular factors in relation to intravascular coagulation. *Diabetologia*, **12**, 237–243

Trachtenberg, M. D., Packey, D. J. and Sweeney, T. (1981) *In vivo* functioning of the Na^+, K^+-activated ATPase. *Current Topics in Cellular Regulation*, **19**, 159–217

Travis, S. F., Morrison, A. D., Clements, R. S. Jr, Winegard, A. I. and Oske, F. A. (1971) Metabolic alterations in the human erythrocyte produced by increases in the glucose concentration: the role of the polyol pathway. *Journal of Clinical Investigation*, **50**, 2104–2112

Tytell, M., Black, M. M., Garner, J. A. and Lasek, R. J. (1981) Axonal transport: each major rate component reflects the movement of distinct macromolecular complexes. *Science*, **214**, 179–181

Vital, C. and Vallat, J. M. (1980) *Ultrastructural Study of the Human Diseased Peripheral Nerve*, pp. 76–80. New York: Masson

Vital, C. I., Vallat, J. M., LeBlanc, M., Martin, F. and Coquet, M. (1973) Les neuropathies peripheriques du diabete sucre: étude ultrastructurale de 12-cas biopsies. *Journal of Neurological Science*, **18**, 381–398

Vlassara, H., Brownlee, M. and Cerami, A. (1981) Non-enzymatic glycosylation of peripheral nerve protein in diabetes mellitus. *Proceedings of the National Academy of Sciences*, **78**, 5190–5192

Wall, P. D. and Gutnick, M. (1974) Properties of afferent nerve impulses originating from a neuroma. *Nature*, **248**, 740–743

Ward, J. D., Barnes, C. G., Fisher, D. J., Jessup, J. D. and Baker, R. W. R. (1971) Improvement in nerve conduction following treatment in newly diagnosed diabetes. *Lancet*, **1**, 428–430

Waxman, S. G. (1982) Diabetic radiculoneuropathy: clinical patterns of sensory loss and distal paresthesias. *Acta Diabetologia Latina*, **19**, 199–207

Waxman, S. G., Brill, M. H., Geschwind, N., Sabin, T. D. and Lettvin, J. Y. (1976) Probability of conduction deficit as related to fiber length in random-distribution models of peripheral neuropathies. *Journal of Neurological Science*, **29**, 39–53

Williams, E., Timperley, W. R., Ward, J. D. and Duckworth, T. (1980) Electron microscopical studies of vessels in diabetic peripheral neuropathy. *Journal of Clinical Pathology*, **33**, 462–470

Williams, I. R. and Mayer, R. F. (1976) Subacute proximal diabetic neuropathy. *Neurology*, **26**, 108–116

Williams, S. K., Howarth, N. L., Devenny, J. J. and Bitensky, M. W. (1982) Structural and functional consequences of increased tubulin glycosylation in diabetes mellitus. *Proceedings of the National Academy of Sciences*, **79**, 6546–6550

Winegrad, A. I., Clements, R. S. Jr and Morrison, A. D. (1972) Insulin-independent pathways of carbohydrate metabolism. In *Handbook of Physiology, Section 7 Volume I*, edited by R. O. Greep, E. B. Astwood, D. F. Steiner, N. Freinkel and S. R. Greiger, pp. 457–471. Baltimore: Waverley Press

Yagihashi, S., Kudo, K. and Nishihira, M. (1979) Peripheral nerve structures of experimental diabetic rats and the effect of insulin treatment. *Tohoku Journal of Experimental Medicine*, **127**, 35–44

Yue, D. K., Hanwell, M. A., Satchell, F. M. and Turtle, J. R. (1982) The effect of aldose reductase inhibition on motor nerve conduction velocity in diabetic rats. *Diabetes*, **31**, 789–794

7
Neuropathy in connective tissue disorders
Robert P. Lisak and Arnold I. Levinson

INTRODUCTION

Involvement of the peripheral nervous system (PNS), including the cranial nerves, is frequently seen in the connective tissue disorders, and may be the first clinical manifestation in some of these diseases. Peripheral nerve disease in patients with connective tissue disorders may be primary, secondary to involvement of other organ systems (uremic or entrapment neuropathies), or a result of therapy (gold neuropathy). Primary involvement of the PNS may be in a pattern of mononeuropathy (mononeuritis including cranial nerves) or mononeuropathy multiplex (mononeuritis including cranial nerves), diffuse polyneuropathy (usually mixed sensory-motor neuropathy) or, rarely, demyelinating neuropathy of Guillain-Barré type.

Certain of the connective tissue disorders are more likely to involve the PNS (i.e. polyarteritis nodosa in comparison with scleroderma) and certain patterns of involvement also are associated with particular collagen vascular diseases (i.e. isolated involvement of the fifth cranial nerve is characteristic of mixed connective tissue disease (MCTD)). Central nervous system (CNS) involvement also tends to occur more frequently and in particular patterns in different disorders (seizures and changes in mental status in systemic lupus erythematosus, spinal cord compression in rheumatoid arthritis).

The pathogenic mechanisms involved in primary involvement of the PNS are complex and may vary with respect to the collagen vascular disease and to the type of involvement (mononeuropathies vs diffuse polyneuropathies vs Guillain-Barré syndrome).

SYSTEMIC LUPUS ERYTHEMATOSUS

Systemic lupus erythematosus (SLE) is a multisystem inflammatory disorder of unknown etiology. It predominantly afflicts women between the second and fifth

154

decades of life. The clinical presentation is heterogeneous with patients presenting with one or more of the following abnormalities: fever, arthralgias or arthritis, mucocutaneous abnormalities, Raynaud's phenomenon, hematologic abnormalities, glomerulonephritis, polyserositis, and neuropsychiatric disturbances. Indeed, several of the above features are included as criteria requisite for the diagnosis of SLE as recently specified by the American Rheumatism Association (*Table 7.1*) (Tan *et al.*, 1982). The natural history of SLE is extremely variable, characterized by a relatively benign course in some and a fulminant progressive or accelerated course in others. Most observers agree that patients with involvement of the CNS or the kidneys have the worst prognosis. Long-term survival has improved markedly in the past two decades, largely due to improvement in general medical care and the advent of corticosteroid therapy and more effective antibiotics.

Pathogenesis

Several of the clinical manifestations of SLE can be attributed to immune-mediated tissue destruction. Patients produce a myriad of autoantibodies including those directed against red cells, white cells, platelets, and nuclear constituents of cells. The interaction of antibody and formed elements of the blood leads to activation of the complement system and removal of sensitized targets by phagocytic cells of the reticuloendothelial system. Antibodies against nuclear determinants, particularly against native (double-stranded) DNA, bind antigen and may be deposited in strategic areas throughout the body. Deposition of such immune complexes with subsequent complement-mediated injury probably accounts for many of the renal and cutaneous manifestations. Characteristic patterns of immune reactants have been observed in the renal glomerulus and dermal/epidermal junction of the skin, respectively. The pathogenesis of the CNS and PNS (*see below*) manifestations is less clear, although immunoglobulin and complement deposition have been observed in the choroid plexes at time of necropsy and some workers report antineuron antibodies in serum and cerebrospinal fluid. Several forms of peripheral neuropathy are seen and are thought to represent the consequences of immune complex mediated vasculitis (vasa nervorum).

The multitude of antibodies may reflect the consequence of polyclonal B-cell activation by an unknown agent or agents. Recent studies have highlighted a number of immunoregulatory aberrations in patients with SLE, particularly impaired functions of the regulatory T-cell network controlling B-cell responses. This is a complex area, however, where distinguishing between primary and secondary pathophysiologic events is often quite difficult. Based on experimental animal models of SLE, disturbances have been observed at multiple levels of this regulatory network. Thus, from an immunopathologic standpoint, it is likely that diverse mechanisms will be incriminated in man as well. The responsible initiating agent is unknown. In certain lupus strains of mice, viral infection seems important but unequivocal evidence for a viral etiology of human lupus is not available. Most observers agree that interactions between environmental and a number of genetically determined host factors provide the framework for the development of SLE (Decker *et al.*, 1979).

156

Table 7.1 The 1982 revised criteria for classification of systemic lupus erythematosus*
(from Tan *et al.*, 1982 courtesy of the Editor and Publishers, *Arthritis and Rheumatism*)

Criterion	Definition
1 Malar rash	Fixed erythema, flat or raised, over the malar eminences, tending to spare the nasolabial folds
2 Discoid rash	Erythematous raised patches with adherent keratotic scaling and follicular plugging: atrophic scarring may occur in older lesions
3 Photosensitivity	Skin rash as a result of unusual reaction to sunlight, by patient history or physician observation
4 Oral ulcers	Oral or nasopharyngeal ulceration, usually painless, observed by a physician
5 Arthritis	Nonerosive arthritis involving two or more peripheral joints, characterized by tenderness, swelling, or effusion
6 Serositis	(a) Pleuritis – convincing history of pleuritic pain or rub heard by a physician or evidence of pleural effusion or (b) Pericarditis – documented by ECG or rub or evidence of pericardial effusion
7 Renal disorder	(a) Persistent proteinuria greater than 0.5 g/day or greater than 3+ if quantitation not performed or (b) Cellular casts – may be red cell, hemoglobin, granular, tubular, or mixed
8 Neurologic disorder	(a) Seizures – in the absence of offending drugs or known metabolic derangements: e.g. uremia, ketoacidosis, or electrolyte imbalance or (b) Psychosis – in the absence of offending drugs or known metabolic derangements, e.g. uremia, ketoacidosis, or electrolyte imbalance
9 Hematologic disorder	(a) Hemolytic anemia with reticulocytosis or (b) Leukopenia – less than $4000 \times 10^6/l$ total on two or more occasions or (c) Lymphopenia – less than $1500 \times 10^6/l$ on two or more occasions or (d) Thrombocytopenia – less than $100\,000 \times 10^6/l$ in the absence of offending drugs
10 Immunologic disorder	(a) Positive LE cell preparation or (b) Anti-DNA: antibody to native DNA in abnormal titer or (c) Anti-Sm: presence of antibody to Sm nuclear antigen or (d) False positive serologic test for syphilis known to be positive for at least 6 months and confirmed by *Treponema pallidum* immobilization or fluorescent treponemal antibody absorption test
11 Antinuclear antibody	An abnormal titer of antinuclear antibody by immunofluorescence or an equivalent assay at any point in time and in the absence of drugs known to be associated with 'drug-induced lupus' syndrome

* The proposed classification is based on 11 criteria. For the purpose of identifying patients in clinical studies, a person shall be said to have systemic lupus erythematosus if any 4 or more of the 11 criteria are present, serially or simultaneously, during any interval of observation

Peripheral nervous system disease

Although involvement of the CNS in patients with SLE is the most common and widely appreciated neurologic manifestation, peripheral nerve and cranial nerve involvement are well recognized, occurring in about 10% of patients (Berry and Hodges, 1965; Dubois, 1966; Johnson and Richardson, 1968; Feinglass *et al.*, 1976). The patterns of PNS involvement seen in such patients are:

(1) symmetric distal sensory-motor neuropathy
(2) mononeuropathy (mononeuritis) multiplex
(3) cranial nerve involvement, and
(4) Guillain-Barré syndrome.

PNS involvement is generally seen in patients with previously diagnosed SLE, in contrast to CNS involvement which may be among the earliest manifestations of disease. Involvement of CNS may make it difficult to establish the concomitant presence of a neuropathy or to distinguish PNS from CNS localization of cranial nerve deficits (Johnson and Richardson, 1968).

Sensory-motor neuropathy

The most common PNS involvement in patients with SLE is a symmetric subacute or chronically progressive symmetric mixed sensory-motor neuropathy with sensory findings predominantly (Johnson and Richardson, 1968; Feinglass *et al.*, 1976). The clinical picture in most would suggest an axonal neuropathy but there are no studies using modern morphologic techniques or clinical electrophysiologic testing to document unequivocally such a pathologic pattern. Studies of the more slowly progressive or subacute neuropathy with a sensory or sensory-motor pattern of neuropathy show changes in both myelin and axons which do not always allow one to decide unequivocally which is primarily involved. The issue is further confused by a clinical continuum with patients exhibiting slightly atypical courses of Guillain-Barré syndrome, including predominant motor involvement, cytoalbuminologic dissociation and a pathologic picture including loss of myelin and perivascular mononuclear cell infiltration without any definite evidence of arteritis (Bailey, Sayre and Clark, 1956; Johnson and Richardson, 1968). Still other patients have what seems to be classic Guillain-Barré syndrome (*see below*).

In addition to loss of myelinated fibers and evidence of loss of axon cylinders, pathologic studies in patients with this type of neuropathy have demonstrated varying degrees of perivascular mononuclear and polymorphonuclear cell infiltration (Lewis, 1965) and changes in the blood vessels ranging from frank vasculitis with inflammatory cells (Bailey, Sayre and Clarke 1956) to vascular changes without inflammation (Hepinstall and Sowry, 1952; Goldberg and Chitanondh, 1959) to normal vessels (Bailey, Sayre and Clark, 1956; Scheinberg, 1956; Lewis, 1965; Johnson and Richardson, 1968). In other cases, fibrinoid material, apparently similar to hematoxylin bodies is found and is thought to compress nerve fibers (Scheinberg, 1956). It has been suggested that such material can cause disease by mechanical effects on nerve fibers. The pathogenic mechanisms in this form of SLE neuropathy are not understood.

Mononeuropathy

Patients with SLE may present with the clinical picture of acute or subacute mononeuropathy, mononeuropathy multiplex or plexopathy (Scheinberg, 1956; Feinglass *et al.*, 1976; Block *et al.*, 1979). Involvement of adjacent major nerves may result in what may appear at first to be a distal symmetric polyneuropathy. Because of the pattern of involvement (single large nerves in an acute or subacute pattern) and the presence of arteritis in some patients, it has been thought that the deposition of immune complexes is responsible for this form of neuropathy in SLE, as well as in other connective tissue disorders.

Cranial nerves

Clinical involvement of one or more cranial nerves is seen in patients with SLE, frequently in association with signs of other peripheral neuropathies or unequivocal CNS disease (Johnson and Richardson, 1968; Ashworth and Tait, 1971; Lundberg and Werner, 1972; Feinglass *et al.*, 1976). In some of these patients it is difficult to distinguish true peripheral nerve disease from involvement due to brainstem or other CNS lesions. As in mononeuropathies of nerves of the limbs or plexus involvement, a vascular pathogenic mechanism is believed to be involved. In other patients weakness of muscles innervated by the cranial nerves may represent simultaneous myasthenia gravis and SLE (Denny and Rose, 1961; Wolf and Barrows, 1966).

Guillain-Barré syndrome

Fairly typical instances of Guillain-Barré syndrome have been reported in patients with SLE (Clark and Bailey, 1956; Feinglass *et al.*, 1976), although in many the course of disease is more subacute and resembles the chronic progressive or recurrent demyelinative polyneuropathies (CRIP) (Goldberg and Chitanondh, 1959; Lewis, 1965; Johnson and Richardson, 1968). In others, the picture merges with that of a rapidly progressive distal sensory-motor neuropathy in which the motor findings predominate. The pathogenic mechanisms of this SLE-associated Guillain-Barré syndrome or CRIP are unknown. In idiopathic Guillain-Barré syndrome and CRIP the pathogenesis is likewise not understood, although a humoral or cell-mediated immunologic reaction to PNS is postulated (Arnason, 1971; Cook and Dowling, 1981; Lisak, Brown and Sumner, 1983). It is possible that a similar mechanism pertains in patients with Guillain-Barré syndrome associated with SLE. Defects in immunologic control mechanisms could allow for the emergence of an organ specific immunopathogenic reaction (to PNS myelin) in the setting of a non-organ specific disorder such as SLE, despite the view that many manifestations of SLE are felt not to be due to antibodies or cell-mediated immunity to self antigens. A second possibility is that the Guillain-Barré syndrome in SLE is vascular in etiology and simply part of a continuum of symmetric neuropathy as discussed earlier. Although idiopathic Guillain-Barré syndrome is clearly demyelinative, there are several features of importance to this discussion:

(1) Circulating immune complexes are found in serum of patients with Guillain-Barré syndrome (Tachovsky *et al.*, 1976; Cook and Dowling, 1981)
(2) While the clinical picture in Guillain-Barré syndrome is bilateral and basically symmetric, the pathology (Asbury, Arnason and Adams, 1969) and the detailed electrophysiology (Brown, Feasby and Yates, 1981; Sumner, personal communication) reveals a multifocal segmental disorder, and
(3) It is possible that non-Ig serum factors such as activated complement could cause demyelination or abnormalities in Schwann cells leading to demyelination (Lisak, Brown and Sumner, 1983).

One could then argue that if multifocal demyelination can lead to the clinically symmetric pattern seen in Guillain-Barré syndrome of the chronic and relapsing demyelinating neuropathies (Lewis and Sumner, 1982), then multiple vascular lesions within the same nerve could result in a Guillain-Barré-like picture in SLE. By extension, one could postulate that many or even all neuropathies in SLE patients (and other connective tissue disorders) are vascular in pathogenesis and that the clinical and pathologic picture seen (diffuse polyneuropathy, typical or atypical Guillain-Barré syndrome, mononeuropathy or plexopathy) is simply the result of the rate of and pattern of lesions. Experimental acute ischemia or infarction does not result in classic PNS demyelination (Parry and Brown, 1981; Parry and Brown, 1982) but subacute or chronic ischemia might: (a) cause demyelination or (b) cause proximal lesions which distally appear diffuse (Parry and Brown, 1981).

Laboratory studies in PNS disease

Clinical neurophysiologic testing, as discussed in Chapter 1, is of great value in establishing the pattern and nature of the involvement of the PNS. Analysis of CSF frequently shows increased total protein, especially in Guillain-Barré or atypical Guillain-Barré cases. Most patients with active PNS involvement show serologic evidence of active SLE but there is no direct correlation between titers of autoantibodies or decrease in complement components and clinical PNS involvement.

Therapy of PNS disease

The treatment of active PNS (and CNS) disease with corticosteroids or immunosuppressive drugs is controversial. Efficacy of these agents has not been substantiated in large controlled series and even enthusiasts of such therapy for CNS disease in SLE express reservations with regard to beneficial effects of this therapy in the neuropathies (Feinglass *et al.*, 1976). Individual case reports are difficult to interpret in SLE which has an unpredictable course. Nonetheless, we recommend treating a rapidly progressive symmetric polyneuropathy resulting in significant disability or mononeuropathy multiplex with corticosteroids or an increase in dosage if the patient is already being treated at doses below 1 mg/kg prednisone equivalent/day. If the patient is already on high doses of corticosteroids, it would be reasonable to add immunosuppressive agents or try pulse therapy with corticosteroids, especially in progressive mononeuropathy multiplex. The literature is not helpful as far as any role for plasmapheresis. In neuropathies in which axonal damage has occurred the first evidence of therapeutic success may be absence of further disease progression.

RHEUMATOID ARTHRITIS

Clinical description

Rheumatoid arthritis (RA) is a chronic inflammatory disorder of the joints which typically has its onset between the ages of 30 and 70 years with peak onset in the fourth decade. The disease affects females approximately three times more often than males. Systemic involvement in RA is not uncommon; pulmonary, cutaneous, hematologic, cardiovascular and neurologic systems are the organ systems most frequently affected. RA commonly presents in an insidious fashion with constitutional signs and symptoms and arthralgias followed by the appearance of frank arthritis which is usually symmetric in distribution. Joints of the hands and feet are most frequently involved, although inflamed knees, elbows, and cervical spine are often seen. The proximal interphalangeal and metacarpophalangeal joints are typically involved in the hands with serious involvement causing classical disfigurations, e.g. volar subluxation and ulnar deviation of the fingers as well as swan-neck deformities. Progressive disease causes severe degrees of limitation of motion and may lead to flexion contractures. Patients characteristically display a jelling phenomenon with marked joint stiffness experienced upon arising in the mornings. Rheumatoid nodules are seen in patients with highly expressed (actively inflamed joints, high rheumatoid factor titers) disease most often around points of pressure. RA runs an unpredictable course characterized by remissions and relapses with variable degrees of severity.

As noted, RA may involve other organs besides the joints as evidenced by the lungs where three different patterns of inflammation may be seen. These include diffuse interstitial fibrosis, pleural effusions, and pulmonary nodules. Clinically manifest cardiac involvement is uncommon, although pericarditis is not uncommonly seen at necropsy. Vasculitis involving small and large vessels may occur in patients with highly expressed disease and usually presents with cutaneous manifestations. Vasculitis of the vasa nervorum causes peripheral neuropathy which may be of the sensory or motor variety. Additional neurologic manifestations include spinal cord compression by the odontoid process secondary to atlanto-axial subluxation and tenosynovitis causing any of several entrapment syndromes (*see below*).

Pathophysiology

The etiology of RA is unknown, although immunologic, genetic and perhaps infectious factors are important. The serologic hallmark of RA is rheumatoid factor which represents an autoantibody directed against the Fc fragment of IgG. The classical rheumatoid factor which is measured in standard serologic testing is an IgM anti-IgG. Anti-globulins of IgG or IgA isotype may also be found, but require specialized technology for their identification. Rheumatoid factors are elaborated in large amounts in the joint where they and their reaction products activate the complement pathway and initiate complement and neutrophil dependent inflammation. However, rheumatoid factors alone are not responsible for joint inflammation. A number of other inflammatory disorders are associated with serum rheumatoid factors, but not joint disease. Furthermore, T-cells account for the majority of lymphocytes infiltrating the synovial tissue and fluid and there is evidence that some of these T-cells are in an 'active state'. Products of lymphocyte activation, such as migration inhibition factor, have been identified in the synovial fluid. A complicated story to explain the pathogenesis of the joint inflammation in RA is emerging which entails interactions between a number of cellular components (including macrophages and synovial cells) as well as the elaboration of injurious humoral factors. Evidence for an infectious etiology has been sought for a number of years. Although several types of organisms have been incriminated, firm evidence for any of them is lacking (Williams, 1979).

Treatment of RA

The mainstay of therapy remains acetylsalicylic acid (aspirin). Patients who cannot tolerate the high levels of drug needed are treated with one of a number of nonsteroidal anti-inflammatory agents. Approaches taken in patients with more severe disease include the use of anti-malarials, gold salts, penicillamine, immunosuppressive agents, or total body irradiation in recent experimental trials. The appropriate mixture of rest and exercise as well as physical therapy are critical adjuncts. Corticosteroids are no longer as widely employed for joint manifestations, but may be useful with or without immunosuppressive agents for certain manifestations of vasculitis, including certain PNS syndromes.

PNS disease

Peripheral neuropathy occurs in 1–10% of patients with rheumatoid arthritis (Johnson *et al.*, 1959; Conn and Dyck, 1975). Several clinical patterns are seen including:

(1) Entrapment neuropathies
(2) A relatively mild distal symmetric neuropathy with predominantly, if not exclusively, sensory involvement
(3) Mononeuritis or mononeuritis multiplex

(4) A severe distal sensorimotor neuropathy which is probably a result from a series of fulminant mononeuropathies. Autonomic dysfunction may also occur (Edmonds *et al.*, 1979).

Entrapment neuropathies

Rheumatoid arthritis patients may have any of several entrapment neuropathies (Nakano, 1978) including:

(1) Median nerve in the carpal tunnel
(2) Digital branches of median or ulnar nerves
(3) Anterior interosseous nerve
(4) Ulnar nerve in Guyton's canal at the wrist or at the elbow
(5) Posterior interosseous nerve syndrome at the elbow
(6) Lower sciatic nerve (with a Baker's cyst in the popliteal fossa affecting posterior tibial, peroneal or both branches of sciatic nerve), and
(7) Tarsal tunnel syndrome, entrapping the posterior tibial nerve in the flexor retinaculum along the medial malleolus of the ankle.

Therapy includes splinting, local corticosteroid injection or surgery.

Distal symmetric polyneuropathy

Patients may have a gradual onset with paresthesias and decreased sensation in lower or upper extremities or both (Pallis and Scott, 1965). Motor symptoms are frequently not present or may be impossible to discern because of deformities (Conn and Dyck, 1975). This type of neuropathy may be slowly progressive, may stabilize or occasionally progress to an extent to cause severe disability. The pathologic mechanisms of this type of rheumatoid arthritis associated neuropathy are poorly understood since most pathologic studies have been of mononeuritis multiplex and severe progressive sensory-motor neuropathy. In one patient segmental demyelination and occasional degeneration of large myelinated fibers were said to be present (Peyronnard *et al.*, 1982). Similar findings have also been described in patients with RA without clinical neuropathy (Beckett and Dinn, 1972). Another patient showed intimal proliferation and Wallerian degeneration with severe fiber loss of myelinated fibers (Beckett and Dinn, 1972). While mild ischemia has been invoked as a possible mechanism in this syndrome, the vessels within the nerves have not always been abnormal at the level examined (Conn and Dyck, 1975) or when abnormal, are often quite mild. In the absence of rapid progression of this variety of RA neuropathy, conservative therapy is suggested.

Mononeuritis

Mononeuritis or mononeuritis multiplex is a well recognized PNS complication of RA. The clinical picture evolves acutely or subacutely and has a tendency to evolve into a severe distal sensory-motor neuropathy. There is little pathologic data on mononeuritis in RA but the course of the neuropathy and the progression to the picture of the more severe distal neuropathy suggests that the pathologic picture and vascular pathogenesis described in that form is present in the more limited mononeuritis or mononeuritis multiplex. Interestingly, cranial nerve mononeuritis which is seen in SLE, MCTD, scleroderma and primary Sjögren's syndrome is rare in classic RA.

Severe distal sensory-motor neuropathy

The severe distal sensory-motor neuropathy evolves rapidly and probably represents a series of mononeuritis multiplexes involving multiple nerves giving a symmetric distal picture. This type of neuropathy and mononeuritis multiplex are most frequently seen in patients with long-standing highly expressed RA exhibiting other signs of vasculitis including rheumatoid nodules, skin vasculitis, weight loss, fever, high titer rheumatoid factor and frequently decreased serum complement (Conn and Dyck, 1975). The development of this neurologic picture often is associated with a poor general outcome (Ferguson and Slocumb, 1961) since it often represents a part of a generalized vasculitis. Earlier it was thought that this neuropathy was associated or even triggered by the use of corticosteroids but similar patterns of PNS involvement have developed in patients with recent reduction in corticosteroid dose and in patients not receiving corticosteroids. The use of corticosteroids may decrease the degree of inflammatory response associated with the vascular lesion.

Examination of the vessels in patients with the severe progressive neuropathies includes any one of a number of patterns of involvement:

(1) Mononuclear perivascular infiltration without associated vascular wall changes
(2) Fibrinoid necrosis with vessel wall infiltration by mononuclear cells, eosinophils and polymorphonuclear cells
(3) Occlusion of the vessel lumen sometimes associated with hemorrhage around the vessel wall
(4) Intimal proliferation with or without media damage, and
(5) Perivascular or arterial wall fibrosis.

Detailed examination of a single nerve may reveal all of these changes (Irby, Adams and Toone, 1958; Weller, Bruckner and Chamberlain, 1970; Conn, McDuffie and Dyck, 1972; Dyck, Conn and Okazaki, 1972; Kim and Collins, 1981; Peyronnard *et al.*, 1982).

Analysis of the nerves reveals segmental demyelination (Beckett and Dinn, 1972). With severe deficits, Wallerian degeneration and fiber degeneration is usually seen, especially in association with extensive vasculitis; true infarction (circumscribed necrosis of all elements) is unusual (Conn and Dyck, 1975). The lesions of ischemia and fiber degeneration tend to be maximal in the mid-arm and thigh and in cross-section are seen in a central fascicular pattern (Dyck, Conn and Okazaki, 1972). This suggests that poor collateral flow in a water-shed area tends to result in greater ischemia (Sladky, Greenberg and Brown, 1983). Examination of a distal nerve may reveal diffuse axonal and myelin loss without any visible vascular changes at that level.

Laboratory evaluation in PNS disease

Serologic studies of patients with RA and neuropathy generally indicate active disease (increased rheumatoid factor, decreased complement), especially in patients with mononeuritis or severe sensory-motor neuropathy. Clinical neurophysiologic testing is useful in helping to establish the pattern of involvement and is especially useful in sorting out entrapment neuropathies. This is very important since several of these are best treated with local injection of corticosteroids or surgical decompression.

Therapy of PNS disease

The development of mononeuritis or severe sensory-motor neuropathy, especially when associated with evidence of generalized vasculitis, should be treated with high dose corticosteroid therapy and, if progressive, cytotoxic immunosuppressive anti-inflammatory drugs, such as cyclophosphamide, should be added. There is no proof, however, that this will lead to arrest of neuropathy with eventual improvement in RA.

SCLERODERMA

Clinical description

Scleroderma is a disorder of collagen which affects the skin and several internal organs including the gastrointestinal tract, heart, lungs, kidneys and rarely the nervous system. Cutaneous involvement represents the most common and usually the earliest manifestation of disease. Early involvement is registered by swelling of the fingers and hands which is followed by a hidebound appearance of the overlying skin with loss of wrinkles. This process frequently extends to involve other parts of the body, including the upper torso and face. Additional cutaneous manifestations include hyperpigmentation with areas of depigmentation and telangiectasias. As noted, cutaneous manifestations frequently antedate visceral involvement; however, skin involvement occasionally is lacking.

Scleroderma frequently affects the gastrointestinal tract, with the esophagus being the site most often involved. Clinically, patients present with retrosternal chest pain, fullness, pyrosis and occasionally regurgitation of stomach contents. These problems can be attributed to impaired gastroesophageal sphincter function and aperistalsis seen in the distal two-thirds of the esophagus in many patients. Abnormal esophageal motility occurs at some time in more than 50% of patients and is frequently associated with antecedent Raynaud's phenomenon. The stomach is infrequently involved, but abnormalities of the small and large intestines are more common. Involvement of the wall of the small intestine may lead to a picture of obstruction and occasionally frank malabsorption. Obstipation is the most common sign of large intestine involvement.

Several types of pulmonary disease including fibrosis, pulmonary hypertension, aspiration pneumonia (secondary to disorders of esophageal motility) and rarely restrictive disease due to chest wall involvement are seen. The clinical picture is signalled by the appearance of a non-productive cough, exertional dyspnea, a restrictive pattern on spirometric testing, reduced diffusion capacity, and arterial desaturation most prominent with exercise.

Primary cardiac involvement by the fibrotic process results in conduction abnormalities, arrhythmia and cardiomyopathy. In addition, cardiac decompensation may occur secondary to pulmonary disease and/or systemic hypertension, a usual concomitant of renal disease. The latter often presents abruptly, manifesting as renal failure, proteinuria, and is frequently associated with a picture of microangiopathic hemolytic anemia. Aggressive management of renal failure, particularly of coexistent malignant hypertension, is essential to prevent a fatal outcome. Renal failure is associated with the worst prognosis (Rodnan, 1979; Subcommittee report, 1980).

Pathogenesis

The etiology of scleroderma is unknown. Most observers feel that the overwhelming fibrotic reaction with variable degrees of mononuclear cell infiltration seen in many organs results from a primary angiopathic disorder which initially affects small arterial vessels. This fibrosis represents an exaggerated repair reaction to the vascular obliterative process. This exaggerated fibrotic reaction is probably due to aberrant regulation of collagen metabolism. An immunopathologic basis has long been considered since scleroderma often occurs in association with other putative autoimmune disorders, e.g. SLE and polymyositis. There is also a high incidence of hypergammaglobulinemia. Antinuclear and antinucleolar antibodies are seen. Recent evidence implicates a role for T-cells and T-cell elaborated lymphokines in the regulation of fibroblast proliferation and collagen synthesis. Furthermore, scleroderma-like lesions have been observed in patients undergoing chronic graft-versus-host disease, a T-cell mediated process.

Treatment of scleroderma

Although therapeutic approaches to the management of the secondary manifestations of scleroderma have been improved over the past few years, e.g. reversal of renal failure with aggressive antihypertensive therapy, as yet no agent has proved efficacious in the treatment of the pulmonary vasculopathic and fibrotic disorders. Corticosteroids may be useful in managing the acute edematous form of disease but do not modify disease outcome. Variable results have been seen with other agents, including D-penicillamine, alkylating drugs and colchicine. In preliminary trials, captopril, an agent used for its potent antihypertensive effects in patients with accelerated renal diseases remarkably has shown a salutary effect on cutaneous involvement.

PNS disease

While myositis is seen in patients with scleroderma, direct involvement of PNS and CNS is most unusual. Peripheral neuropathy is rare (Kibler and Rose, 1960; Conn and Dyck, 1975) and not prominent, although trigeminal neuropathy has been described (Beighton, Gumpel and Carnes, 1968; Ashworth and Tait, 1971; Teasdall, Frayha and Shulman, 1980). Whether any of the patients with trigeminal neuropathy had mixed connective tissue disease (MCTD) or whether MCTD is a separate entity (*see below*) is not clear. Pathologic examination in one case of peripheral neuropathy demonstrated: (1) thickened blood vessels with intimal proliferation and perivascular fibrosis; and (2) an increase in perineural connective tissue (Richter, 1954). It has been suggested that neuropathy can result from an increase in collagen within the nerve. While active vasculitis was not seen, this picture is not dissimilar to that seen in some patients with RA and chronic neuropathy. Kibler and Rose (1960) reported a patient with scleroderma and a picture of mononeuritis multiplex, but nerve biopsy could not be obtained. We have seen a patient with scleroderma with a picture of severe mononeuritis multiplex who had active vasculitis and increased connective tissue on sural nerve biopsy. After failing to respond to corticosteroids, her neuropathy stabilized and then gradually improved with the addition of cyclophosphamide. Carpal tunnel syndrome has also been reported (Teasdall, Frayha and Shulman, 1980).

MIXED CONNECTIVE TISSUE DISEASE (MCTD)

Mixed connective tissue disease (MCTD) is a syndrome that includes features of SLE, scleroderma and polymyositis. As originally described by Sharp *et al.* (1972), this overlap presentation was associated with a characteristic antinuclear antibody directed against the ribonucleoprotein component of an extractable nuclear antigen. This condition was thought to be relatively benign and to respond to modest doses of corticosteroids. Characteristic clinical features included arthralgias with or without a mild non-deforming arthritis, Raynaud's phenomenon, abnormal esophageal motility, and myositis. Noteworthy in the original description was the absence of cerebral, pulmonary, and renal involvement. Laboratory features which distinguished patients from those with SLE included normal serum complement and the absence of antibodies directed against native DNA. Subsequent reports as well as follow-up reports of the original cohort of patients have necessitated revamping the definition of this syndrome. It is now clear that 10% or more patients will develop renal disease, including immune complex glomerulopathy. A smaller number develop neuropsychiatric disturbances including cranial nerve neuropathy, peripheral neuropathy, seizures, and aseptic meningitis. More than 80% of patients have pulmonary disease. Furthermore, complement abnormalities as well as low titers of anti-DNA antibodies have been seen in patients who present with features of an overlap syndrome. Moreover, the serologic hallmark of this syndrome is also seen in SLE. Whether MCTD deserves to be separated out as a unique syndrome is beyond the scope of this chapter. Clearly, patients do present with features of more than one rheumatic syndrome and occasionally they present with or develop neuropathy.

PNS disease

Although polymyositis was clearly identified as a common neurologic manifestation of MCTD (Sharp *et al.*, 1972), it has become apparent that other neuropsychiatric problems are seen in patients with this entity. Among these are involvement of the PNS including trigeminal sensory neuropathy, a distal neuropathy and rarely carpal tunnel syndrome (Bennett, Bong and Spargo, 1978; Vincent and van Houzen, 1980). Indeed, trigeminal sensory neuropathy may be the first manifestation of disease (Ashworth and Tait, 1971; Searles, Mladinick and Messner, 1978). Although it is assumed that involvement of the vasculature of the PNS is responsible for clinical manifestations, there is no documentation of this in MCTD. Patients with other overlap syndromes not fitting into the 'classic pattern' of MCTD may also have PNS disease in any of the patterns described in SLE and MCTD and indeed may present with neurologic disease as the first manifestation of disease. It is not clear whether therapy of PNS manifestations of MCTD with corticosteroids is of any benefit despite the widely held view that other aspects of MCTD respond to corticosteroids.

VASCULITIS

The vasculitides represent a spectrum of disorders characterized by inflammation and destruction of blood vessel walls. Vascular inflammation may occur on a primary basis or may occur as part of an underlying disease process. Examples in the latter category are the vasculitis occurring in SLE, rheumatoid arthritis, Sjögren's syndrome, or mixed cryoglobulinemia. In general, attempts have been made to classify vasculitic syndromes according to characteristic clinical and pathologic features. Such attempts are useful in that certain vasculitic presentations are associated with characteristic clinical courses and characteristic responses to therapeutic intervention. It should be emphasized, however, that considerable degrees of overlap exist within such a clinicopathologic spectrum. From a pathologic standpoint, investigators have focused on the size of the vessel wall, the nature of the inflammatory infiltrate, and the presence of granulomas, to name just a few distinguishing features. For example, involvement of small and medium sized muscular arteries is classically seen in the polyarteritis group of systemic necrotizing vasculitis. Included in this group are classical polyarteritis nodosa and allergic granulomatosis (Churg-Strauss vasculitis). Post-capillary venules represent the targets of hypersensitivity or leukocytoclastic vasculitides. The latter are typically associated with polymorphonuclear cell infiltration, pyknotic nuclei, extravasation of erythrocytes and fibrinoid necrosis. Further classification of vasculitic syndromes is described by Kohler and Claman (1981).

Vascular damage may affect any organ producing multisystem signs and symptoms of vascular compromise (*Table 7.2*). As noted, characteristic clinical presentations are seen in some of these disorders. Wegener's granulomatosis is characterized by granulomatous vasculitis involving the upper and lower respiratory tracts in association with glomerulonephritis. These patients typically

Table 7.2 Clinical manifestations of vasculitis
(modified from Fan *et al.*, 1980)

Cutaneous
  Rash

Nervous
  Polyneuropathy
  Mononeuritis multiplex
  Cerebrovascular accident
  Headache
  Organic brain syndrome

Respiratory
  Septal perforation
  Epistaxis
  Sinusitis
  Pulmonary infiltrates
  Asthma

Cardiovascular
  Myocardial infarction
  Congestive heart failure
  Aortic insufficiency
  Claudication
  Hypertension

Gastrointestinal
  Abdominal pain
  Hematochezia

Genitourinary
  Glomerulonephritis

Musculoskeletal
  Arthralgia – arthritis
  Myalgia – myositis

---

present with a history of sinusitis, pulmonary infiltrates, nasal septal perforation, and hematuria. As is true of most vasculitic disorders, other systems including the stomach, gastrointestinal tract, and neurologic system may be involved. Churg-Strauss vasculitis, also associated with granulomas, is characterized by asthma and eosinophilia along with other systemic features. Polyarteritis nodosa is often associated with aneurysm formation in medium sized vessels, e.g. the renal and celiac vessels. The leukocytoclastic or hypersensitivity vasculitides most frequently involve the skin, although any organ may be affected. Cutaneous involvement most frequently takes the form of palpable purpura. Fever, malaise, arthralgias and occasionally frank arthritis can be seen in any of these syndromes.

Pathogenesis

It is generally accepted that polyarteritis nodosa and certain of the leukocytoclastic vasculitides are caused by immune-complex mediated destruction of vessel walls.

Evidence rests largely on the finding of immune reactants in the vessel wall in some patients and the development of similar clinical problems during the course of immune-complex mediated disease in experimental animal models. Although drugs and infectious micro-organisms have occasionally been implicated, in most instances an etiologic agent cannot be identified. Hepatitis B virus has been emphasized in certain series as an important agent. The etiology of the granulomatous forms of vasculitis is unknown.

Treatment of vasculitis

Treatment entails identification and removal of the offending antigen if possible. When vasculitis occurs as part of an underlying systemic process, treatment should be directed at that process. Corticosteroids are frequently used as a first line agent for their anti-inflammatory effect and should be tapered as symptoms allow. It is not clear, however, whether they modify disease outcome. Cytotoxic therapy, i.e. cyclophosphamide, should be reserved for patients with Wegener's granulomatosis and fulminant vasculitis of the polyarteritis nodosa group. Indeed, it is now clear that these two disorders, formerly associated with a high incidence of fatal outcome, can be controlled and cured by careful therapy with cyclophosphamide.

PNS disease

Involvement of peripheral nervous system is common in patients with vasculitis, whether in association with other connective tissue diseases (i.e. rheumatoid arthritis with active vasculitis) or in the group of 'essential' vasculitides including mixed cryoglobulinemia (Kernohan and Woltman, 1938; Lovshin and Kernohan, 1948; Churg and Strauss, 1951; Rose and Spencer, 1957; Russell, 1959; MacFayden, 1960; Ford and Siekert, 1965; Warrell, Godfrey and Olsen, 1968; Citron *et al.*, 1970; Conn and Dyck, 1975; Stern, 1975; Fauci, Haynes and Katz, 1978). Indeed, in some of these disorders such as polyarteritis (periarteritis) nodosa, as many as 50% of patients will have PNS involvement, often extensive and frequently as the initial manifestation of disease (Frohnert and Sheps, 1967). The classical involvement of PNS in this group of disorders is an acute or subacute rapid development of mononeuritis or mononeuritis multiplex or, perhaps more commonly, such extensive and rapid evolution of multiple nerves that a 'symmetric' neuropathy is seen (Bleehen, Lovelace and Cotton, 1963; Lovelace, 1964). Ischemic lesions involving central fascicles (*Figure 7.1*), similar to vasculitis of RA and experimental vascular occlusion (Parry and Brown, 1981; Sladky, Greenberg and Brown, 1983), are seen along with evidence of vasculitis involving vasa nervorum (*Figure 7.1*) (Bleehan, Lovelace and Cotton, 1963; Lovelace, 1964; Winkelman and Moore, 1950). Biopsy of distal portions of the PNS may only reveal loss of nerve fibers and Wallerian degeneration (*Figure 7.3*).

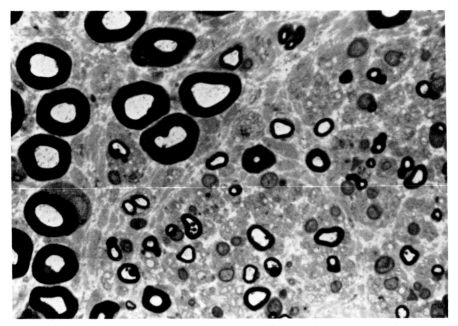

Figure 7.1 Nerve biopsy of a patient with vasculitis and neuropathy demonstrating loss of fibers in the central portion of the nerve (right side of figure) with relative sparing of the more lateral portion (left side of figure) (courtesy of Dr Mark J. Brown)

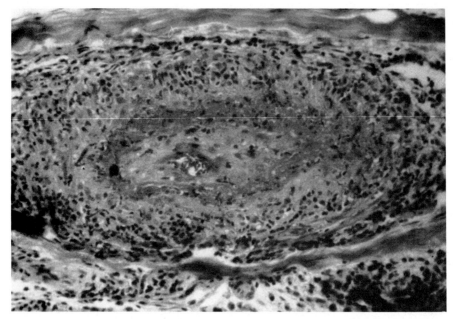

Figure 7.2 Nerve biopsy of a patient with polyarteritis nodosa and neuropathy demonstrating a severe obliterative arteritis with marked inflammatory response within the vessel wall (courtesy of Dr Mark J. Brown)

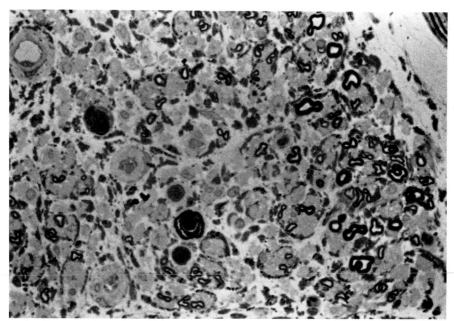

Figure 7.3 Sural nerve biopsy of a patient with an overlap connective tissue disease syndrome and mononeuritis multiplex demonstrating marked loss of nerve fibers and myelin ovoids (Wallerian degeneration) (courtesy of Dr Mark J. Brown)

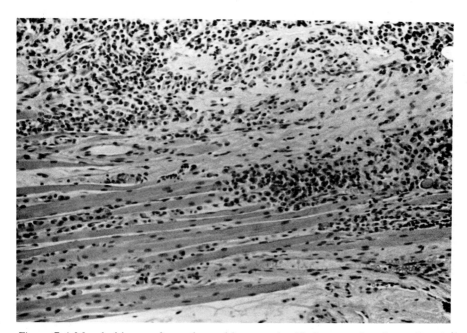

Figure 7.4 Muscle biopsy of a patient with an unclassified connective tissue disorder with mononeuritis multiplex demonstrating muscle fiber necrosis, fibrosis and mononuclear cell infiltration with many plasma cells. Bone marrow was normal

Laboratory tests in PNS disease

Electrical studies are helpful in establishing the pattern of involvement and biopsy of peripheral nerve (*Figure 7.2*) and muscle (*Figure 7.4*) are often the best way to establish tissue diagnosis in patients presenting with PNS disease as part of the early stages of disease. The decision as to which sural or superficial sensory radial nerve to biopsy can be guided by electrophysiologic testing. It is better to avoid biopsying a muscle after EMG since focal necrosis and inflammation can result from the EMG needle. Blood tests and X-rays are of some use in defining the different syndromes (cryoglobulinemia, eosinophilia, pulmonary involvement, etc.) but do not always point to active PNS disease.

Therapy of PNS disease

Therapy for PNS is controversial, as it is for vasculitis in general. Treatment with corticosteroids has probably improved survival in several vasculitides including polyarteritis nodosa and it has been suggested by several groups that the early addition of a cytotoxic agent such as cyclophosphamide or azathioprine further improves the outlook (Fauci *et al.*, 1979; Leib, Restivo and Paulus, 1979; Zweiman, 1979). Wegener's granulomatosis is said to be particularly responsive to cyclophosphamide therapy (Wolff *et al.*, 1974; Fauci *et al.*, 1983). Attempting to assess the effect of such therapy on PNS involvement is even more difficult. Lack of further progression or new nerve involvement may be the first or only sign of 'improvement' and actual increase in neurologic function may be delayed. It seems reasonable to consider the neuropathy as part of the active disease processes and signs of progression of PNS involvement certainly would indicate the need for further or different therapy.

CRYOGLOBULINEMIA

Cryoglobulins are serum immunoglobulin molecules which reversibly precipitate when exposed to cold temperatures. Three major types of cryoglobulins have been identified including:

(1) Monoclonal proteins primarily observed in patients with plasma cell dyscrasias
(2) Mixed monoclonal-polyclonal in which the mononclonal component is directed against polyclonal immunoglobulin activity, and
(3) Mixed polyclonal in which polyclonal immunoglobulins are directed against polyclonal immunoglobulins.

Cryoglobulins of the latter two types demonstrate rheumatoid factor activity and are frequently observed in connective tissue disorders where they behave *in vivo* as immune complexes. Accordingly, they may be a cause of immune-complex mediated disease, e.g. vasculitis, in these disorders. In addition, mixed cryoglobulinemia may occur on an idiopathic basis (mixed essential cryoglobulinemia). This syndrome is associated with clinical features which include palpable purpura, arthritis, and glomerulonephritis and other signs of a vasculitis process (Brouet *et al.*, 1974).

Peripheral neuropathy has been described in patients with cryoglobulinemia whether in association with other disorders or in essential mixed cryoglobulinemia (Ravenna and Testa, 1972; Abramsky and Slavin, 1974; Gorevic *et al.*, 1980; Chad *et al.*, 1982; Konishi *et al.*, 1982). Both mononeuropathy and distal neuropathy have been reported. The neuropathy may be acute or subacute in evolution and varies in extent from mild paresthesias to marked motor and sensory involvement of all four extremities. Pathologic studies have revealed Wallerian degeneration, demyelination, and vascular changes have shown active and healed vasculitis, perineuritis and perivascular mononuclear cell infiltrates (Cream *et al.*, 1974; Vallat *et al.*, 1980; Chad *et al.*, 1982; Konishi *et al.*, 1982). Some immunofluorescent studies have demonstrated the same Ig isotype as the serum cryoglobulins in vessel walls, and IgG, IgM and complement have been found in skin and inflamed glomeruli (Gorevic *et al.*, 1980) and fibrinogen in vessels within a damaged medium-sized artery in muscle (Gorevic *et al.*, 1980). Several mechanisms have been suggested as being important in the pathogenesis of neuropathy in mixed cryoglobulinemia including:

(1) Interference with local microcirculation by intravascular deposition, and
(2) Vasculitis and perivascular infiltrates with cryoglobulins acting as immune complexes activating complement.

There is little information on the specific effect of corticosteroid or cytotoxic drugs on PNS manifestations in patients with cryoglobulinemia. It has been suggested that plasma exchange may be of some help.

SJÖGREN'S SYNDROME

Clinical presentation

Sjögren's syndrome is a disorder of unknown etiology, predominantly affecting middle-aged women. The syndrome encompasses a triad of keratoconjunctivitis sicca (dry eyes), xerostomia (dry mouth) and chronic arthritis which most commonly is accounted for by rheumatoid arthritis. Two of these features are necessary to make this diagnosis. Clinically, patients with Sjögren's syndrome frequently manifest signs and symptoms of reduced secretions along other mucosal surfaces including the respiratory tract, the gastrointestinal and genitourinary tracts. Excessive dental caries, bronchitis and pneumonitis are not infrequent problems. Parotid gland enlargement occurs in approximately one-half of the patients. Lymphodermopathy is sometimes quite prominent, raising the spectre of malignant symptoms when seen. Indeed, a spectrum of lymphoid infiltration is seen running from benign infiltration of glands to pseudolymphoma and to the less common malignant lymphoma. Other extraglandular manifestations include vasculitis, liver disease, renal tubular acidosis, and peripheral neuropathy.

Pathogenesis

Impaired glandular secretion is due to the infiltration of mononuclear cells – lymphocytes, plasma cells and monocytes. The mechanisms by which these cells destroy or interfere with the secretory process are unclear, although both antibody and cell mediated mechanism have been postulated. A number of putative autoantibodies have been reported including rheumatoid factor (more than 90% of patients), antisalivary duct antibodies, and certain antinuclear antibodies.

PNS disease

Involvement of the PNS is not uncommon in patients with Sjögren's syndrome, whether it is primary or as part of the picture of rheumatoid arthritis. Indeed, the spectrum of neuropathy is essentially that as seen in rheumatoid arthritis, being predominantly a mild distal sensory neuropathy in most patients with asymmetric mononeuropathy or the less common mononeuropathy multiplex (Kaltreider and Talal, 1969; Alexander *et al.*, 1982; Peyronnard *et al.*, 1982). Entrapment is unusual in the sicca syndrome not accompanied by RA, whereas cranial neuropathy, especially trigeminal involvement, is more frequently seen in the sicca syndrome than RA. It is believed that the pathogenesis of neuropathy is related to involvement of blood vessels within the nerve and, indeed, vasculitis and perivascular infiltrates are seen in pathologic studies along with evidence of demyelination (Kaltreider and Talal, 1969). However, these findings are not demonstrable in every instance. Examination of muscle frequently demonstrates active or healed vasculitis in addition to lesions of denervation.

RELAPSING POLYCHONDRITIS

Relapsing polychondritis is a rare disorder which presents as recurrent episodes of inflammation of cartilaginous structures. Patients most frequently present with involvement of the ears, which are inflamed and ultimately become thickened and floppy. Arthritic complaints are common and involvement is quite variable with symmetric rheumatoid arthritis-like presentations as well as asymmetric joint presentations. Inflammation in the larynx, trachea and bronchi is seen and also of the eyes and heart. The latter is characterized by valvular insufficiency, particularly of the aortic valve. Diagnosis rests on the demonstration of inflamed cartilaginous structures in at least two organs, involvement of an organ of special sense and a biopsy revealing inflammation of cartilage. The natural history and prognosis of this disorder are not clearly resolved. The syndrome is characterized by recurrent episodes which appear to be responsive to therapy with corticosteroids. However, fatal outcomes have followed tracheobronchial collapse or ruptured aortic aneurysm.

PNS disease

The PNS may be affected in relapsing polychondritis with cranial nerves characteristically involved including VI, VII and VIII. CNS involvement is also seen, as is involvement of organs of special sensation (Hughes *et al.*, 1972; McAdam *et al.*, 1976; Sundaram and Rajput, 1983). PNS involvement is acute or subacute in evolution and the mononeuropathy or mononeuropathy multiplex and the frequent multifocal pattern of CNS involvement suggest that vasculitis is important in the pathogenesis of lesions. While there is evidence of vasculitis in other organs and tissues, there is no proof of vasculitic involvement in the PNS and CNS. As is true for most of the connective tissue disorders, proof of efficacy of corticosteroid therapy is lacking. Nonetheless, therapy with high doses of corticosteroids or increasing the current level of therapy is worth an attempt.

REITER'S DISEASE

As originally described, Reiter's disease was a syndrome of polyarthritis, conjunctivitis and urethritis. Although children and females may be rarely affected, this disorder has a predilection for men in their third and fourth decades. The syndrome has now been expanded to an hexad with the addition of mucosal ulcerations, circinate balanitis, and keratoderma blennorrhagica. Non-gonococcal urethritis is usually the first manifestation of this disorder and is followed shortly by polyarthritis and conjunctivitis. However, the temporal relationship between these features may be quite variable. The arthritis, which may range from mild to severe, is characteristically asymmetric, involving the joints of the lower extremities most frequently, particularly the knees. Sacroiliitis is also seen, particularly in patients who have had the illness for more than 5 years. Additional rheumatic presentations include tendinitis and painful heels. The arthritic process tends to be self-limited with spontaneous resolution in the usual case. Ocular involvement includes conjunctivitis which presents most frequently with purulent discharge and photophobia. However, mild conjunctivitis may not be accompanied by obvious signs and requires careful history taking and physical examination. Iritis is an infrequent concomitant of the initial presentation, although it is seen more frequently during chronic or severe forms of disease. Urethritis is characterized by mucopurulent discharge, but may be asymptomatic. Keratodermia blennorrhagica refers to a self-limited eruption of hyperkeratotic lesions on the palms and soles of the feet which heal with scaling. Subungual lesions may also be observed. Balanitis circinata presents as penile erythema and ulceration in a perimeatal distribution. Mucosal lesions include asymptomatic palatal and buccal mucosa ulcerations.

Additional less common features of Reiter's syndrome include aortitis with aortic insufficiency, A-V conduction abnormalities and central and peripheral nervous system disease (*see below*).

Pathogenesis

The pathogenesis of Reiter's syndrome is unknown. Most cases in men follow a venereal contact. An infectious etiology has long been sought with numerous organisms having been incriminated. Reiter's-like syndrome sometimes is preceded by dysentery. In these instances, Yersinia, Salmonella, and Shigella infections have been identified and the arthritis is thought to represent an unusual host reaction to these organisms. A genetic predisposition is signalled by the high incidence of HLA-B27 seen in patients with this disease.

Treatment

The mainstay of therapy for arthritic and axial skeletal complaints is non-steroidal anti-inflammatory agents or aspirin. Based on clinical experience, indomethacin appears to be particularly efficacious. Local injections of corticosteroids have a place in symptomatic control and palliation, but systemic corticosteroids are generally not indicated. D-penicillamine and gold do not appear to be particularly effective in patients with severe forms of arthritis. Encouraging results have accompanied the use of methotrexate and azathioprine, but further studies are needed.

PNS disease

Involvement of the PNS has been reported in Reiter's disease, although it is not common. Some instances (radicular syndromes and 'sciatica') may result from arthritis of the spine and others (meralgia paresthetica) may be coincidental or related to changes in body weight. There are, however, reports of plexopathy and polyneuropathy as well (Good, 1974).

DRUG-INDUCED NEUROPATHIES

Many medications are capable of causing neuropathies (Manigand, 1982). It is not our purpose to review here all medications known to produce disease of the PNS, but to emphasize a few that are of special concern because of their relatively frequent use in patients with connective tissue diseases.

Gold neuropathy

It is clear that therapy with intramuscular gold for rheumatoid arthritis can be associated with an acute or subacute symmetric polyneuropathy which may progress rapidly and be associated with significant disability (Walsh, 1970; Katrak *et al.*, 1980). Focal or diffuse myokymia is common and progression may occur for a time, despite discontinuation of therapy (Katrak *et al.*, 1980). Evidence for both axonal degeneration and demyelination, and segmental remyelination is seen and similar lesions can be produced in hens in a dose related manner. The mechanisms responsible for the neuropathy are not known, but the neuropathy need not be seen concomitantly with signs of gold hypersensitivity. The clinical pattern of PNS involvement and the clinical setting in individual patients also suggests that this neuropathy is not due to vasculitis of the PNS associated with rheumatoid arthritis.

Indomethacin

Four patients were reported to have developed a distal symmetric polyneuropathy while receiving indomethacin (Eade *et al.*, 1975). Two of these subjects had inflammatory arthritis (neither had classical seropositive RA), one had osteoarthritis and one subject had myalgias of uncertain cause. Only the patient with osteoarthritis had received indomethacin alone, but the others were not receiving other agents associated with induction of PNS disease. Discontinuing indomethacin was associated with clinical improvement in all four patients. Neuropathy was mentioned as occurring in two other patients (one with rheumatoid arthritis and one with osteoarthritis) but details were not available.

Chloroquine

The appearance of a vacuolar myopathy in patients treated with chloroquine is well described. However, some patients also develop symptoms and signs of PNS disease as well (Begg and Simpson, 1964; Kastorp, Ferngren and Lundberg, 1973; Godeau *et al.*, 1976). While some of these patients had SLE and one could implicate the underlying disorder as the cause of the PNS disease, others had been receiving chloroquine as malaria prophylaxis (Kastorp *et al.*, 1973).

Corticosteroids

The use of corticosteroids in patients with RA has been implicated as playing a role in the production of a severe neuropathy (Hart, Golding and MacKenzie, 1957; Bleehan, Lovelace and Cotton, 1963; Lovelace, 1964). It is more likely, however, that such an association simply indicates the severity of the disease. Similar neuropathies associated with vascular changes have been described in patients not receiving corticosteroids, although such therapy could conceivably alter or modify the histologic and immunopathologic features at biopsy (Conn and Dyck, 1975). In a patient with diabetes mellitus and a connective tissue disease, further deterioration in control of hyperglycemia secondary to corticosteroid administration could result in accentuation of diabetic neuropathy.

Cimetidine

Two asthmatic patients who received cimetidine and corticosteroids for a short period of time developed a reversible motor polyneuropathy felt to be axonal (by clinical electrophysiologic criteria) in the one subject so studied (Walls, Pearce and Venables, 1980). A single lumbar puncture was performed in each with no abnormalities detected. It was felt that this did not represent Guillain-Barré syndrome but that diagnosis was not fully eliminated in either patient.

Isoniazid (INH) and hydralazine

Both of these agents may be used in patients with connective tissue disorders; INH in patients with positive PPD skin test receiving immunosuppressive therapy and hydralazine for hypertension. Although hydralazine has been associated with production of a lupus-like syndrome, it is more probable that polyneuropathy with hydralazine, like that associated with INH, is due to pyridoxine (B_6) deficiency (Kirkendall and Page, 1958; Raskin and Fishman, 1965; Koch-Weser, 1976). Many INH preparations contain B_6, but the appearance of a neuropathy in a patient receiving either of these two agents should raise the question of pyridoxine deficiency neuropathy.

Acknowledgements

We would like to thank Tracy Rhodes for assistance in preparing the manuscript and Dr Mark Brown for some of the illustrations.

References

Abramsky, O. and Slavin, S. (1974) Neurologic manifestations in patients with mixed cryoglobulinemia. *Neurology (Minneapolis)*, **24**, 245–249

Alexander, E. L., Provost, T. T., Stevens, M. B. and Alexander, G. E. (1982) Neurologic complications of primary Sjögren's syndrome. *Medicine*, **61**, 247–257

Arnason, B. G. W. (1971) Idiopathic polyneuritis (Landry-Guillain-Barré-Strohl syndrome) and experimental allergic neuritis: a comparison. *Research Publications Association for Research in Nervous and Mental Disorders*, **49**, 156–175

Asbury, A. K., Arnason, B. G. W. and Adams, R. D. (1969) The inflammatory lesion in idiopathic polyneuritis. *Medicine*, **48**, 173–215

Ashworth, B. and Tait, G. B. W. (1971) Trigeminal neuropathy in connective tissue diseases. *Neurology (Minneapolis)*, **21**, 609–614

Bailey, A. A., Sayre, G. P. and Clark, E. C. (1956) Neuritis associated with systemic lupus erythematosus. *Archives of Neurology and Psychiatry*, **75**, 251–259

Beckett, V. L. and Dinn, J. J. (1972) Segmental demyelination in rheumatoid arthritis. *Quarterly Journal of Medicine*, **91**, 71–80

Begg, T. B. and Simpson, J. A. (1964) Chloraquine neuropathy. *British Medical Journal*, **1**, 770

Beighton, R., Gumpel, J. M. and Carnes, N. G. M. (1968) Prodromal trigeminal sensory neuropathy in progressive systemic sclerosis. *Annals of Rheumatic Diseases*, **27**, 367–369

Bennett, R. M., Bong, D. M. and Spargo, B. H. (1978) Neuropsychiatric problems in mixed connective tissue disease. *American Journal of Medicine*, **65**, 955–961

Berry, R. G. and Hodges, J. H. (1965) Nervous system involvement in systemic lupus erythematosus. *Transactions of the American Neurological Association*, **90**, 231–233

Bleehen, S. S., Lovelace, R. E. and Cotton, R. E. (1963) Mononeuritis multiplex in polyarteritis nodosa. *Quarterly Journal of Medicine*, **32**, 193–209

Block, S. L., Jarrett, M. P., Swerdlow, M. and Grayzel, A. I. (1979) Bracheal plexus neuropathy as the initial presentation of systemic lupus erythematosus. *Neurology (New York)*, **29**, 1633–1634

Brouet, J. C., Clauvel, J. P., Danon, F., Klein, M. and Seligman, M. (1974) Biologic and clinical significance of cryoglobulin: a report of 86 cases. *American Journal of Medicine*, **57**, 775–788

Brown, W. F., Feasby, T. E. and Yates, S. K. (1981) Conduction block and denervation in Guillain-Barré polyneuritis. *Annals of Neurology*, **10**, 86

Chad, D., Pariser, K., Bradley, W. G., Adelman, L. S. and Penn, V. W. (1982) The pathogenesis of cryoglobulinemic neuropathy. *Neurology (New York)*, **32**, 725–729

Churg, J. and Strauss, L. (1951) Allergic granulomatosis, allergic angiitis and periarteritis nodosa. *American Journal of Pathology*, **27**, 277–301

Citron, B. P., Halpern, M., McCarron, M. *et al.* (1970) Necrotizing angiitis in drug addicts. *New England Journal of Medicine*, **283**, 1003–1011

Clark, E. C. and Bailey, A. A. (1956) Neurologic and psychiatric signs associated with systemic lupus erythematosus. *Journal of the American Medical Association*, **160**, 455–457

Conn, D. L. and Dyck, P. J. (1975) Angiopathic neuropathy and connective tissue diseases. In *Peripheral Neuropathy*, edited by P. J. Dyck, P. K. Thomas and E. H. Lambert, pp. 1149–1165. Philadelphia: W. B. Saunders

Conn, D. L., McDuffie, F. C. and Dyck, P. J. (1972) Immunopathologic study of sural nerves in rheumatoid arthritis. *Arthritis and Rheumatism*, **15**, 135–143

Cook, S. D. and Dowling, P. C. (1981) The role of autoantibody and immune complexes in the pathogenesis of Guillain-Barré syndrome. *Annals of Neurology*, **9**, 70–79

Cream, J. J., Hern, J. E. C., Hughes, R. A. C. and MacKenzie, I. C. K. (1974) Mixed or immune complex cryoglobulinemia and neuropathy. *Journal of Neurology, Neurosurgery and Psychiatry*, **37**, 82–87

Decker, J. L., Steinberg, A. D., Reinertsen, J. L., Plotz, P. H., Balow, J. E. and Klippel, J. H. (1979) Systemic lupus erythematosus: evolving concepts. *Annals of Internal Medicine*, **91**, 587–604

Denny, D. and Rose, R. L. (1961) Myasthenia gravis followed by systemic lupus erythematosus. A case report. *Neurology (Minneapolis)*, **11**, 710–713

Dubois, E. L. (1966) The clinical picture of systemic lupus erythematosus. In *Systemic Lupus Erythematosus*, edited by E. L. Dubois, pp. 207–208. New York: McGraw Hill

Dyck, P. J., Conn, D. L. and Okazaki, H. (1972) Necrotizing angiopathic neuropathy: three-dimensional morphology of fiber degeneration related to sites of occluded vessels. *Mayo Clinic Proceedings*, **47**, 461–475

Eade, O. E., Acheson, E. D., Cuthbert, M. F. and Hawkes, C. H. (1975) Peripheral neuropathy and indomethacin. *British Medical Journal*, **1**, 66–67

Edmonds, M. E., Jones, T. C., Saunders, W. A. and Sturrack, R. D. (1979) Autonomic neuropathy in rheumatoid arthritis. *British Medical Journal*, **2**, 173–175

Fan, P. T., Davis, J. A., Somer, T., Kaplan, L. and Bluestone, R. (1980) A clinical approach to systemic vasculitis. *Seminars in Arthritis and Rheumatism*, **9**, 248–304

Fauci, A. S., Haynes, B. F. and Katz, P. (1978) The spectrum of vasculitis. Clinical, pathologic, immunologic and therapeutic considerations. *Annals of Internal Medicine*, **89**, 660–676

Fauci, A. S., Katz, P., Haynes, B. F. and Wolff, S. (1979) Cyclophosphamide therapy of severe systemic necrotizing vasculitis. *New England Journal of Medicine*, **301**, 235–238

Fauci, A. S., Haynes, B. F., Katz, P. and Wolff, S. M. (1983) Wegener's granulomatosis: prospective clinical and therapeutic experience with 85 patients for 21 years. *Annals of Internal Medicine*, **98**, 76–85

Feinglass, E. J., Arnett, F. C., Dorsch, C. A., Zizic, T. M. and Stevens, M. B. (1976) Neuropsychiatric manifestations of systemic lupus erythematosus: diagnosis, clinical spectrum, and relationship to other features of the disease. *Medicine*, **55**, 323–339

Ferguson, R. H. and Slocumb, C. H. (1961) Peripheral neuropathy in rheumatoid arthritis. *Bulletin of Rheumatologic Diseases*, **11**, 251–254

Ford, R. G. and Siekert, R. G. (1965) Central nervous system manifestations of periarteritis nodosa. *Neurology*, **15**, 114–122

Frohnert, P. P. and Sheps, S. G. (1967) Long-term follow-up study of polyarteritis nodosa. *American Journal of Medicine*, **43**, 8–14

Godeau, P., Herreman, G., Himmich, H., Godet-Guillain, J., Chevallay, M. and Fordeau, M. (1976) Neuromyopathie due à la chiloraquine au cours du lupus érythémateux. *Annals Medicine Interne*, **127**, 544–551

Goldberg, A. J. and Chitanondh, H. (1959) Polyneuritis with albumino-cytologic dissociation in systemic lupus erythematosus. *American Journal of Medicine*, **27**, 342–350

Good, A. E. (1974) Reiter's disease: a review with special attention to cardiovascular and neurologic sequelae. *Seminars in Arthritis and Rheumatism*, **3**, 253–286

Gorevic, P. D., Kassab, H. J., Levo, Y. *et al.* (1980) Mixed cryoglobulinemia: clinical aspects and long-term follow-up of 40 patients. *American Journal of Medicine*, **69**, 287–308

Hart, F. D., Golding, J. R. and Mackenzie, D. H. (1957) Neuropathy in rheumatoid disease. *Annals of the Rheumatic Diseases*, **16**, 471–480

Hepinstall, R. H. and Sowry, G. S. C. (1952) Peripheral neuritis in systemic lupus erythematosus. *British Medical Journal*, **1**, 525–527

Hughes, R. A. C., Berry, C. L., Seifert, M. and Lessof, M. H. (1972) Relapsing polychondritis: three cases with a clinicopathologic study and literature review. *Quarterly Journal of Medicine*, **41**, 363–380

Irby, R., Adams, R. A. and Toone, E. C. Jr (1958) Peripheral neuritis associated with rheumatoid arthritis. *Arthritis and Rheumatism*, **1**, 44–53

Johnson, R. L., Smyth, C. J., Holt, G. W., Lubchemo, A. and Valentine, E. (1959) Steroid therapy and vascular lesions in rheumatoid arthritis. *Arthritis and Rheumatism*, **2**, 224–249

Johnson, R. T. and Richardson, E. P. (1968) The neurological manifestations of systemic lupus erythematosus. *Medicine*, **47**, 337–369

Kaltreider, H. B. and Talal, N. (1969) The neuropathy of Sjögren's syndrome. Trigeminal involvement. *Annals of Internal Medicine*, **70**, 751–762

Kastorp, A., Ferngren, H. and Lundberg, P. (1973) Neuromyopathy during malaria suppression with chloraquine. *British Medical Journal*, **4**, 736

Katrak, S. M., Pollock, M., O'Brien, C. P. *et al.* (1980) Clinical and morphological features of gold neuropathy. *Brain*, **103**, 671–693

Kernohan, J. W. and Woltman, H. W. (1938) Periarteritis nodosa: a clinical pathologic study with special reference to nervous system. *Archives of Neurology and Psychiatry*, **39**, 655–684

Kibler, R. F. and Rose, F. C. (1960) Peripheral neuropathy in the 'collagen diseases'. A case of scleroderma neuropathy. *British Medical Journal*, **1**, 1751–1784

Kim, R. C. and Collins, G. H. (1981) The neuropathology of rheumatoid disease. *Human Pathology*, **12**, 5–15

Kirkendall, W. M. and Page, E. B. (1958) Polyneuritis occurring during hydralazine therapy. *Journal of the American Medical Association*, **167**, 427–432

Koch-Weser, J. (1976) Drug therapy: hydralazine. *New England Journal of Medicine*, **295**, 320–323

Kohler, P. F. and Claman, H. N. (1981) Systemic vasculitis. In *Clinical Immunology Update*, edited by E. C. Franklin, pp. 293–316. New York: Elsevier-North Holland

Konishi, T., Saida, K., Ohnishi, A. and Nishitani, H. (1982) Perineuritis in mononeuritis multiplex with cryoglobulinemia. *Muscle and Nerve*, **5**, 173–177

Lewis, D. C. (1965) Systemic lupus and polyneuropathy. *Archives of Internal Medicine*, **116**, 518–521

Lewis, R. A. and Sumner, A. J. (1982) The electrodiagnostic distinctions between chronic familial and acquired demyelinative neuropathies. *Neurology (New York)*, **32**, 592–596

Lieb, E. S., Restivo, C. and Paulus, H. E. (1977) Immunosuppressive and corticosteroid therapy of polyarteritis nodosa. *American Journal of Medicine*, **67**, 941–947

Lisak, R. P., Brown, M. J. and Sumner, A. J. (1983) Abnormal serum factors in Guillain-Barré syndrome. *Italian Journal of Neurologic Science* (in press)

Lovelace, R. E. (1964) Mononeuritis multiplex in polyarteritis nodosa. *Neurology (Minneapolis)*, **14**, 434–442

Lovshin, L. L. and Kernohan, J. W. (1948) Peripheral neuritis in periarteritis nodosa: a clinical pathologic study. *Archives of Internal Medicine*, **82**, 321–338

Lunberg, P. O. and Werner, I. (1972) Trigeminal sensory neuropathy in systemic lupus erythematosus. *Acta Neurologica Scandinavica*, **48**, 330–340

MacFayden, D. J. (1960) Wegener's granulomatosis with discrete lung lesions and peripheral neuritis. *Canadian Medical Association Journal*, **83**, 760–764

Manigand, G. (1982) Accidents neurologiques des medicaments. II. Neuropathies peripheriques. Accidents ototoxiques. Blocs neuromusculaires. *Therapie*, **37**, 225–248

McAdam, L. P., O'Hanlan, M. A., Bluestone, R. and Pearson, C. M. (1976) Relapsing polychondritis. A prospective study of 23 patients and a review of the literature. *Medicine*, **55**, 193–215

Nakano, K. K. (1978) The entrapment neuropathies. *Muscle and Nerve*, **1**, 264–279

Pallis, C. A. and Scott, J. R. (1965) Peripheral neuropathy in rheumatoid arthritis. *British Medical Journal*, **1**, 1141–1147

Parry, G. J. and Brown, M. J. (1981) Arachidonate-induced experimental nerve infarction. *Journal of the Neurological Sciences*, **50**, 123–133

Parry, G. J. and Brown, M. J. (1982) Selective fiber vulnerability in acute ischemic neuropathy. *Annals of Neurology*, **11**, 147–154

Peyronnard, J.-M., Charron, L., Beaudet, F. and Couture, F. (1982) Vasculitic neuropathy in rheumatoid disease and Sjögren's syndrome. *Neurology (New York)*, **32**, 839–845

Raskin, N. H. and Fishman, R. A. (1965) Pyridoxine deficiency neuropathy due to hydralazine. *New England Journal of Medicine*, **273**, 1182–1185

Ravenna, C. and Testa, G. F. (1972) Polyneuritis in essential cryoglobulinemia: a clinical, immunoelectrophoretic and electromyographic study with report of a case. *European Neurology*, **7**, 241–248

Richter, R. B. (1954) Peripheral neuropathy and connective tissue disease. *Journal of Neuropathology and Experimental Neurology*, **13**, 168–180

Rodnan, G. P. (Ed.) (1979) Systemic sclerosis. In *Clinics in Rheumatic Diseases*, pp. 1–302. Philadelphia: W. B. Saunders

Rose, G. A. and Spenser, H. (1957) Polyarteritis nodosa. *Quarterly Journal of Medicine*, **26**, 30–43

Russell, R. W. R. (1959) Giant-cell arteritis: a review of 35 cases. *Quarterly Journal of Medicine*, **28**, 471–489

Scheinberg, L. (1956) Polyneuritis in systemic lupus erythematosus. *New England Journal of Medicine*, **255**, 416–421

Searles, R. P., Mladinick, K. and Messner, R. P. (1978) Isolated trigeminal sensory neuropathy: early manifestation of mixed connective tissue disease. *Neurology (New York)*, **28**, 1286–1289

Sharp, G. C., Irvin, W. S., Tan, E. M., Gould, R. G. and Holman, H. R. (1972) Mixed connective tissue disorder disease – an apparently distinct rheumatic disease syndrome associated with a specific antibody to an extractable nuclear antigen (ENA). *American Journal of Medicine*, **52**, 148–159

Sladky, J. T., Greenberg, J. H. and Brown, M. J. (1983) Regional blood flow in normal and ischemic rat sciatic nerve. *Neurology (New York)*, **33** (Suppl. 2), 101

Stern, G. M. (1975) The peripheral nerves in Wegener's granulomatosis. In *Handbook of Clinical Neurology*, edited by P. J. Vinken and G. W. Bruyn, Vol. 8, pp. 112–117. Amsterdam: North-Holland

Subcommittee for Scleroderma Criteria of the American Rheumatism Association, Diagnostic and Therapeutic Committee (1980) Preliminary criteria for the classification of systemic sclerosis (scleroderma). *Arthritis and Rheumatism*, **23**, 581–590

Sundaram, M. B. M. and Rajput, A. H. (1983) Nervous system complications of relapsing polychondritis. *Neurology*, **33**, 513–515

Tachovsky, T. G., Lisak, R. P., Koprowski, H., Theofilopoulos, A. N. and Dixon, F. J. (1976) Circulating immune complexes in multiple sclerosis and other neurological diseases. *Lancet*, **2**, 997–999

Tan, E. M., Cohen, A. S., Fries, J. F. *et al.* (1982) The 1982 revised criteria for the classification of systemic lupus erythematosus. *Arthritis and Rheumatism*, **25**, 1271–1277

Teasdall, R. D., Frayha, R. A. and Shulman, L. E. (1980) Cranial nerve involvement in systemic sclerosis (scleroderma): a report of 10 cases. *Medicine*, **59**, 149–159

Vallat, J. M., Desprages-Gotteron, R., Leboutet, M. J., Loubet, A., Gaulde, N. and Treves, R. (1980) Cryoglobulinemic neuropathy: a pathologic study. *Annals of Neurology*, **8**, 179–185

Vincent, F. M. and van Houzen, R. N. (1980) Trigeminal sensory neuropathy and bilateral carpal tunnel syndrome: the initial manifestation of mixed connective tissue disease. *Journal of Neurology, Neurosurgery and Psychiatry*, **43**, 458–460

Walls, T. J., Pearce, G. J. and Venables, G. S. (1980) Motor neuropathy associated with cimetidine. *British Medical Journal*, **281**, 974–975

Walsh, J. C. (1970) Gold neuropathy. *Neurology (Minneapolis)*, **20**, 455–458

Warrell, D. A., Godfrey, S. and Olsen, E. G. J. (1968) Giant-cell arteritis with periperal neuropathy. *Lancet*, **1**, 1010–1013

Weller, R. O., Bruckner, F. E. and Chamberlain, M. A. (1970) Rheumatoid neuropathy: a histologic and electrophysiological study. *Journal of Neurology, Neurosurgery and Psychiatry*, **33**, 592–604

Williams, R. C. Jr (1979) Rheumatoid arthritis. *Hospital Practice*, **14**, 57–63

Winkelman, N. W. and Moore, M. T. (1950) Disseminated necrotizing periarteritis (periarteritis nodosa). A clinical pathologic report. *Journal of Neuropathology and Experimental Neurology*, **9**, 60–77

Wolff, S. M. and Barrows, H. S. (1966) Myasthenia gravis and systemic lupus erythematosus. *Archives of Neurology*, **14**, 254–258

Wolff, S. M., Fauci, A. S., Horn, R. G. and Dale, D. C. (1974) Wegener's granulomatosis. *Annals of Internal Medicine*, **81**, 513–525

Zweiman, B. (1979) A new therapeutic strategy in systemic vasculitis? *New England Journal of Medicine*, **301**, 266–267

8

Toxic neuropathies

Pamela M. Le Quesne

GENERAL ASPECTS

Diagnosis

Many cases of toxic neuropathy result from a single massive exposure occurring either accidentally or in a suicide or murder attempt, in which case the cause is obvious. It is usually possible to determine whether a potentially toxic drug is being taken. When exposure occurs at work, several people are likely to be similarly affected and epidemiological studies will elicit the cause. In other instances, exposure to a toxic substance may only be revealed after careful consideration of the patient's habits and way of life.

The relative degree of motor and sensory involvement, the distribution of muscle weakness, the extent of tendon reflex loss, the presence of paraesthesiae, pain or autonomic disturbances vary in different toxic conditions. Concurrent involvement of parts of the central nervous system (e.g. pyramidal tracts, optic nerves or cerebellum) sometimes occurs. There may be abnormalities of other systems. The characteristic features of various toxic neuropathies are summarized in *Tables 8.1* and *8.3*. Some or all of these features should be recognized before ascribing peripheral neuropathy to a particular toxic substance.

The pattern of electrophysiological involvement may be characteristic. Axonal degeneration occurs in most toxic neuropathies (*see* Chapter 1) and so little slowing of conduction velocity is to be expected. However, segmental demyelination occurs in a few, e.g. following perhexilene, and secondary demyelination is marked in hexacarbon neuropathy and considerable reduction in velocity is often found. In some instances particular pathological features may be identified in peripheral nerve biopsies.

With the recent improvement in analytical techniques, biochemical diagnosis of some conditions has become more certain. The increase in accuracy and sensitivity of detection of elements by atomic absorption spectrophotometry has been a notable advance. The detection of compounds by chromatographic techniques,

Table 8.1 Features of various occupational and environmental toxic neuropathies

	Acrylamide	Arsenic	Carbon disulphide	Hexacarbons	Lead	Organophosphates	Thallium
Motor	++	++	+	Distal	++	++	++
Reflex	Widespread loss	AJ-	Widespread loss	AJ- ? Increased during recovery	-	AJ- Others increased	AJ- Others increased
Sensory	++	++	++	+	-	-	++
Pain	-	+	+	-	-	-	++
Autonomic	Sweating ++ Sphincters						
CNS	Ataxia Drowsiness Severe - encephalopathy		Optic neuropathy Headache Depression Psychosis Parkinsonism	Mild spasticity during recovery	Encephalopathy in children	Spastic paraparesis	Optic neuropathy Abnormal movements Confusion Abnormal EEG
Other systems	Weight loss Red, desquamating hands and feet	Acute-circulatory failure GI disturbance Hyperkeratosis Mee's lines Raindrop pigmentation			Anaemia Colic Blue line	Acute - GI	Acute - GI Alopecia (after 3-4 weeks)
Pathology	AD Neurofilaments	AD	AD Fusiform neurofilamentous swellings	AD Neurofilaments SD over dilatations	Man - AD Animals - SD	AD	AD Beaded swellings due to swollen mitochondria
Treatment		BAL			Penicillamine	Atropine or cholinesterase reactivators for acute	Potassium salts Prussian blue

AJ = ankle jerk; AD = axonal degeneration; BAL = British anti-Lewisite; SD = segmental demyelination particularly high pressure liquid chromatography, has been particularly useful in studying drug toxicity. Blood levels can often be monitored and found to be above the recognized therapeutic range in those with toxic manifestations, either due to excessive intake or to unusual metabolic patterns due to disease or genetic factors.

Treatment

Removal from exposure is often all that is necessary or indeed possible. In the following sections treatment will only be mentioned when specific measures are available.

Prognosis

Improvement, sometimes continuing for several years, is expected when exposure to a toxic substance ceases. In some instances, first signs of recovery are delayed for several weeks, as with perhexilene, and patients intoxicated by hexacarbon solvents may actually continue to worsen for 4–6 weeks after cessation of exposure. The speed and extent of eventual recovery is related to the severity of neuropathy, with some residual abnormalities if it was severe. Concomitant CNS abnormalities may be permanent.

Some substances produce neuropathy after a single exposure. In these cases there is usually a latent interval of a few days or weeks before neurological abnormalities develop, which then progress for several days or weeks. Recovery is then similar to that after chronic exposure.

In the following sections prognosis will only be considered when it differs from the above description.

Pathology

Many types of toxic neuropathy have characteristic pathological features which will be described in the relevant sections. Axonal degeneration is common. Primary myelin damage resulting in segmental demyelination occurs in only a few toxic conditions. Initial predegenerative changes within axons differ. Thus, there may be axonal dilatation due to accumulation of neurofilaments or of swollen mitochondria. The type of fibre showing earliest changes also varies, as does the exact site of damage (terminal, preterminal or paranodal).

Recently it has been increasingly appreciated that pathological changes due to toxic substances are rarely confined to peripheral nerves. Spencer and Schaumburg (1977) have proposed the concept of central-peripheral distal axonopathy. Thus, most toxic substances cause distal degeneration of nerve fibres, spreading proximally with continuing intoxication. However, the relative degree of damage to peripheral and central axons varies in different conditions. In some intoxications CNS damage may be clinically important from the onset, while in others signs may only become manifest as peripheral nerves recover or pathologically recognizable damage may be insufficient to produce clinically detectable signs.

INDUSTRIAL AND ENVIRONMENTAL TOXINS

Acrylamide

EXPOSURE

One of the most important uses of acrylamide is as a grouting agent for stabilizing soil in mining and engineering works; polymerization is made to occur *in situ* by a catalytic process after the monomer has been pumped into the soil. The polymer is also extensively used for cleaning and separating suspensions from solution.

Acrylamide monomer is neurotoxic but the polymer is not. Symptoms of intoxication have been reported in men handling the monomer in the polymerization process (Garland and Patterson, 1967) or when pumping it into the soil preparatory to polymerization for grouting (Kesson, Baird and Lawson, 1977).

CLINICAL FEATURES

The nature of the neurological disorder varies with the severity of exposure. When chronic neuropathy develops after several months' exposure, sensory loss without paraesthesiae is usually the first symptom. Distal weakness follows. Widespread loss of tendon reflexes occurs, even when other evidence of neuropathy is mild. Difficulties with micturition and profuse sweating suggest autonomic nerve involvement. If exposure is more severe, sleep disturbances and daytime drowsiness may occur before the onset of neuropathy. Ataxia is also a prominent feature and sphincter disturbances are more marked.

Encephalopathy has been reported as the initial manifestation of toxicity in several members of one family following heavy exposure due to contaminated well water (Igisu *et al.*, 1975). They became confused, disorientated and had hallucinations with ataxia and retention of urine. Peripheral neuropathy developed about 1 week later.

Redness and desquamation of the skin of the hands are common, probably due to a direct toxic effect of acrylamide on the skin. Weight loss out of proportion to the severity of the neurological disorder is usual and is often an early sign of toxicity.

ELECTROPHYSIOLOGY

The findings are typical of axonal neuropathy with signs of denervation and little or no slowing of motor conduction velocity (Fullerton, 1969). More marked reduction of velocity has been found in animals, probably because intoxication was more severe (Fullerton and Barnes, 1966; Hopkins and Gilliatt, 1971).

Reduction in sensory nerve action potential amplitude is the most sensitive indication of nerve abnormality in humans (Takahashi, Ohara and Hashimoto, 1971).

PATHOLOGY

Acrylamide produces a typical dying-back neuropathy affecting particularly the largest fibres (Fullerton and Barnes, 1966). It has been shown in animal experiments, both physiologically and pathologically, that initial damage is to the primary annulospiral endings of the muscle spindles (Sumner and Asbury, 1975; Schaumburg, Wisniewski and Spencer, 1974), hence the sensitivity of tendon reflexes to acrylamide intoxication. Neurofilaments accumulate within axons before they degenerate completely, causing dilatation of paranodal regions above the site of degeneration and at motor nerve terminals (Tsujihata, Engel and Lambert, 1974).

Pathological changes have also been demonstrated in the cerebellum of intoxicated rats (Cavanagh and Nolan, 1982). Cerebellar changes in man, perhaps coupled with proprioceptive deficit, may account for the ataxia observed.

Arsenic

EXPOSURE

Arsenic is no longer used therapeutically or as a pigment. It is still present in some insecticides and weed killers. Occupational exposure occurs in smelters, but is usually slight. Intoxication usually occurs accidentally or deliberately in suicide or murder attempts.

CLINICAL FEATURES

Following a single large exposure, hypotension, vomiting and loss of consciousness due to circulatory failure may occur. If the patient survives, peripheral neuropathy develops after a latent interval of 2–3 weeks. Sensory disturbances and pain are prominent. The severity of weakness is variable. Deterioration occurs for 1–2 weeks. Even in the presence of severe neuropathy, it is rare to find widespread supression of reflexes.

Following repeated exposure to smaller amounts of arsenic a distal, symmetrical sensorimotor neuropathy develops in which pain and sensory manifestations predominate. Gastrointestinal symptoms may occur or there may be no history of systemic disturbance.

Mees' lines appear on the nails and move distally as the nails grow. Hyperkeratosis of the palms of the hands and soles of the feet are common following chronic exposure and patchy 'raindrop' pigmentation may be seen, particularly over the abdomen.

BIOCHEMICAL DIAGNOSIS

Normal values and those to be expected following intoxication are given in *Table 8.2*. Analysis of pubic hair gives more reliable data than of head hair because it is less liable to environmental and cosmetic contamination. Many hair dyes and tonics contain arsenic. It is important to weigh the hair sample prior to sending it for analysis to ensure that it is adequate. The value of nail analysis is limited because the only part that can be sampled reflects the state at one particular time many weeks earlier.

Table 8.2 Normal and hazardous levels of arsenic and thallium in various tissues

	Blood		Urine		Hair	
	Normal	Hazardous	Normal	Hazardous	Normal	Hazardous
Arsenic	$<30\,\mu g/l$	$>50\,\mu g/l$	$<40\,\mu g/l$	$>200\,\mu g/l$	$<1\,mg/kg$	$>1\,mg/kg$ may be up to $50\,mg/kg$
Thallium (with survival)	$<10\,\mu g/l$ Adults: up to 1 mg/l Children: up to 8 mg/l	$>50\,\mu g/l$	$<20\,\mu g/l$ up to 4 mg/l up to 20 mg/l	$>200\,\mu g/l$		

TREATMENT

Chelation therapy may be life-saving following acute massive exposure. British anti-Lewisite (BAL) is the most effective agent. If given within a few hours of exposure, BAL may prevent or reduce the severity of neuropathy. There is no evidence that it has any effect if given at a later stage. However, since degeneration can continue for several months after a single exposure, there are good theoretical reasons for giving a course of BAL even at a later stage. Likewise, in chronic neuropathy it seems prudent to reduce the body burden of arsenic. Until there is more evidence that chelation is ineffective, a course of treatment is recommended.

PATHOLOGY

Since it has not been possible to reproduce arsenic neuropathy in animals, few details of the pathological process have been elucidated. Biopsy studies of affected subjects have shown axonal degeneration. Continuing degeneration was recognized some months after acute exposure in some affected individuals, suggesting either that residual arsenic was still neurotoxic or that the time course of degeneration was more prolonged than during acute traumatic Wallerian degeneration (Le Quesne and McLeod, 1977).

Carbon disulphide

EXPOSURE

Exposure to carbon disulphide is now an occupational problem only in the viscose rayon industry. Industrial hygienic standards are usually such that clinical problems are rare. The present threshold limit value (TLV) in most countries is $30\,mg/m^3$.

CLINICAL AND ELECTROPHYSIOLOGICAL FEATURES

Peripheral neuropathy follows long continued low level exposure. Paraesthesiae and painful muscles occur first. Distal weakness follows if exposure continues. The only evidence of neuropathy may be absent reflexes. Cranial nerves may be involved with absent corneal reflexes. Optic neuropathy has been described.

In the past, when heavier exposure occurred, headaches and psychiatric manifestations were common with mood changes, particularly depression (Vigliani, 1954). Frank psychotic manifestations with hallucinations have been described and also Parkinsonism.

PATHOLOGY

There have been no detailed pathological descriptions of peripheral nerves in humans. Scattered CNS degenerative changes have been attributed to primary vascular damage by some authors and to a direct toxic effect by others.

Following chronic experimental exposure of rabbits and rats, para- and internodal fusiform swellings filled with neurofilaments develop in the distal parts of peripheral nerves and also at the distal ends of long fibre tracts in the CNS (Seppalainen and Haltia, 1980). There is thinning of myelin sheaths over the swelling and often distal degeneration of axons below them, similar to changes in hexacarbon neuropathy (*see below*).

Hexacarbons

EXPOSURE

Many different hexacarbon solvents are used industrially and in domestic products, e.g. glue. Although probably all hexacarbons have addictive potential for their euphoriant effect, only two are known to cause peripheral neuropathy; n-hexane and methyl butyl ketone. They are converted to a common neurotoxic metabolite, 2,5 hexanedione. Large quantities are used under normal working conditions without evidence of toxicity. Peripheral neuropathy only develops after high levels of exposure.

An outbreak of peripheral neuropathy due to methyl butyl ketone affected 86 workers in a coated-fabrics plant in Columbus, Ohio in 1973 and drew attention to the potential toxicity of this substance (Allen *et al.*, 1975). For many years polyneuropathy was common amongst Italian shoemakers. n-Hexane is now recognized as the cause (Cianchetti *et al.*, 1976). More severe neuropathy has been described in sniffers of glue in which n-hexane was the solvent (Korobkin *et al.*, 1975; Altenkirch *et al.*, 1977).

CLINICAL AND ELECTROPHYSIOLOGICAL FEATURES

Although sensory symptoms occur first these remain mild. With continuing exposure, distal weakness develops which can become profound before proximal muscles are involved. It is rare for reflexes other than ankle jerks to be lost.

Neuropathy may progress for several months after exposure ceases. This unusual course must be appreciated to avoid diagnostic problems before recovery starts.

As peripheral neuropathy improves, spasticity may become evident, revealing CNS damage. However, this is not sufficiently severe to be functionally important.

Severe slowing of motor nerve conduction velocity has been reported. This is to be expected since pathological changes of paranodal myelin retraction and demyelination have been described.

PATHOLOGY

The descriptive term 'giant axonal neuropathy' highlights the salient feature. Accumulations of neurofilaments produce axonal dilatations which are most marked at the proximal sides of nodes of Ranvier (Spencer *et al.*, 1975). Secondary myelin breakdown occurs over the swellings. These changes precede complete degeneration of the axon and are widespread. They have been seen in sural nerve biopsies from affected subjects and are thus of diagnostic importance.

Giant axonal swellings also occur in nerve tracts in the spinal cord, medulla and cerebellum (Spencer and Schaumburg, 1977). In these situations, however, complete nerve fibre degeneration is less common than in the peripheral nerves.

Lead

EXPOSURE

Lead neuropathy was common in the early part of the century following heavy occupational exposure. Exposure is now well controlled in storage battery manufacture and smelting where lead is encountered. Neuropathy is therefore rare. Lead glazed pottery is still used in some primitive communities and can provide a substantial source of lead. General environmental contamination is not sufficient to produce neuropathy. Childhood lead poisoning will not be considered here.

CLINICAL AND ELECTROPHYSIOLOGICAL FEATURES

Weakness particularly affects the most exercised muscles, e.g. wrist drop was common in painters using lead based paints. There are usually no sensory abnormalities.

Anaemia and colic are early manifestations of lead intoxication. A lead line may develop on the gums.

There has been little opportunity for extensive electrophysiological study. Buchthal and Behse (1979) found no reduction in nerve conduction velocity in one patient with lead neuropathy. This is in contrast to the findings in animal nerves where gross slowing of conduction may occur (Fullerton, 1966) and reflects the difference in pathology in man and animals.

A number of studies of workers with elevated blood lead levels in the range 1.5–3.5 μmol/l (30–70 μg/100 ml) suggest that slight reduction in velocity may occur without clinical abnormalities. In some instances a dose-response effect has been detected (Araki and Honma, 1976; Seppalainen, Hernberg and Kock, 1979) whereas in another study minor changes were unrelated to blood lead levels (Buchthal and Behse, 1979).

PATHOLOGY

Although segmental demyelination is present in experimental lead neuropathy in animals (Fullerton, 1966), this type of change has not been described in human nerves. Older studies describe axonal degeneration and this was confirmed in a more recent study (Buchthal and Behse, 1979).

Organophosphates

EXPOSURE

Organophosphorus (OP) compounds are widely used as insecticides. Some are used as plasticizers and in lubricating oils. Their toxic properties vary considerably. Practically all organophosphates are acetylcholinesterase inhibitors and have the expected acute toxic effects which have been responsible for many fatalities (Namba *et al.*, 1971). This aspect of their toxicity will not be considered further. No OP compounds in current use have caused peripheral neuropathy following their use as insecticides. Occasional cases of neuropathy have followed suicide attempts, most commonly with trichlorphon (Dipterex) (Hierons and Johnson, 1978). Treatment with atropine has enabled the patients to survive long enough to develop neuropathy.

Tri-ortho-cresyl phosphate (TOCP), used in lubrication oil and as a degreaser, has been responsible for most cases of OP neuropathy. Epidemics have followed accidental contamination of cooking oil (Smith and Spalding, 1959).

CLINICAL AND ELECTROPHYSIOLOGICAL FEATURES
Intoxication has usually followed accidental ingestion of a single dose. Following initial gastrointestinal symptoms and possibly other evidence of acute acetyl-cholinesterase inhibition, such as fasciculations and meiosis, there is a latent interval of 1–3 weeks before the onset of neurological symptoms.

Paraesthesiae may occur at the onset but are always mild and other sensory changes are minimal or absent. Weakness progresses rapidly for some days. The relative involvement of peripheral and central motor pathways varies in different subjects. Spasticity and upper motor neurone weakness may be present at the onset or only become manifest as the peripheral nerves recover. Ankle reflexes are always absent but other tendon reflexes may be either absent or increased.

Normal motor nerve conduction velocity has been described in the presence of severe weakness in both humans and animals (Hierons and Johnson, 1978; Hern, 1973). This is because large diameter fibres are not selectively affected (*see* acrylamide neuropathy). Sensory nerve action potentials may be reduced in amplitude or absent even when there is no significant sensory loss (Hierons and Johnson, 1978).

Treatment with atropine and cholinesterase reactivators (e.g. pralidoxime) control effects of acute acetylcholinesterase inhibition. However, they have no influence on the development of neuropathy.

Functional recovery may be poor with residual spastic paraparesis because of irrecoverable damage to the central nervous system.

PATHOLOGY
Dying-back axonal degeneration occurs in both peripheral and central nerve fibres (Cavanagh, 1954), with some increase of tubulo-vesicular profiles in the axoplasm of affected axons (Prineas, 1969).

BIOCHEMICAL LESION
The development of neuropathy is related to the inhibition of a specific 'neurotoxic' esterase (Johnson, 1975). Its chemical composition has not been elucidated, but its activity can be measured in brain tissue. Thus, the neurotoxicity of any particular OP compound can be predicted by an *in vitro* test.

There is no *in vivo* method of detecting 'neurotoxic' esterase inhibition. Measurement of acetyl (erythrocyte) and pseudo (plasma) cholinesterase activity in the blood will reveal exposure to an OP compound during the preceding few weeks. Treatment of acute cholinergic effects with atropine has no effect on cholinesterase activity, but cholinesterase reactivators such as pralidoxime cause an immediate return of acetylcholinesterase activity to the normal range.

Thallium

EXPOSURE

At one time thallium salts were used therapeutically, particularly in the treatment of ringworm and cosmetically as a depilatory agent. They have also been widely used as rodenticides, but their sale is now restricted in many parts of the world. Intoxication has most often followed ingestion of a thallium salt either accidentally or deliberately in suicide or murder attempts; 1–2 g are lethal to adults.

CLINICAL AND ELECTROPHYSIOLOGICAL FEATURES

After massive exposure gastrointestinal symptoms occur, followed by a latent interval of 1–7 days before the onset of neurological abnormalities, which may then progress rapidly.

Clinical features have been reviewed by Cavanagh *et al.* (1974). Motor and sensory systems are involved. Painful paraesthesiae and pain in muscles and joints are common. Ankle reflexes are lost early but other reflexes may be preserved for a time or even increased. Cranial nerves including optic nerves may be involved early. Choreiform movements, particularly around the mouth, are often seen. In severe intoxication, confusion, sleep disturbances and frank psychosis may occur. Diffuse slow waves are seen on the EEG.

Abnormal liver function tests are common. Loss of head and body hair with sparing of the inner third of the eyebrows occurs after about 2–3 weeks. Mees' lines on the nails are similar to those following arsenic intoxication.

Following chronic exposure the course of the disease is slower. Gastrointestinal symptoms may be absent, but alopecia usually occurs.

Electrophysiological findings are characteristic of axonal degeneration. Denervation with little or no reduction in conduction velocity and reduction in amplitude of sensory nerve action potentials are found.

The levels of thallium to be expected in various tissues following intoxication are shown in *Table 8.2*.

TREATMENT

Administration of potassium will assist in displacing thallium from its intracellular site and is an important first line of treatment.

Some types of chelation therapy are contraindicated because mobilization of thallium can result in a dangerous increase in brain thallium. Potassium ferric cyano-ferrate II (Prussian blue) by mouth (10 g twice daily) is effective therapy. Normally, thallium is reabsorbed after excretion in the bile. This cycle may be broken by Prussian blue, the potassium being replaced by thallium which is then excreted.

PATHOLOGY

Axonal degeneration of nerve fibres may be confined to the most distal parts of the peripheral nerves (Cavanagh *et al.*, 1974). Before degenerating, bead-like swellings, due to accumulations of swollen degenerating mitochondria, develop along the nerves (Spencer *et al.*, 1973).

DRUG-INDUCED PERIPHERAL NEUROPATHIES

Only those drugs which unequivocally produce peripheral neuropathy will be considered. The toxic dose level and other characteristic features are shown in *Table 8.3*. Other drugs have been implicated occasionally but either the incriminating evidence is doubtful or the complication is too rare to merit inclusion here.

Amiodarone

Sensorimotor neuropathy has been described in a few patients following 400 mg/day for one or more years. CSF protein is raised. Both axonal degeneration

Table 8.3 Drug-induced neuropathies

Drug	Toxic dose	Clinical features	Special features
Amiodorone	400 mg/day for a year		Raised CSF protein Lipid storage
Dapsone	200–500 mg/day for months	Mainly motor	? in slow acetylators
Disulfiram	1.0–1.5 g/day		
Gold	Variable		
Isoniazid	5–20 mg/kg/day		Pyridoxine deficiency in slow acetylators
Metronidazole	400 mg t.d.s. for months	Sensory	CNS lesions like B_1 deficiency
Misonidazole	More than 6 g/m^2/week	Sensory	CNS lesions like B_1 deficiency
Perhexilene	300–400 mg/day for months	Papilloedema Postural hypotension	Raised CSF protein Segmental demyelination with slow conduction Lipid storage
Platinum	Several courses of 75–100 mg/m^2	Tinnitus High frequency hearing loss Renal toxicity	
Thalidomide	200–400 mg/day	Proximal weakness	Poor recovery
Vincristine	Mild with 2 mg twice monthly		

and segmental demyelination are present in the nerves. Lysosomal dense bodies have been identified in Schwann cells and also in fibroblasts and perineural cells (Meier *et al.*, 1979). The changes are similar to those in perhexilene neuropathy.

Meier *et al.* (1979) found that the iodine content of nerve and muscle was increased, suggesting that the stored lipid was related to accumulation of the drug (which contains iodine) or its metabolites. Amiodarone neuropathy tends to be dose-dependent (Martinez-Arizala *et al.*, 1983).

Dapsone

The most important use of dapsone is in the treatment of leprosy when it is administered at a dose of 25–300 mg weekly. At much higher doses (up to 400 mg daily) it is occasionally used to treat various skin diseases such as dermatitis herpetiformis, pyoderma gangrenosum and cystic acne.

Pure or predominantly motor neuropathy has been reported occasionally following high doses (Gutman, Martin and Welton, 1976; Helander and Partanen, 1978).

Reduction of motor nerve conduction velocity is slight even in the presence of severe denervation, suggesting primary axonal pathology.

Dapsone is acetylated by N-acetyl transferase, as is isoniazid. Koller *et al.* (1977) found slow acetylation of isoniazid in one patient with dapsone neuropathy. Because of the rarity of the condition it has not been established whether neuropathy only occurs in slow acetylators.

Disulfiram

Disulfiram (tetraethylthiuram disulphide) is used in the treatment of alcoholism and so toxic effects of the drug must be distinguished from alcoholic neuropathy. The incidence of neuropathy is low and is dose related, most commonly occurring after 1.0–1.5 g daily, although occasionally 500 mg daily for several months has been responsible (Moddel *et al.*, 1978; Mokri, Ohnishi and Dyck, 1981).

Sensory abnormalities predominate although considerable weakness may occur if administration of the drug continues after symptoms develop. Optic neuritis has been described, not always in association with peripheral neuropathy (Gardner-Thorpe and Benjamin, 1971).

Only slight changes in motor nerve conduction velocity occur. Reduction in amplitude of sensory nerve action potentials is also a feature.

Axonal degneration has been the most common finding in biopsied sural nerves. However, segmental demyelination was found to predominate in one nerve examined by Nukada and Pollock (1981). The reasons for the different findings are not known.

Gold

Sodium aurothiomalate is still occasionally used in the treatment of rheumatoid arthritis, although less commonly than before the introduction of steroid and other anti-inflammatory drugs. Peripheral neuropathy is a rare complication and is not clearly dose related. It has been described following a small total dose: 85 mg in the patient described by Walsh (1970); or after higher doses: over 1.3 g in two cases described by Katrak *et al.* (1980).

Both motor and sensory systems are involved, although sensory abnormalities are sometimes more marked. Myokymia was prominent in two of three patients reported by Katrak *et al.* (1980).

Fever, rashes and renal abnormalities are commoner complications than neuropathy. The nature of these reactions and sudden onset of neuropathy in some instances has led to the suggestion that an immunological response to the drug may be involved. This has not been proved.

Sural nerves obtained at biopsy have shown either axonal degeneration affecting fibres of all diameters (Walsh, 1970) or a mixture of axonal degeneration and segmental demyelination (Katrak *et al.* 1980).

Katrak *et al.* (1980) produced a dose related neuropathy in rats by giving sodium aurothiomalate, suggesting that the drug has a direct toxic effect on the nerves. Again both types of pathological lesion were found.

Isoniazid

EXPOSURE
Isoniazid was introduced for the treatment of tuberculosis in the early 1950s and it soon became apparent that peripheral neuropathy was a common complication of high dose therapy. Symptoms occurred in about 20% of patients treated with 5 mg/kg daily and 40% of those treated with 20 mg/kg.

PREDISPOSING FACTORS
After absorption, isoniazid is acetylated in the liver by the enzyme acetyl transferase. The rate of acetylation varies in different subjects. Neuropathy is more likely to develop in slow acetylators who have higher blood levels of free isoniazid for a longer time than rapid acetylators. The amount of acetyl transferase in the liver is genetically determined, slow inactivation (low acetyl transferase) being an autosomal recessive trait.

CLINICAL FEATURES
Numbness and painful burning paraesthesiae occur in the extremities. Deep sensation is less affected. Distal weakness with cramps and painful muscles occur at a later stage.

BIOCHEMICAL LESION
Isoniazid induces pyridoxine deficiency by inhibiting pyridoxal phosphate kinase and also combines with pyridoxal phosphate.

TREATMENT AND PROGNOSIS
Administration of pyridoxine prevents the development of neuropathy without interfering with the antituberculous action of isoniazid. It is a wise precaution to

give pyridoxine to patients who are slow acetylators (assessed by measuring blood levels of isoniazid 6 hours after an oral dose) and who require treatment with high doses of isoniazid. Pyridoxine has no effect on the rate of recovery, which depends on the time taken for regeneration of nerve fibres.

PATHOLOGY

In human nerves axonal degeneration affects myelinated and unmyelinated fibres and regeneration is prominent (Ochoa, 1970).

One day after a single high dose to rats, Jacobs *et al.* (1979) found focal periaxonal vacuoles within myelin sheaths and increased prominence of smooth endoplasmic reticulum.

Metronidazole

Metronidazole is used in the treatment of various protozoal and some anaerobic infections. It has also been used in Crohn's disease. Sensory neuropathy has been described occasionally following treatment for several months with 400 mg three times daily (Coxon and Pallis, 1976; Bradley, Karlsson and Rassol, 1977).

Following high doses, encephalopathy and cerebellar ataxia have been described in addition to sensory neuropathy (Kusumi *et al.*, 1980).

A single report of a sural nerve biopsy (Bradley, Karlsson and Rassol, 1977) suggests that primary axonal changes occur.

Cerebellar and brain stem lesions have been described in rats following high doses (Rogulja, Kovac and Schmid, 1973), similar to those described following misonidazole administration to rats (*see below*).

Misonidazole

EXPOSURE

Misonidazole is used to sensitize radioresistant hypoxic cells to the effects of radiotherapy. Neurotoxicity is dose limiting. A single dose should not exceed 4 g/m^2 and no more than 6 g/m^2 should be given in 1 week.

CLINICAL AND ELECTROPHYSIOLOGICAL FEATURES

Neuropathy is predominantly or entirely sensory, with painful paraesthesiae, sensory loss and clumsiness (Dische *et al.*, 1977). After high doses convulsions have occurred.

Decrease in sural nerve action potential amplitude has been described during treatment with little effect on velocity of motor or sensory fibres (Mamoli *et al.*, 1979).

PATHOLOGY

Urtasun *et al.* (1978) described a mixture of segmental demyelination and axonal degeneration with increase in neurofilaments in one biopsied sural nerve.

However, teased fibres were not examined and the incidence of demyelination was not established. The electrophysiological findings suggest that primary axonal changes are likely to be more important.

Griffin *et al.* (1979) have demonstrated changes in the central nervous system in rats following administration of misonidazole. Spongy degenerative changes with extracellular oedema and swelling of astroglial processes were found in certain specific nuclear groups in the brain stem, such as the lateral, superior and spinal vestibular nuclei and the superior olives. These and other localized haemorrhagic lesions are very similar to lesions induced by thiamine deficiency, suggesting a similar basic underlying abnormality. However, administration of thiamine has not prevented misonidazaole toxicity in either rats or humans.

Perhexilene

EXPOSURE

Neurotoxic effects have usually occurred after several month's treatment with 300–400 mg/day (Lhermitte *et al.*, 1976).

It has been shown that oxidation of a number of drugs is under genetic control and that speed of oxidation can be determined by measurement of oxidation of the drug debrisoquine. Shah *et al.* (1982) found that the rate of oxidation of debrisoquine was slower in patients with neuropathy than in those who had taken similar amounts of perhexilene without developing neuropathy. The difference did not correlate with abnormalities of liver function. Therefore speed of perhexilene metabolism and thus likelihood of developing neuropathy appears to be genetically determined.

CLINICAL AND ELECTROPHYSIOLOGICAL FEATURES

Painful paraesthesiae and sensory loss occur first. Weakness follows and although predominantly distal, some patients have also had marked proximal weakness.

Papilloedema has been reported in a number of patients and has been ascribed to raised CSF protein content which is usually over 1 g/l. Values up to 4.9 g/l have been described. Postural hypotension suggesting autonomic nerve involvement occasionally occurs. Marked weight loss independent of the severity of the neuropathy is a recognized complication. Abnormalities of liver function also occur. Marked slowing of motor nerve conduction velocity is characteristic, suggesting the presence of segmental demyelination in affected nerves. Values below 20 m/s are often found.

There may be a delay of several weeks before any improvement occurs after administration of the drug is stopped.

PATHOLOGY

Sural nerve biopsies from affected subjects have confirmed the presence of segmental demyelination as the predominant finding. A variable degree of axonal degeneration is also present (Lhermitte *et al.*, 1976; Said, 1978). However, the most characteristic finding is the presence of lipid inclusions, not only in Schwann cells where they are prominent, but also in endothelial cells, perineurial cells, fibroblasts and phagocytes. An increased content of gangliosides but not other glycolipids has been found on chemical analysis of affected nerves (Pollett *et al.*, 1977).

Platinum

Platinum is given in the form of cisplatin (*cis*-diamminedichloroplatinum) as a chemotherapeutic agent in a number of solid neoplastic tumours. Sensory peripheral neuropathy is a complication of high doses (several courses of 75–100 mg/m^2). Ototoxicity, manifest as tinnitus and high frequency hearing loss, is commoner and occurs at lower doses. However, renal toxicity is dose-limiting and peripheral neuropathy is now rarely seen.

Thalidomide

EXPOSURE

Although thalidomide neuropathy is now mainly of historical interest, it is important to be aware of the condition since the drug is still used in the management of certain forms of leprosy and certain rare skin conditions such as Hutchinson's summer prurigo and prurigo nodularis. Although carefully sought, neuropathy has not been described as a complication of the use of the drug in leprosy. This may be because lower doses are used than when the drug was used as a hypnotic.

In the early 1960s thalidomide was extensively used in a number of countries and neuropathy was a common complication of high doses (200–400 mg/night) or long duration administration. Since discovery of its teratogenic effects it has no longer been available as a hypnotic.

Glutethimide, which is still available, is structurally similar to thalidomide but is much less toxic. A few cases of mild sensory neuropathy have been described in people taking high doses for many months.

CLINICAL FEATURES

Distal painful paraesthesiae with numbness occurred first. If the drug was continued, weakness, which was often proximal, developed. Cramps were common. Although ankle jerks were sometimes absent, other reflexes were usually increased, indicating CNS damage (Fullerton and Kremer, 1961).

Redness of the palms of the hands and brittle, broken finger and toe nails occurred.

One of the disturbing features was the persistence of distressing painful paraesthesiae in about half the patients after the drug was stopped (Fullerton and O'Sullivan, 1968).

PATHOLOGY

Marked loss of large diameter fibres was found in sural nerves as long as 2–6 years after stopping the drug (Fullerton and O'Sullivan, 1968). Increase in number of small diameter fibres indicating attempted regeneration was only found in two of six nerves. The clinical and pathological findings suggested that regeneration is particularly poor after this toxic insult.

Vinca alkaloids

EXPOSURE

Vinblastine was the first vinca alkaloid to be introduced for the treatment of leukaemia and lymphomas. Its use is limited by bone marrow toxicity. Vincristine use is limited by neurotoxicity. Vindesine is toxic to both bone marrow and peripheral nerves.

Vincristine is frequently used in multiple chemotheraphy regimes, $1.4\,mg/m^2$ (maximum 2 mg) being given intravenously on days one and eight of a monthly cycle. Mild neuropathy develops in all those thus treated and more severe neuropathy if the drug is given more frequently. A higher dose is rarely used.

CLINICAL AND ELECTROPHYSIOLOGICAL FEATURES

Experience of the clinical syndrome was gained when vincristine was given more frequently after it was first introduced (Casey *et al.*, 1973). Widespread loss of reflexes occurs early, followed by distal numbness and paraesthesiae. Sensory loss rarely becomes severe or extensive, even in those who develop marked weakness.

Weakness is usually first manifest as clumsiness of the hands. This is followed by weakness at the ankles and then proximally. Predilection for extensor muscles of the finger and wrist may occur. Weakness may progress rapidly, particularly in older patients, unless treatment is stopped immediately. Thus, weakness rather than sensory abnormalities is the indication for reducing treatment. Muscle cramps may occur, particularly for a few days after treatment.

Constipation and occasionally paralytic ileus suggest that autonomic nerves are also involved. Prophylactic laxatives are usually given to avoid these complications.

Alopecia follows high or frequent doses. It is not a problem with current dose schedules.

Sensory nerve action potentials are reduced in amplitude. Motor nerve conduction velocity is little reduced even in the presence of considerable reduction in muscle action potential amplitude.

On stopping treatment paraesthesiae always disappear and sensory loss will recover unless it has been extensive. Ankle jerks remain absent but other reflexes usually return. If treatment is stopped when weakness is mild, recovery will be complete. However, if severe weakness develops full power may not return.

PATHOLOGY

In man, vincristine produces a dying-back neuropathy. However, myopathic changes predominate in the animal models studied (rats and guinea-pigs).

Degeneration is associated with the formation of spheromembranous bodies containing mitochondrial remnants, smooth-profiled vesicles and irregular dense bodies (Anderson, Song and Slotwiner, 1967). Similar changes have been described in human muscles (Bradley *et al.*, 1970).

In human CNS, neurofilamentous proliferation is prominent in anterior horn cells, spinal ganglia, medulla and pons (Schochet, Lampert and Earle, 1968). Crystalline osmiophilic masses also develop in neurons. *In vitro* studies have shown that vinca alkaloids interact with tubulin to produce the crystalline arrays. Polymerization of microtubules is inhibited.

References

Allen, N., Mendell, J. R., Billmaier, J., Fontaine, R. E., and O'Neill, J. (1975) Toxic polyneuropathy due to methyl n-butyl ketone. *Archives of Neurology*, **32**, 209–218

Altenkirch, H., Mager, J., Stoltenburg, G. and Helmbrecht, J. (1977) Toxic polyneuropathies after sniffing a glue thinner. *Journal of Neurology*, **214**, 137–152

Anderson, P. J., Song, S. K. and Slotwiner, P. (1967) The fine structure of spheromembranous degeneration of skeletal muscle induced by vincristine. *Journal of Neuropathology and Experimental Neurology*, **26**, 15–24

Araki, S. and Honma, T. (1976) Relationships between lead absorption and peripheral nerve conduction velocities in lead workers. *Scandinavian Journal of Work Environment and Health*, **4**, 225–231

Bradley, W. G., Karlsson, I. J. and Rassol, C. G. (1977) Metronidazole neuropathy. *British Medical Journal*, **2**, 610–611

Bradley, W. G., Lassman, L. P., Pearce, G. W. and Walton, J. N. (1970) The neuromyopathy of vincristine in man. Clinical, electrophysiological and pathological studies. *Journal of the Neurological Sciences*, **10**, 107–131

Buchthal, F. and Behse, F. (1979) Electrophysiology and nerve biopsy in men exposed to lead. *British Journal of Industrial Medicine*, **36**, 135–147

Casey, E. B., Jelliffe, A. M., Le Quesne, P. M. and Millett, Y. L. (1973) Vincristine neuropathy – clinical and electrophysiological observations. *Brain*, **96**, 69–86

Cavanagh, J. B. (1954) The toxic effects of tri-ortho-cresyl phosphate on the nervous system. *Journal of Neurology, Neurosurgery and Psychiatry*, **17**, 163–172

Cavanagh, J. B., Fuller, N. H., Johnson, H. R. M. and Rudge, P. (1974) The effects of thallium salts, with particular reference to the nervous system changes. *Quarterly Journal of Medicine*, **43**, 293–319

Cavanagh, J. B. and Nolan, C. C. (1982) Selective loss of Purkinje cells from the rat cerebellum caused by acrylamide and the responses of β-glucuronidase and β-galactosidase. *Acta Neuropathologica*, **58**, 210–214

Cianchetti, C., Abbritti, G., Perticoni, G., Siracusa, A. and Curradi, F. (1976) Toxic polyneuropathy of shoe-industry workers. *Journal of Neurology, Neurosurgery and Psychiatry*, **39**, 1151–1161

Coxon, A. and Pallis, C. A. (1976) Metronidazole neuropathy. *Journal of Neurology, Neurosurgery and Psychiatry*, **39**, 403–405

Dische, S., Saunders, M. I., Lee, M. E., Adams, G. E. and Flockhart, I. R. (1977) Clinical testing of the radiosensitizer Ro07-0582: experience with multiple doses. *British Journal of Cancer*, **35**, 567–579

Fullerton, P. M. (1966) Chronic peripheral neuropathy produced by lead poisoning in guinea-pigs. *Journal of Neuropathology and Experimental Neurology*, **25**, 214–236

Fullerton, P. M. (1969) Electrophysiological and histological observations on peripheral nerves in acrylamide poisoning in man. *Journal of Neurology, Neurosurgery and Psychiatry*, **32**, 186–192

Fullerton, P. M. and Barnes, J. M. (1966) Peripheral neuropathy in rats produced by acrylamide. *British Journal of Industrial Medicine*, **23**, 210–221

Fullerton, P. M. and Kremer, M. (1961) Neuropathy after intake of thalidomide (Distaval). *British Medical Journal*, **2**, 855–858

Fullerton, P. M. and O'Sullivan, D. J. (1968) Thalidomide neuropathy: a clinical, electrophysiological, and histological follow-up. *Journal of Neurology, Neurosurgery and Psychiatry*, **31**, 543–551

Gardner-Thorpe, C. and Benjamin, S. (1971) Peripheral neuropathy after disulfiram administration. *Journal of Neurology, Neurosurgery and Psychiatry*, **34**, 253–259

Garland, T. O. and Patterson, M. W. H. (1967) Six cases of acrylamide poisoning. *British Medical Journal*, **4**, 134–138

Griffin, J. W., Price, D. L., Kuethe, D. O. and Goldberg, A. M. (1979) Neurotoxicity of misonidazole in rats. I. Neuropathology. *Neurotoxicology*, **1**, 299–312

Gutman, L., Martin, J. D. and Welton, W. (1976) Dapsone motor neuropathy – an axonal disease. *Neurology*, **26**, 514–516

Helander, I. and Partanen, J. (1978) Dapsone-induced distal axonal degeneration of the motor neurons. *Dermatologia*, **156**, 321–324

Hern, J. E. C. (1973) Tri-ortho-cresyl phosphate neuropathy in the baboon. In *New Developments in Electromyography and Clinical Neurophysiology*, Vol. 2, edited by J. E. Desmedt, pp. 181–187. Basel: Karger

Hierons, R. and Johnson, M. K. (1978) Clinical and toxicological investigations of a case of delayed neuropathy in man after acute poisoning by an organophosphorus pesticide. *Archives of Toxicology*, **40**, 279–284

Hopkins, A. P. and Gilliatt, R. W. (1971) Motor and sensory nerve conduction velocity in the baboon: normal values and changes during acrylamide neuropathy. *Journal of Neurology, Neurosurgery and Psychiatry*, **34**, 415–426

Igisu, H., Goto, I., Kawamura, Y., Kato, M., Izumi, K. and Kuroiwa, Y. (1975) Acrylamide encephaloneuropathy due to well water pollution. *Journal of Neurology, Neurosurgery and Psychiatry*, **38**, 581–584

Jacobs, J. M., Miller, R. H., Whittle, A. and Cavanagh, J. B. (1979) Studies on the early changes in acute isoniazid neuropathy in the rat. *Acta Neuropathologica*, **47**, 85–92

Johnson, M. K. (1975) Organophosphorus esters causing delayed neurotoxic effects. Mechanism of action and structure/activity studies. *Archives of Toxicology*, **34**, 259–288

Katrak, S. M., Pollock, M., O'Brien, C. P. *et al.* (1980) Clinical and morphological features of gold neuropathy. *Brain*, **103**, 671–693

Kesson, C. M., Baird, A. W. and Lawson, D. H. (1977) Acrylamide poisoning. *Postgraduate Medical Journal*, **53**, 16–17

Koller, W. C., Gehlmann, L. K., Malkinson, F. D. and Davis, F. A. (1977) Dapsone-induced peripheral neuropathy. *Archives of Neurology*, **34**, 644–646

Korobkin, R., Asbury, A. K., Sumner, A. J. and Nielsen, S. L. (1975) Glue-sniffing neuropathy. *Archives of Neurology*, **32**, 158–162

Kusumi, R. K., Plouffe, J. F., Wyatt, R. H. and Fass, R. J. (1980) Central nervous system toxicity associated with metronidazole therapy. *Annals of Internal Medicine*, **93**, 59–60

Le Quesne, P. M. and McLeod, J. G. (1977) Peripheral neuropathy following a single exposure to arsenic. Clinical course in four patients with electrophysiological and histological studies. *Journal of the Neurological Sciences*, **32**, 437–451

Lhermitte, F., Fardeau, M., Chedru, F. and Mallecourt, J. (1976) Polyneuropathy after perhexiline and maleate therapy. *British Medical Journal*, **1**, 1256

Mamoli, B., Wessely, P., Kogelnik, H. D., Muller, M. and Rathkolb, O. (1979) Electroneurographic investigations of misonidazole polyneuropathy. *European Neurology*, **18**, 405–414

Martinez-Arizala, A., Sobol, S. M., McCarty, G. E., Nichols, B. R. and Rakita, L. (1983) Amiodarone neuropathy. *Neurology*, **33**, 643–645

Meier, C., Kauer, B., Muller, U. and Ludin, H. P. (1979) Neuromyopathy during chronic amiodarone treatment. A case report. *Journal of Neurology*, **220**, 231–239

Moddel, G., Bilbao, J. M., Payne, D. and Ashby, P. (1978) Disulfiram neuropathy. *Archives of Neurology*, **35**, 658–660

Mokri, B., Ohnishi, A. and Dyck, P. J. (1981) Disulfiram neuropathy. *Neurology*, **31**, 730–735

Namba, T., Nolte, C. T., Jackrel, J. and Grob, D. (1971) Poisoning due to organophosphate insecticides. *American Journal of Medicine*, **50**, 475–492

Nukada, H. and Pollock, M. (1981) Disulfiram neuropathy – a morphometric study of sural nerve. *Journal of the Neurological Sciences*, **51**, 51–67

Ochoa, J. (1970) Isoniazid neuropathy in man: quantitative electron microscope study. *Brain*, **93**, 831–850

Pollet, S., Hauw, J. J., Escourolle, R. and Baumann, N. (1977) Peripheral nerve lipid abnormalities in patients on perhexiline maleate. *Lancet*, **1**, 1258

Prineas, J. (1969) The pathogenesis of dying-back polyneuropathies. Part I. An ultrastructural study of experimental tri-ortho-cresyl phosphate intoxication in the cat. *Journal of Neuropathology and Experimental Neurology*, **28**, 571–597

Rogulja, P. V., Kovac, W. and Schmid, H. (1973) Metronidazole-encephalopathie der Ratte. *Acta Neuropathologica*, **25**, 36–45

Said, G. (1978) Perhexiline neuropathy: a clinicopathological study. *Annals of Neurology*, **3**, 223–228

Schaumburg, H. H., Wisniewski, H. M. and Spencer, P. S. (1974) Ultrastructural studies of the dying-back process. I. Peripheral nerve terminal and axon degeneration in systemic acrylamide introxication. *Journal of Neuropathology and Experimental Neurology*, **33**, 260–284

Schochet, S. S., Lampert, P. W. and Earle, K. M. (1968) Neuronal changes induced by intrathecal vincristine sulfate. *Journal of Neuropathology and Experimental Neurology*, **27**, 645–657

Seppalainen, A. M. and Haltia, M. (1980) Carbon disulfide. In *Experimental and Clinical Neurotoxicology*, edited by P. S. Spencer and H. H. Schaumburg, pp. 356–373. Baltimore: Williams and Wilkins

Seppalainen, A. M., Hernberg, S. and Kock, B. (1979) Relationship between blood lead levels and nerve conduction velocities. *Neurotoxicology*, **1**, 313–332

Shah, R. R., Oates, N. S., Idle, J. R., Smith, R. L. and Lockhart, J. D. F. (1982) Impaired oxidation of debrisoquine in patients with perhexiline neuropathy. *British Medical Journal*, **284**, 295–299

Smith, H. V. and Spalding, J. M. K. (1959) Outbreak of paralysis in Morocco due to ortho-cresyl phosphate poisoning. *Lancet*, **2**, 1019–1021

Spencer, P. S., Peterson, E. R., Madrid, R. and Raine, C. S. (1973) Effects of thallium salts on neuronal mitochondria in organotypic cord-ganglia-muscle combination cultures. *Journal of Cell Biology*, **58**, 79–95

Spencer, P. S. and Schaumburg, H. H. (1977) Ultrastructural studies of the dying-back process. IV. Differential vulnerability of PNS and CNS fibers in experimental central-peripheral distal axonopathies. *Journal of Neuropathology and Experimental Neurology*, **36**, 300–320

Spencer, P. S., Schaumburg, H. H., Raleigh, R. L. and Terhaar, J. (1975) Nervous system degeneration produced by the industrial solvent methyl n-butyl ketone. *Archives of Neurology*, **32**, 219–222

Sumner, A. J. and Asbury, A. K. (1975) Physiological studies of the dying-back phenomenon. Muscle stretch afferents in acrylamide neuropathy. *Brain*, **98**, 91–100

Takahashi, M., Ohara, T. and Hashimoto, K. (1971) Electrophysiological study of nerve injuries in workers handling acrylamide. *Internationales Archiv für Arbeits-und Umweltmedizin*, **28**, 1–11

Tsujihata, M., Engel, A. G. and Lambert, E. H. (1974) Motor end-plate fine structure in acrylamide dying-back neuropathy: a sequential morphometric study. *Neurology*, **24**, 849–856

Urtasun, R. C., Chapman, J. D., Feldstein, M. L. *et al.* (1978) Peripheral neuropathy related to misonidazole: incidence and pathology. *British Journal of Cancer*, **37**, Suppl. III, 271–275

Vigliani, E. C. (1954) Carbon disulphide poisoning in viscose rayon factories. *British Journal of Industrial Medicine*, **11**, 235–244

Walsh, J. C. (1970) Gold neuropathy. *Neurology*, **20**, 455–458

9
Genetically determined neuropathies
A. E. Harding and P. K. Thomas

The inherited neuropathies are a complex, heterogeneous group of disorders. In some syndromes abnormal function of peripheral nerve is the only manifestation of the underlying gene mutation; in others peripheral neuropathy is one feature of a multisystem disease. As in the classification of most genetic disorders, it is convenient to separate neuropathies with a known metabolic basis or other defect from those of unknown aetiology. As knowledge advances, conditions from the second category can be transferred to the first. A classification of the genetically determined neuropathies is outlined in *Tables 9.1* and *9.2*. The clinical features of these disorders will be briefly described in the first part of this chapter. The

Table 9.1 Classification of hereditary neuropathies: neuropathies with specific metabolic or other defects

---

Hereditary amyloidoses
   Type I   (Andrade)
   Type II (Rukavina)
   Type III (van Allen)
   Type IV (Meretoja)

Porphyrias
   Acute intermittent
   Variegate
   Hereditary coproporphyria

Disorders of lipid metabolism
   Metachromatic leucodystrophy (sulphatide lipidosis)
   Globoid cell leucodystrophy (galactosylceramide lipidosis, Krabbe's disease)
   Adrenoleucodystrophy and adrenomyeloneuropathy
   Cockayne syndrome
   Hereditary high density lipoprotein deficiency (Tangier disease)
   Abetalipoproteinaemia (Bassen-Kornzweig disease)
   Phytanic acid storage disease (Refsum's disease)
   α-Galactosidase A deficiency (Fabry's disease)

Disorders associated with defective DNA repair
   Ataxia telangiectasia
   Xeroderma pigmentosum

Table 9.2 Classification of hereditary neuropathies: neuropathies of unknown cause

---

Hereditary motor and sensory neuropathies
    Type I   (hypertrophic form)
    Type II (neuronal form)
    Type III (Dejerine-Sottas disease, congenital hypomyelination neuropathy)

Hereditary sensory and autonomic neuropathies
    Type I   (dominantly inherited sensory neuropathy)
    Type II (congenital sensory neuropathy)
    Type III (Riley-Day syndrome, familial dysautonomia)
    Type IV (congenital sensory neuropathy with anhidrosis)
    Other types of congenital sensory neuropathy
    Sensory neuropathy associated with hereditary spastic paraplegia

Neuropathy associated with hereditary ataxias
    Friedreich's ataxia
    Dominantly inherited cerebellar ataxia
    Marinesco-Sjögren syndrome
    Glutamate dehydrogenase deficiency
    Ramsay Hunt syndrome of ataxia and myoclonus
    Dominantly inherited Parkinsonism and ataxia

Miscellaneous disorders
    Giant axonal neuropathy
    Chediak-Higashi disease
    Chorea-acanthocytosis syndrome
    Hereditary liability to pressure palsies

---

subsequent sections will discuss the recognition, differential diagnosis and management of inherited neuropathies. Hereditary motor neuronopathies (spinal muscular atrophies) have not been included.

NEUROPATHIES ASSOCIATED WITH SPECIFIC METABOLIC OR OTHER DEFECTS

Hereditary amyloidoses

There are four varieties of inherited neuropathy in which deposition of amyloid occurs. It appears that these are genetically distinct, although this is not entirely certain for types I and III. All are of autosomal dominant inheritance. The pathogenesis of neuropathy in amyloidosis is not absolutely clear, but it is likely to be related to the presence of amyloid deposits both in peripheral nerve and in sensory and autonomic ganglia. Degeneration of axons may occur before amyloid is detectable histologically in nerve biopsies and this led to the suggestion that amyloid deposition was a later event (Coimbra and Andrade, 1971). Absence of amyloid in distal nerve biopsies, however, does not preclude its presence more proximally. Amyloid deposits are usually seen initially within the endoneurium or around the vasa nervorum. Their distribution is widespread in peripheral nerve trunks, and sympathetic and dorsal root ganglia. The diagnosis of amyloid neuropathy is often suggested by a characteristic clinical picture, but it may be confirmed by peripheral nerve biopsy.

TYPE I (ANDRADE)

This condition was first described in northern Portugal by Andrade (1952) but it has also been observed in Brazil, Japan (Araki *et al.*, 1968) and elsewhere. It is the commonest form of hereditary amyloid neuropathy. Onset is usually in the third and fourth decades, with the insidious development of loss of pain and temperature sensation in the legs. This is often associated with pain and sometimes paraesthesiae. Sensory disturbance in the upper limbs eventually appears, and loss of joint position and vibration sense, distal wasting and weakness and tendon areflexia are late features of the disease. Autonomic failure, comprising impotence, postural hypotension, distal anhidrosis, abnormal pupils, and bladder and bowel involvement, often gives rise to early symptoms. The loss of pain sensation in the feet may lead to neuropathic arthropathy and skin ulceration. Amyloid deposition also occurs in the ocular vitreous, kidneys and heart. The disorder is progressive and patients generally die about 10 years after onset.

TYPE II (RUKAVINA)

This variant has been described in two families in the USA (Rukavina *et al.*, 1956; Mahloudji *et al.*, 1969). It often presents with the carpal tunnel syndrome in early middle life. Symptoms and signs of more generalized sensory and autonomic neuropathy follow, and visceral deposition of amyloid occurs. The disease is, again, slowly progressive.

TYPE III (VAN ALLEN)

The clinical features of type III hereditary amyloid neuropathy are similar to those of type I but autonomic features are less conspicuous (van Allen, Frohlich and Davis, 1969). There is a high incidence of duodenal ulcer amongst affected individuals.

TYPE IV (MERETOJA)

This condition is characterized by cranial neuropathy, lattice corneal dystrophy and skin laxity. Onset, with corneal opacities, is usually in the third decade of life. Signs of neuropathy in the limbs may develop later (Boysen *et al.*, 1979). The disease was first described by Meretoja and Teppo (1971) in Finland.

Porphyria

Peripheral neuropathy occurs in acute intermittent and variegate porphyria, and also in hereditary coproporphyria. All three are of autosomal dominant inheritance. The clinical features of the neuropathy are similar. Onset is subacute, over days or weeks, and there are usually prodromal or accompanying abdominal symptoms and psychiatric disturbances. Muscle weakness may be generalized, proximal, distal or asymmetrical, and is sometimes more prominent in the arms than the legs. Paradoxical retention of the ankle jerks with loss of the knee jerks may also be observed. Autonomic features, including vomiting, abdominal pain, tachycardia, hypertension and retention of urine, are frequent. Recovery usually occurs but is slow. Cutaneous photosensitivity often precedes acute episodes of neuropathy by a number of years in variegate porphyria.

Outside South Africa, acute intermittent porphyria is the most commonly encountered type. Its exact prevalence is difficult to assess because of the large number of asymptomatic cases. The incidence of the disorder in Sweden and England has been estimated at 1:13 000 and 1:18 000 (Wetterberg, 1967; Hierons, 1957). Females are more likely to have acute attacks than males. Variegate porphyria occurs in about 3 per 1000 of the white South African population. It is rare elsewhere in the world, apart perhaps from Finland (Mustajoki, 1980). Introduction of the gene mutation into South Africa can be traced to a Dutch couple who emigrated in 1688. The disease has only become a significant medical problem with widespread use of drugs. Hereditary coproporphyria is extremely rare.

Haem synthesis is defective in the porphyrias. In acute intermittent porphyria, there is a deficiency of uroporphyrinogen I synthetase which gives rise to a block in the synthetic pathway for haem and accumulation of δ-aminolaevulinic acid (ALA) and porphobilinogen (PBG) (Strand *et al.*, 1970; Watson *et al.*, 1973). In acute attacks, excess amounts of ALA and PBG are excreted in the urine. This also occurs to a lesser extent in variegate porphyria, although the exact metabolic defect in this disorder is unknown. Hereditary coproporphyria is due to a deficiency of coproporphyrin oxidase (Elder *et al.*, 1976). Coproporphyrin and protoporphyrin are excreted in large amounts in the faeces in variegate porphyria. The precipitation of acute attacks of acute intermittent porphyria by a number of drugs, particularly barbiturates, is thought to result from induction of a hepatic cytochrome which increases demands for haem and thus induces ALA synthetase activity. The reason for development of neuropathy in the porphyrias is not known. Porphyric neuropathy is also discussed briefly in Chapter 5.

Neuropathies associated with disorders of lipid metabolism

Metachromatic leucodystrophy

Metachromatic leucodystrophy (MLD) is genetically heterogeneous and comprises at least five distinct autosomal recessive disorders. In all of them, galactosyl sulphatide accumulates in glia, Schwann cells and macrophages, and stains metachromatically. Demyelination occurs in the central and peripheral nervous systems.

A deficiency of aryl sulphatase A occurs in the infantile, juvenile and late onset forms of MLD, whereas multiple sulphatase deficiencies exist in a further rare variant. Heterozygotes for the three types of aryl sulphatase A deficiency have reduced enzyme activity, usually about 50% of normal but occasionally extending into the homozygote range (Dubois, Harzer and Baumann, 1977). This has been explained on the basis of segregation of more than one mutant allele for the structural gene of aryl sulphatase A within the population (Langenbeck *et al.*, 1977). Recently, an additional variety has been described, the AB variant, in which aryl sulphatase activity is normal (Hahn *et al.*, 1981, 1982). This is possibly the result of a deficiency of activator enzyme. The cause of the demyelination in MLD is not fully understood: there is not a great deal of correlation between the amount of storage material and degree of demyelination. Sulphatide storage could potentially interfere with Schwann cell function, or an abnormal composition of myelin may give rise to instability (O'Brien, 1964). Motor nerve conduction velocity in peripheral nerves is reduced, and sensory nerve action potentials are reduced in amplitude or absent (Fullerton, 1964; Yudell *et al.*, 1967). Extensive segmental demyelination is seen in nerve biopsies, together with metachromatically staining material within Schwann cells and macrophages (Norman, Urich and Tingey, 1960; Dayan, 1967). Ultrastructurally, inclusions comprising myelin figures, prismatic inclusions, zebra bodies and 'tuffstone' bodies are seen in peripheral nerve (Bischoff, 1975; Thomas *et al.*, 1977). The metachromasia is related to the presence of lamellar material with a 5.8 nm periodicity.

LATE INFANTILE METACHROMATIC LEUCODYSTROPHY

This is by far the commonest form of MLD. Onset is usually between the ages of 1 and 2 years, but may occur up until the fourth year of life. Antecedent development is normal. Irritability and poor feeding are noticed early in the course of the disease. These are followed by difficulties in walking, sitting and crawling due to ataxia, weakness and hypotonia. The tendon reflexes are usually depressed or absent. In the second stage of the illness, muscle tone increases and weakness and ataxia are more obvious. There is dysarthria and dementia. The latter is progressive and eventually the child is quadriplegic, deaf and blind due to optic atrophy. Opisthotonus and myoclonic jerks occur. The tendon reflexes usually remain depressed but the plantar responses are extensor. Patients die at about the age of 6 years (Hagberg, 1963).

JUVENILE METACHROMATIC LEUCODYSTROPHY

This form of MLD develops between the ages of 3 and 20, but usually during the first decade. The incidence of the disease is about one quarter that of the late infantile type. The clinical features are similar, but rather more variable in the juvenile onset cases. The first symptoms are most commonly behavioural and gait disturbances. Most, but not all, patients have depressed or absent tendon reflexes. Choreoathetoid movements may occur. The disease is relentlessly progressive, but survival to the seventh decade has been reported (Schutta *et al.*, 1966; Austin *et al.*, 1968; Dulaney and Moser, 1978; Gordon, 1978).

ADULT ONSET METACHROMATIC LEUCODYSTROPHY

Less than 20 patients with this syndrome have been described. Onset is usually in the late second and third decades, so distinction of late juvenile and early adult onset cases is somewhat arbitrary. The diagnosis should be considered in any adult with a combination of dementia and peripheral neuropathy; Bosch and Hart (1978) described a patient who first developed symptoms at the age of 62 years. The clinical features are similar to those of the juvenile type, with a variable mixture of cerebellar and pyramidal signs, dementia, optic atrophy and peripheral neuro-pathy. The last may be clinically unobtrusive. The disorder is again slowly progressive (Pilz, 1972; Pilz *et al.*, 1977; Percy, Kaback and Herndon, 1977).

MULTIPLE SULPHATASE DEFICIENCY

This disorder, sometimes referred to as the O variant, is characterized biochemically by deficiencies of arylsulphatases A, B and C. Clinically it resembles the late infantile form of MLD but additional features, including ichthyosis, flaring of the ribs and hepatosplenomegaly, are present. Death occurs between the ages of 3 and 12 years (Austin, 1965; Rampini *et al.*, 1970; Moser *et al.*, 1972).

AB VARIANT

A further variant of MLD has recently been recognized in which the activity of arylsulphatase A and B is normal. It has therefore been termed the AB variant (Hahn *et al.*, 1981, 1982). Onset has been in early childhood with a protracted course. The changes in peripheral nerve are similar to those of the classical form of MLD.

Globoid cell leucodystrophy (Krabbe's disease)

This rare disease is caused by a deficiency of galactosylceramide β-galactosidase. Inheritance is autosomal recessive. The name of the condition arose from the finding of multinucleate globoid cells (macrophages) containing prismatic and tubular inclusions composed of cerebroside, in cerebral white matter. Globoid cells are not present in peripheral nerve, but similar inclusions are found in Schwann cells and endoneurial macrophages. Demyelination and axonal loss are demonstrable (Bischoff and Ulrich, 1969).

Onset is between 3 and 6 months. Arrest and deterioration of motor and intellectual development occurs associated with generalized hypertonus, optic atrophy, deafness, tonic seizures and intermittent fever. Loss of tendon reflexes is often noted about 6 months after onset (Dunn *et al.*, 1969), and the presence of peripheral neuropathy may be confirmed by the use of nerve conduction studies. Patients die between the ages of 18 and 24 months (Wilson, Lake and Dunn, 1970). Reports of later onset cases suggest that globoid cell leucodystrophy is genetically heterogenous (Liu, 1970; Crome *et al.*, 1973). The patients described to date have had an age of onset between 2 and 6 years, and a clinical picture characterized by dementia, blindness due to optic atrophy and cortical lesions, and spasticity. Peripheral nerve involvement is not invariable.

Adrenoleucodystrophy and adrenomyeloneuropathy

Adrenoleucodystrophy is an X-linked recessive disorder. The exact metabolic defect has not been identified but an increased ratio of C26 to C22 fatty acids can be demonstrated in the skin fibroblasts of patients and carriers (Moser *et al.*, 1980; O'Neill, Moser and Saxena, 1981). The disease gives rise to progressive dementia, quadriplegia, seizures, blindness and adrenal insufficiency in childhood. Elongated inclusions in macrophages are seen in cerebral white matter, the adrenal cortex and Schwann cells (Powers and Schaumburg, 1974; Schaumburg *et al.*, 1975). It is likely that adrenomyeloneuropathy is caused by the same gene mutation, as both syndromes have been reported in members of the same family. Adreno-myeloneuropathy is characterized clinically by spastic paraplegia, distal muscle weakness and sensory loss (Griffin *et al.*, 1977). These features develop in adolescence or adult life and are usually preceded by hypoadrenalism, and sometimes hypogonadism. Female carriers may have mild spastic paraparesis and adrenal insufficiency.

Cockayne syndrome

This syndrome comprises growth retardation, progeria, ataxia, pigmentary retinopathy, deafness, photosensitivity and mental retardation. Hyporeflexia, slow motor nerve conduction velocities and loss of myelinated fibres together with segmental demyelination in nerve have been described (Moosa and Dubowitz, 1970; Lewis, Grunnet and Zimmerman, 1982). The central nervous system changes are those of primary white matter disease and the disorder is thus probably classifiable as a leucodystrophy.

Hereditary high density lipoprotein deficiency (Tangier disease)

Tangier disease is rare; less than 30 cases have been reported to date. It is of autosomal recessive inheritance. High density α-lipoproteins are markedly reduced in the plasma of affected individuals; plasma cholesterol is also low, whereas triglyceride levels may be normal or increased. Cholesteryl esters are deposited in several tissues, including the spleen, tonsils, bone marrow, intestine and skin (Herbert, Gotto and Fredrickson, 1978; Yao *et al.*, 1978). About half of the patients reported with Tangier disease have had peripheral nerve involvement. Pathologically, this manifests as degeneration of unmyelinated and small myelinated nerve fibres, with the accumulation of neutral lipids and cholesteryl esters in Schwann cells (Kocen *et al.*, 1973; Dyck *et al.*, 1978). The aetiology of this neuropathy is unknown.

Onset of neurological symptoms is either in childhood or adult life. Two syndromes are observed (Pollock *et al.*, 1983). The first is the occurrence of transient mononeuropathies. The second is a generalized neuropathy with a curious combination of weakness of the facial and small hand muscles, depressed or absent tendon reflexes and extensive dissociated loss of pain and temperature sensation. This often spares the distal parts of the limbs and resembles the sensory disturbance seen in syringomyelia (*Figure 9.1*). A clue to the diagnosis is the presence of enlarged, yellow pigmented tonsils due to the deposition of cholesteryl esters (Kocen *et al.*, 1967; Haas, Austad and Bergin, 1974; Dyck *et al.*, 1978).

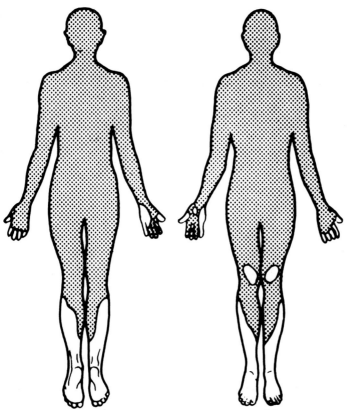

Figure 9.1 Tangier disease. Shaded areas show distribution of reduced pain and temperature sensation. (From Kocen *et al.*, 1967, courtesy of the Editor and Publishers, *The Lancet*)

Abetalipoproteinaemia (Bassen-Kornzweig disease)

This is another autosomal recessive disorder which has been described most frequently amongst the Ashkenazi Jewish population. It is characterized biochemically by hypocholesterolaemia, low levels of circulating phospholipids, free fatty acids and chylomicrons, and the absence of low density lipoproteins. It is likely that the disease is caused by failure of synthesis of apoprotein B. This substance, which is important in the transport of triglyceride from intestinal cells into plasma, is absent in abetalipoproteinaemia.

The disorder usually presents with symptoms of fat malabsorption in infancy, but these may not be severe and often subside with age. Symptoms of neurological dysfunction, of which the first is usually ataxia, occur during the first decade in one third of cases, and nearly always by the age of 20. Depressed or absent tendon reflexes may be found before symptoms develop. The clinical features are similar to those of Friedreich's ataxia, with dysarthria, cerebellar ataxia, areflexia, proprioceptive loss, pes cavus and scoliosis. However, muscle weakness tends to be generalized rather than pyramidal in distribution and extensor plantar responses are not universal. Also, loss of touch, pain and temperature sensation occur, and pigmentary retinal degeneration is common. Acanthocytes are found in peripheral blood smears. Motor nerve conduction velocity is normal or slightly reduced and sensory nerve action potentials are reduced in amplitude or absent. Sural nerve biopsy shows loss of myelinated fibres (Herbert, Gotto and Fredrickson, 1978; Miller *et al.*, 1980).

There is an increasing amount of evidence to suggest that the neurological complications of abetalipoproteinaemia are secondary to deficiency of vitamin E. The disease is associated with very low or absent serum vitamin E levels from birth (Muller, Lloyd and Bird, 1977).

Phytanic acid storage disease (Refsum's disease)

Refsum's disease is uncommon and only about 100 cases have been reported. It has been suggested that the original mutation arose in Scandinavia, and that the disorder was disseminated by the Vikings; the majority of patients have been described in Norway, Sweden, Germany, France, UK and Ireland (Richterich, Rosen and Rossi, 1965). Inheritance is autosomal recessive and there is an increased incidence of parental consanguinity.

The neurological disorder is probably directly related to accumulation of phytanic acid (3,7,11,15-tetramethylhexadecanoic acid) in the peripheral and central nervous systems (Refsum *et al.*, 1975). Phytanic acid is a metabolic product of phytol which is present in the diet as a component of plant and animal lipids. In Refsum's disease, normal alpha oxidation of phytanic acid to α-hydroxyphytanic acid is blocked, leading to high serum and tissue levels of phytanic acid (Refsum *et al.*, 1975; Kahlke, 1964). A partial defect of phytanic acid oxidation has been shown in skin fibroblasts from heterozygotes (Herndon, Steinberg and Uhlendorf, 1969).

The major clinical feature of the disease is that of a chronic distal sensorimotor neuropathy. Symptoms usually develop between the ages of 10 and 30 years, but occasionally in childhood or middle life. Cerebellar ataxia and atypical pigmentary retinal degeneration are usual. Other associated abnormalities include cataract, sensorineural deafness, anosmia, pupillary changes, skeletal deformities and ichthyosis. Cardiomyopathy occurs and may lead to sudden death (Refsum *et al.*, 1975). The course is usually slowly progressive but remissions and relapses are not uncommon.

The neuropathy is of demyelinating type and the peripheral nerves may be palpably thickened. Nerve conduction velocities are sometimes, but not always, markedly reduced (Salisachs, 1982). This is probably due to the fact that demyelination, with hypertrophic changes, is most marked in the proximal parts of the peripheral nerves and in the roots (Refsum *et al.*, 1975).

Alpha-galactosidase A deficiency (Fabry's disease)

Alpha-galactosidase is a lysosomal hydrolase and deficiency results in impaired breakdown of some glycosphingolipids and their deposition in the tissues, including peripheral nerve (Kint, 1970). Fabry's disease is of X-linked recessive inheritance and linkage to the Xg blood group locus has been demonstrated (Opitz *et al.*, 1965; Johnston *et al.*, 1968). Antenatal diagnosis is possible (Brady *et al.*, 1971). The characteristic systemic manifestation of the disorder is the presence of angiokeratoma corporis diffusum. These are scaly telangiectatic skin lesions which are seen over the trunk, particularly in the 'bathing trunks' area. Other features include corneal dystrophy, dilated conjunctival blood vessels, multifocal cerebral ischaemia, cardiac murmurs and renal failure.

Pain is the major neurological symptom, and is due to a sensory neuropathy. Pain generally develops in childhood or adolescence, and may be the presenting symptom of the disease. There is often a constant aching in the limbs with episodic severe burning pain in the extremities which may be triggered by emotional stress and other factors. Neurological examination is usually normal (Bischoff *et al.*, 1968). Pathologically there is loss of small unmyelinated and myelinated fibres in peripheral nerves related to loss of small dorsal root ganglion cells. Deposits of lamellated glycosphingolipids are seen in perineurial and vascular endothelial cells in nerve (Bischoff *et al.*, 1968; Kocen and Thomas, 1970; Ohnishi and Dyck, 1974). Female carriers very occasionally exhibit all the features of the disease, but more often have mild clinical involvement, such as asymptomatic corneal dystrophy, or none at all. They have reduced activity of α-galactosidase in leucocytes and skin fibroblasts, but this is not generally as severe as the deficiency found in affected males.

Disorders associated with defective DNA repair

Ataxia telangiectasia

This autosomal recessive disorder first gives rise to symptoms in early childhood. The cardinal clinical features are cerebellar ataxia, oculomotor dyspraxia, oculocutaneous telangiectasia, and immunological incompetence. The tendon reflexes are depressed and eventually disappear. Sensory loss (mainly of proprioception) and distal weakness develop late in the evolution of the disease. Nerve conduction studies show small or absent sensory action potentials and slight slowing of motor nerve conduction velocity in older patients, and there may be evidence of denervation in distal muscles on electromyography. There is loss of large myelinated fibres in peripheral nerve (Goodman *et al.*, 1969; Dunn, 1973). DNA repair following gamma irradiation is defective in ataxia telangiectasia (Taylor *et al.*, 1975)

Xeroderma pigmentosum

This syndrome is characterized by hypersensitivity to u.v. light and primarily manifests itself as a dermatological disorder. Skin malignancies are common. Excision repair of damaged DNA is defective. The disorder is heterogeneous and cell hybridization and complementation studies have identified six genetically distinct subgroups.

Depressed or absent tendon reflexes are common in xeroderma pigmentosum, and may be the only neurological manifestation of the disorder. Others include microcephaly, mental retardation, seizures, spasticity, cerebellar ataxia and choreoathetosis. Nerve conduction studies may show abnormal sensory nerve action potentials, and loss of large myelinated fibres has been described in peripheral nerve (Robbins *et al.*, 1974; Thrush *et al.*, 1974). Inheritance is autosomal recessive.

NEUROPATHIES OF UNKNOWN CAUSE

Hereditary motor and sensory neuropathy

The hereditary motor and sensory neuropathies are the most common of the disorders that give rise to the peroneal muscular atrophy syndrome, or Charcot-Marie-Tooth disease (*Figure 9.2*). Peroneal muscular atrophy is merely a syndrome, and not a diagnosis in itself. The classification of the hereditary motor and sensory neuropathies was somewhat confused until recently, but the advent of peripheral nerve electrophysiological and histological investigations, together with family studies, has clarified this issue to a large extent. The historical development of our understanding of these disorders, and the somewhat confusing nomenclature attached to them, have recently been reviewed (Harding and Thomas, 1980a).

Genetic and clinical studies of a considerable number of families with hereditary motor and sensory neuropathy have mostly shown that there are two groups of cases, one in which motor nerve conduction velocity in the upper limbs is usually less than about 38 m/s, and another in which conduction velocity is normal or only slightly reduced. Intrafamilial concordance for motor conduction velocity is high, and statistical analyses support the suggestion of genetic heterogeneity. Nerve biopsies from patients with reduced conduction velocity show evidence of segmental demyelination, sometimes accompanied by hypertrophic changes, with 'onion bulb' formation. Those from cases with slightly reduced or normal motor nerve conduction velocity show axonal degeneration with little in the way of segmental demyelination. These two groups have been termed the hypertrophic (or demyelinating) and the neuronal (or axonal) types of Charcot-Marie-Tooth disease respectively, or hereditary motor and sensory neuropathy (HMSN) types I and II (Dyck and Lambert, 1968a, b; Thomas, Calne and Stewart, 1974; Buchthal and Behse, 1977; Harding and Thomas, 1980a). The peroneal muscular atrophy phenotype is also observed as a manifestation of hereditary distal spinal muscular atrophy (Harding and Thomas, 1980b). In addition to HMSN types I and II, there exists a severe demyelinating neuropathy which presents with abnormal motor development in infancy. This is known as HMSN type III.

The division of HMSN types I and II on the basis of upper limb motor nerve conduction velocity as described above has been agreed upon by the majority of authors but objections to this classification have been raised by Humberstone (1972) and Salisachs (1974) who have reported random distributions of conduction velocity in HMSN. Davis, Bradley and Madrid (1978) proposed the existence of an

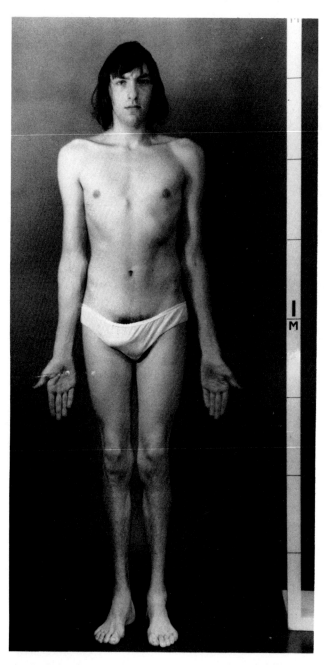

Figure 9.2 Adolescent male at time of presentation with peroneal muscular atrophy showing distal wasting in legs and pes cavus. He was a member of a family with hereditary motor and sensory neuropathy type II

intermediate group on the basis of neurophysiological and pathological studies. Some families are difficult to classify with certainty because, for example, velocities ranging from 30–50 m/s may be recorded from their members. Even greater difficulties may be encountered if only one family member is available for study. This is not surprising, for motor conduction velocity is an indirect and crude disease parameter for HMSN and it would be naive to suggest that it should be a universally reliable marker of the genotype. Motor conduction velocity can be used to divide large series of cases of HMSN statistically and discrimination is good in the majority of patients. Substantial discordance for conduction within families is rare in practice and sometimes may be explicable in terms of recording or diagnostic difficulties. The genetic distinction of types I and II HMSN is confirmed by the demonstration of linkage between dominantly inherited type I HMSN and the Duffy blood group locus. HMSN type II is not linked to Duffy (Bird, Ott and Giblett, 1980; Guiloff *et al.*, 1982).

There is evidence for further genetic heterogeneity within the types I and II disease categories delineated above. Inheritance may be autosomal dominant or autosomal recessive in both. Dominant inheritance is more common, but about 10% of cases of both types are confined to a single sibship and have normal parents (Harding and Thomas, 1980c, d). The incidence of parental consanguinity is increased in these families. It should be stressed that autosomal recessive inheritance cannot be assumed in either disorder unless both parents have been examined clinically and electrophysiologically. X-linked recessive inheritance of HMSN is extremely rare, if it exists at all. A number of families have been reported as having X-linked HMSN (Herringham, 1889; Church, 1906; Bell, 1935; Allan, 1939; Woratz, 1964; Skre, 1974) but it is likely that in most, if not all, inheritance was autosomal dominant with incomplete expression in the females (Harding and Thomas, 1980d).

Autosomal dominant HMSN type I

Worldwide, this is probably the commonest form of HMSN. Two-thirds of patients develop symptoms in the first decade and one-quarter in the second. Onset is rare over the age of 30 years. The most frequent presenting symptoms are difficulties in walking or running and foot deformity. Slowly progressive distal weakness and wasting of the lower limbs are usually the most prominent features, with relatively severe involvement of the peroneal and anterior tibial muscles. Similar involvement of the upper limbs occurs later in most patients. The tendon reflexes are all absent in nearly 60% of cases; depressed or absent ankle jerks are virtually universal. The plantar responses are most often flexor or absent, but occasionally extensor. Sensory impairment, particularly in the legs, occurs in about 70%. Vibration sense is the most frequently affected modality, followed by pain and touch appreciation. Proprioceptive loss is found in about one-half of patients with the disease. Peripheral nerve hypertrophy is clinically detectable in one third. Pes cavus is present in more than two thirds, and tends to be more severe in early onset cases. Scoliosis, usually of mild or moderate degree, is found in 14%. Rare features include facial and bulbar weakness and pupillary abnormalities (Dyck and Lambert, 1968a; Buchthal and Behse, 1977; Harding and Thomas, 1980a).

Special mention should be made here of the so-called Roussy-Lévy syndrome. This eponym tends to be applied to cases of HMSN with prominent ataxia or tremor. These features are found, in varying severity, in about 30% of patients with HMSN type I. Ataxia may be absent, mild or marked within members of the same family (Harding and Thomas, 1980a). The neurophysiological features of HMSN type I and the Roussy-Lévy syndrome are identical (Lapresle and Salisachs, 1973). There is thus good evidence that the Roussy-Lévy syndrome is a phenotypic expression of the gene for HMSN type I. It is certainly not a *forme fruste* of Friedreich's ataxia, and there is no genetic relationship between Friedreich's ataxia and HMSN (Harding, 1981).

HMSN type I varies considerably in severity. A few patients lose the ability to walk, but rarely before the age of 50; 10% never have symptoms but are clinically affected. Males, on average, tend to be slightly more severely affected than females. The disease is very slowly progressive and often appears to be relatively static after the growth period has ceased (Harding and Thomas, 1980a).

Motor nerve conduction velocity in HMSN type I is usually between 10 and 35 m/s in the upper limbs. The small foot muscles are often denervated. Sensory nerve conduction is similarly always abnormal and sensory nerve action potentials are usually unrecordable percutaneously. *See also* Chapter 3 on chronic demyelinating neuropathy.

Autosomal recessive HMSN type I

The clinical features of the autosomal recessive form of HMSN type I are similar to the dominant variety, although there is an impression that the recessive cases are rather more severe. The mean age of onset is about 10 years, with symptoms developing in childhood or early adolescence. Motor milestones may be slightly delayed. The incidence of muscle weakness, ataxia, sensory loss, tendon areflexia and scoliosis is higher in the recessive group. Motor nerve conduction velocity is, on average, lower than in the dominant cases, with values often less than 20 m/s. Peripheral nerve thickening is common and this is reflected histologically by extensive hypertrophic changes. This disorder is often confused clinically with Friedreich's ataxia, but the two are easily distinguished electrophysiologically. The prognosis in autosomal recessive HMSN type I is much better than that for Friedreich's ataxia, although probably not as good as the dominant form of HMSN type I (Dyck and Lambert, 1968a; Davis, Bradley and Madrid, 1978; Harding and Thomas, 1980c).

Autosomal dominant HMSN type II

This form of HMSN tends to give rise to symptoms later than type I. About 30% of cases present in the first decade of life. Peak onset is in the second decade but a considerable number are asymptomatic until much later, sometimes up to the age of 60 years or more. The disease is similar to HMSN type I and the two cannot be distinguished clinically with certainty (*Figure 9.2*). The upper limbs are affected in only 50% of patients with type II HMSN, which is less than in type I. Ataxia and tremor occur much less frequently in type II, and reflex changes are not so severe. About 50% do not have clinical sensory loss. Pes cavus is present in only half, which presumably reflects the later onset of the disorder. Scoliosis is unusual. Type II HMSN is slowly progressive and few patients lose the ability to walk. Females are, again, less severely affected than males; 20% of patients of both sexes are asymptomatic (Harding and Thomas, 1980a).

Motor nerve conduction velocity in the upper limbs may be in the normal range but is usually between 38 and 58 m/s. It is slower in the lower limbs. Sensory conduction is always abnormal, but sensory nerve action potentials are detectable using percutaneous recording in about one quarter of patients. Pathologically, type II HMSN is characterized by axonal degeneration with little evidence of segmental demyelination (Dyck and Lambert, 1968b).

Autosomal recessive HMSN type II

This form of HMSN is rare, and has been described in less than 10 families. It may be a heterogeneous syndrome as severe early onset and relatively mild, later onset cases have been reported (Harding and Thomas, 1980c; Hagberg and Lyon 1981; Ouvrier *et al.*, 1981). The age of onset is most commonly before the age of 5 years, and rarely after the second decade. This differs markedly from the dominant form of HMSN type II. Muscle weakness is more severe in the recessive cases and may involve proximal muscles. The patients described by Ouvrier *et al.* (1981) had severe paralysis of the hands and feet by the age of 20 years and a number were unable to walk in their teens. Ataxia of the upper limbs is present in a small proportion of patients and sensory loss is common. The tendon reflexes are all absent in about 50%. Pes cavus and scoliosis are relatively rare. Some of the severely affected patients reported by Ouvrier *et al.* (1981) had claw hands and joint contractures. Motor nerve conduction velocities range from 35 m/s to the upper part of the normal range. The small foot muscles may be denervated. Sensory nerve action potentials are small or unobtainable. The pathological changes are those of an axonal degeneration, but there is greater reduction of myelinated fibre density and involvement of unmyelinated fibres than in the dominant form of type II HMSN (Ouvrier *et al.*, 1981).

HMSN type III

This is a rare autosomal recessive syndrome and may well be heterogenous. It includes severe cases of genetically-determined demyelinating neuropathy which have sometimes been referred to as Dejerine-Sottas disease in the past. Motor milestones are delayed and normal development is never achieved. Scoliosis is often severe. Motor nerve conduction velocity is usually less than 10 m/s (Dyck and Lambert, 1968a), and the CSF protein content is often increased. The pathological changes include hypomyelination as well as demyelination (*Figure 9.3*) and cases of congenital hypomyelination are probably best classified as HMSN type III (Lyon,

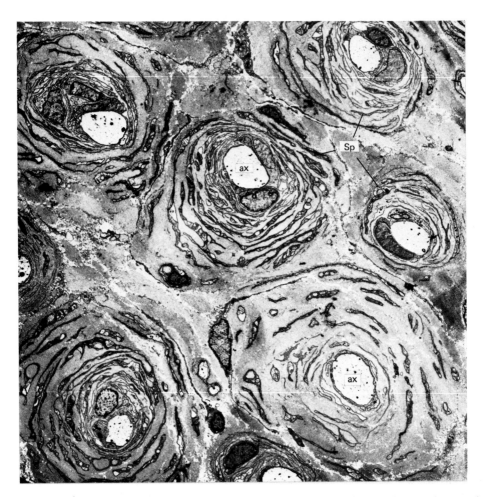

Figure 9.3 Hereditary motor and sensory neuropathy, type III. Electron micrograph showing amyelinate axons (ax) surrounded by proliferated Schwann cell processes (×2500)

1969; Dyck *et al.*, 1971; Anderson *et al.*, 1973; Kennedy, Sung and Berry, 1977; Guzzetta, Ferrière and Lyon, 1982). Early suggestions of a disturbance of ceramide hexosides and hexoside sulphates in this disorder (Dyck *et al.*, 1970) have not been confirmed (Yao and Dyck, 1981). It is of interest that the homozygous expression of the gene for HMSN type I gives rise to a clinical picture similar to that of HMSN type III (Killian and Kloepfer, 1979). It is not known whether similar histological appearances occur.

Other forms of HMSN

There have been a number of reports describing patients with HMSN and other neurological features. These are rare and include optic atrophy and deafness (Rosenberg and Chutorian, 1967; Iwashita *et al.*, 1970), deafness (Satya-Murti, Cacace and Hanson, 1979), optic atrophy (McLeod, Low and Morgan, 1978) and pigmentary retinal degeneration (Massion-Verniory, Dumont and Potvin, 1946). Those with optic atrophy combined with deafness, and pigmentary retinopathy were of autosomal recessive inheritance but the others were autosomal dominant. There is a further disorder giving rise to the peroneal muscular atrophy syndrome in which pyramidal features occur (Dyck and Lambert, 1968b; Harding and Thomas, 1984). Tone tends to be increased in the legs and the knee jerks are usually brisk, although the ankle jerks are depressed or absent. The plantar responses are extensor, and this finding runs true in families. Sensory nerve conduction may be abnormal. The X-linked recessive form of bulbospinal muscular atrophy is generally thought of as a form of spinal muscular atrophy but electrophysiological evidence of sensory neuropathy is frequent in this disorder. Affected males have proximal neurogenic muscle weakness, hyporeflexia, fasciculation of the face and tongue together with dysphagia and dysarthria, postural upper limb tremor and gynaecomastia. Symptoms develop in the third to sixth decades of life (Kennedy, Alter and Sung, 1968; Harding *et al.*, 1982).

Hereditary sensory and autonomic neuropathies

This category includes a number of disorders characterized by a prominence of sensory loss without corresponding motor involvement, by autonomic features or by a combination of the two. At present it is possible to identify dominantly and recessively inherited forms of hereditary sensory neuropathy, hereditary sensory neuropathy with anhidrosis, and the Riley-Day syndrome, together with a number of less well categorized syndromes.

Dominantly inherited sensory neuropathy

The recognition of this condition as a sensory neuropathy was originally made by Denny-Brown (1951) under the title of hereditary sensory radicular neuropathy in a family previously reported as hereditary perforating ulcers of the feet (Hicks, 1922). It constitutes hereditary sensory and autonomic neuropathy type I (HSAN I) in the classification proposed by Dyck (1983). Onset is commonly during the second decade with loss of pain and temperature sensation distally in the lower limbs and later in the upper limbs. Other sensory modalities are affected subsequently and there may be slight distal motor signs. Spontaneous pains, mainly in the legs, are often a troublesome feature. These take the form of a generalized aching or of sharp lightning pains. Autonomic symptoms are not a feature.

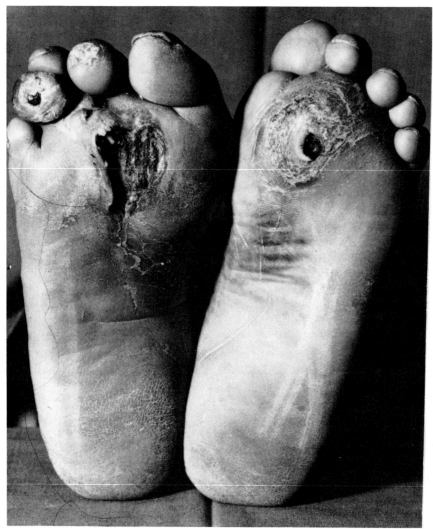

Figure 9.4 Chronic ulceration of feet in dominantly inherited sensory neuropathy

Neuropathic joint degeneration and persistent foot ulceration (*Figure 9.4*) are often troublesome complications. The condition is very slowly progressive. In the early stages, there is a selective loss of small myelinated fibres (Sluga, 1974), with later involvement of all myelinated fibres.

Recessively inherited sensory neuropathy

In this form evidence of neuropathy is present from birth. It has been categorized as hereditary sensory neuropathy type II (HSN II, Ohta *et al.*, 1973) or HSAN II

(Dyck, 1983). There is sensory loss for all sensory modalities, touch-pressure being more severely affected than pain and temperature sensibility (Ohta *et al.*, 1973). The sensory loss is distal in distribution and frequently leads to a mutilating acropathy with neuropathic joint degeneration, tissue destruction and loss of digits. Physiological investigation has failed to demonstrate significant autonomic involvement (Johnson and Spalding, 1964). Although it has been considered that the neuropathy, as distinct from the secondary development of acropathy, is substantially nonprogressive (Murray, 1973), it is probably slowly progressive (Johnson and Spalding, 1964; Ohta *et al.*, 1973; Nukada, Pollock and Haas, 1982).

Nerve biopsies have demonstrated almost total absence of myelinated fibres and a reduction in the unmyelinated fibre population (Ohta *et al.*, 1973).

Riley-Day syndrome (familial dysautonomia)

Occurring most often in Jewish children, this autosomal recessive condition gives rise to difficulty in feeding in infancy, recurrent vomiting and pulmonary infections. There are prominent disturbances of autonomic function including diminished lachrymation, defective temperature regulation, episodes of hypertension and postural hypotension, together with skin blotching and excessive sweating provoked by emotional stimuli. The tendon reflexes are absent and a failure to respond to painful stimuli is evident from the time of birth. The fungiform papillae of the tongue fail to develop. Kyphoscoliosis may appear later in childhood. The clinical and genetic features have been reviewed by Mahloudji, Brunt and McKusick (1970). It constitutes HSAN type III in the classification of Dyck (1983).

The peripheral nerves show a severe depletion in unmyelinated axons and a less severe reduction in the numbers of small myelinated axons (Aguayo, Nair and Bray, 1971). The numbers of neurons in the dorsal root, trigeminal and autonomic ganglia are also reduced (Pearson, Budzilovich and Finegold, 1971). The neurological disorder is non-progressive and probably represents a neuronal aplasia.

Congenital sensory neuropathy with anhidrosis

This is a rare autosomal recessive disorder which becomes manifest within a few months of birth. Retardation of motor development is accompanied by episodes of unexplained pyrexia and a failure to respond normally to painful stimuli. Widespread loss of pain and temperature sensation is demonstrable and cutaneous ulceration, bone fractures and occasionally self-mutilation may be encountered (Swanson, Buchan and Alvord, 1965; Pinsky and DiGeorge, 1966; Vassella *et al.*, 1968). There is a selective loss of small myelinated fibres in sensory nerves and in Lissauer's tract and a virtual absence of unmyelinated axons (Swanson, Buchan and Alvord, 1965; Goebel, Veit and Dyck, 1980). Survival is usually limited. It has been classified as HSAN type IV (Dyck, 1983).

Other forms of hereditary sensory and autonomic neuropathy

Low, Burke and McLeod (1978) and Dyck *et al.* (1983) have recently described two similar cases that probably represent a separate variant of congenital sensory neuropathy. They have been designated HSAN type V (Dyck *et al.*, 1983). Both displayed a selective loss for pain sensibility which was universal in the latter case and distal in distribution in the former. Sweating was possibly impaired in the case of Dyck *et al.* The distinctive feature was a virtually selective loss of small myelinated fibres with preservation of unmyelinated and large myelinated fibres. Both were single cases with no family history of a similar disorder.

Nordborg *et al.* (1981) have also described what is probably a further separate variant consisting of children with a non-progressive sensory neuropathy and dysautonomia with an almost total loss of myelinated fibres in peripheral nerve. Family history was again lacking.

Finally, a severe autosomal recessive sensory neuropathy leading to a mutilating acropathy may occur in association with hereditary spastic paraplegia (Cavanagh *et al.*, 1979). A more benign variant of this syndrome is inherited as a dominant trait (Koenig and Spiro, 1970).

Neuropathy associated with hereditary ataxias

Abnormal sensory nerve conduction is virtually universal in patients with Friedreich's ataxia. Clinically this is associated with loss of vibration and joint position sense and areflexia. Distal muscle wasting is not uncommon in the late stages of the disease. There is loss of the larger dorsal root ganglion cells and sensory nerve fibres and, less frequently, of anterior horn cells (McLeod, 1971; Dyck, Lambert and Nichols, 1972). Peripheral neuropathy has also been reported in association with the Marinesco-Sjögren syndrome (Serratrice, Gastaut and Dubois-Gambarelli, 1973), dominantly inherited cerebellar ataxia (McLeod and Evans, 1981), glutamate dehydrogenase deficiency (Duvoisin *et al.*, 1983), the Ramsay Hunt syndrome of ataxia and myoclonus (Bird and Shaw, 1978), and dominantly inherited Parkinsonism with ataxia (Ziegler *et al.*, 1972; Byrne, Thomas and Zilkha, 1982).

Miscellaneous disorders

Giant axonal neuropathy

This is a rare autosomal recessive disorder. Less than 10 cases have been described and the parental consanguinity rate is high. The disease is characterized by a slowly progressive sensorimotor neuropathy with onset in early childhood. Variable features include optic atrophy, nystagmus, pyramidal signs in the limbs and abnormal eye movements. Most affected children reported to date have had similar facies and tightly curled hair (Asbury *et al.*, 1972; Berg, Rosenberg and Asbury,

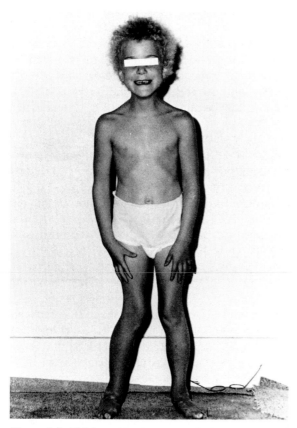

Figure 9.5 Child aged 6 with giant axonal neuropathy showing tightly curled hair and typical facies. (From Berg, Rosenberg and Asbury, 1972, courtesy of the Editor and Publishers, *Pediatrics*. Copyright American Academy of Pediatrics, 1972)

1972; Carpenter *et al.*, 1974; Jones, Nigro and Barre, 1979; Kirkham, Guitton and Coupland, 1980; *Figure 9.5*). The peripheral nerves show large focal axonal swellings which contain an excess number of neurofilaments (Asbury *et al.*, 1972). There is thought to be a generalized disorder of intermediate-size filaments.

Chediak-Higashi disease

This autosomal recessive syndrome is also extremely rare. It comprises defective hair pigmentation, pancytopenia and mental retardation, together with an increased incidence of infection and lymphoreticular maligancy (Blume and Wolff, 1972). Onset is in early childhood. There may be an associated peripheral neuropathy (Lockman, Kennedy and White, 1967), with accumulation of giant lysosomes in Schwann cells.

Chorea-acanthocytosis syndrome

With onset in adult life, this disorder gives rise to chorea, depressed tendon reflexes and variable neurogenic atrophy and sensory loss in the legs. Acanthocytes may be present on peripheral blood smear but this is not invariable. Histologically, there is loss of larger myelinated fibres in the peripheral nerves (Ohnishi *et al.*, 1981). Inheritance appears to be either autosomal dominant or recessive (Estes *et al.*, 1967; Bird *et al.*, 1978).

Hereditary liability to pressure palsies

Predisposition to traction injuries and compression of peripheral nerves may be inherited as an autosomal dominant trait. The condition has recently been reviewed by Meier and Moll (1982). The majority of patients have their first episode of mononeuropathy before the age of 20 years. The peroneal and ulnar nerves are most frequently affected. The brachial plexus and cranial nerves may be involved. Recovery is usually good. Mild slowing of motor and sensory nerve conduction velocity (Earl *et al.*, 1964) indicates a generalized abnormality of peripheral nerve and pathologically there is dysmyelination, with sausage-shaped expansions (tomaculi) where convoluted layers of myelin lamellae thicken the myelin sheath (Behse *et al.*, 1972; Meier and Moll, 1982). Neuralgic amyotrophy has been reported in several members of a few families (Jacob, Andermann and Robb, 1961; Geiger *et al.*, 1974); it is not clear whether these are distinct from those with hereditary liability to pressure palsies.

DIFFERENTIAL DIAGNOSIS

Difficulty in diagnosis of inherited neuropathies most often arises in single cases without a family history, although even in isolated cases the clinical picture may be distinctive. Thus associated features such as the tightly curled hair of children with giant axonal neuropathy (*Figure 9.5*), the enlarged yellow-orange tonsils of Tangier disease, or the characteristic rash of Fabry's disease, may provide a strong indication as to the diagnosis. The neurological picture may also be distinctive as in Refsum's disease, with a combination of sensorimotor neuropathy, ataxia and pigmentary retinal degeneration. Nevertheless, acquired neuropathies that are phenocopies of inherited disorders may be a source of confusion. This may partly explain the male excess in isolated cases of HMSN type II (Harding and Thomas, 1980d). In such cases without a family history, it can be difficult to decide whether they are examples of inherited or acquired disease. Thus sporadic cases of amyloid neuropathy may only be recognized as being of genetic origin when a second family member becomes affected, with consequent implications for disease transmission in this dominantly inherited disorder.

In the clinical recognition of genetic neuropathies, it is convenient to separate those arising in childhood from those with onset in adult life. A genetic basis accounts for a high proportion of childhood neuropathies, particularly where there is evidence of multisystem involvement. Thus neuropathy with ataxia as a prominent associated feature raises the possibility of Friedreich's ataxia, Refsum's disease, abetalipoproteinaemia, ataxia telangiectasia, xeroderma pigmentosum and the Roussy-Lévy variant of HMSN type I. In combination with mental retardation and spasticity, Krabbe's disease, metachromatic leucodystrophy and adreno-leucodystrophy require consideration.

Diagnostic difficulty is most often encountered in relation to motor and sensorimotor neuropathy with no distinctive features. In cases of demyelinating neuropathy with markedly reduced nerve conduction velocity, the diagnosis, after exclusion of Refsum's disease, usually lies between HMSN types I and III and acquired idiopathic inflammatory polyneuropathy. Careful examination, both clinically and with nerve conduction studies, of parents and siblings, may be revealing, as HMSN type I may be transmitted by asymptomatic individuals, particularly females (Harding and Thomas, 1980d). Nerve biopsy is sometimes helpful by demonstrating cellular infiltration if the disorder has an inflammatory basis. Cases of HMSN type III have severely reduced nerve conduction velocity and distinctive nerve biopsy findings (*Figure 9.3*), with hypertrophic appearances in association with uniformly hypomyelinated or amyelinate fibres.

Most sensory neuropathies in childhood (with the exception of leprosy) are inherited. In the past, there have been descriptions of cases designated as congenital indifference to pain (Arbuse, Cantor and Barenberg, 1949; Boyd and Nie, 1949), congenital pure analgesia (Dearborn, 1932), congenital universal insensitivity to pain (McMurray, 1950; Baxter and Olszewski, 1960) and 'asymbolia' for pain (Schilder and Stengel, 1931). Such individuals did not experience pain and did not show the normal physiological responses to noxious stimuli. Postmortem studies failed to demonstrate structural abnormalities in the central or peripheral nervous systems, but the peripheral nerves were not examined by the more sensitive techniques now available. Selective small fibre loss may not have been detected. Their nature is thus uncertain and some may have been instances of congenital sensory neuropathy (Dyck *et al.*, 1983).

In adult life, some inherited neuropathies have distinctive features, such as those related to amyloidosis, Refsum's disease, adrenomyeloneuropathy, Fabry's disease and Tangier disease. HMSN is typified by a lack of distinctive features. Positive symptoms such as paraesthesiae are uncommon and the severity of the weakness and wasting found on examination is often surprisingly great in comparison with the symptoms admitted by the patient, probably because of their insidious onset. The presence of foot or spinal deformity would indicate that the disease started before the cessation of the growth period and thus favour HMSN as the explanation. Difficulty may again arise in distinguishing between cases of HMSN type I with a late onset of symptoms and instances of chronic progressive idiopathic inflammatory polyneuropathy. As in childhood cases, nerve biopsy may be useful in demonstrating cellular infiltrates in chronic inflammatory polyneuropathy.

Amongst cryptogenic neuropathies with onset in adult life, cases with a slowly progressive predominantly motor axonal neuropathy are an important category. Some of these represent late onset HMSN type II. In such cases, skeletal deformity is unlikely to be present. Careful assessment of relatives may detect other family members in whom the presence of neuropathy was unrecognized. Dyck, Oviatt and Lambert (1981) found that 42% of a series of cases of undiagnosed neuropathy were examples of inherited disease after careful scrutiny of the family history and examination of relatives.

Intermittent or recurrent neuropathies constitute an interesting category and amongst hereditary neuropathies are best exemplified by porphyria. A relapsing course may also be observed in Refsum's disease, possibly related to fluctuations in the dietary intake of phytol. Recurrent mononeuropathies are a feature of hereditary liability to pressure palsies and may occur in Tangier disease (Pollock *et al.*, 1983). Familial recurrent brachial plexus palsy may be a separate entity (Jacob, Andermann and Robb, 1961) or related to hereditary liability to pressure palsies (Bradley *et al.*, 1975).

TREATMENT OF GENETICALLY-DETERMINED NEUROPATHIES

Regrettably, few curative treatments are available for the inherited neuropathies. Nevertheless, supportive and symptomatic therapies play an important role in their management, and these should not be neglected.

Prevention of attacks of neuropathy in the porphyrias is possible if administration of drugs known to precipitate them is avoided. These drugs include althesin, barbiturates, bemegride, carbamazepine, carbromal, chloramphenicol, chlorpropamide, chloroquine, dichloralphenazone, ergot preparations, ethanol, ethosuximide, glutethimide, griseofulvin, imipramine, meprobamate, methyldopa, nikethamide, oestrogens, including the oral contraceptives, pentazocine, phenytoin and other hydantoins, pyrazinamide, rifampicin, spironolactone, sulphonamides, theophylline derivatives, tolbutamide and troxidone (Brodie, 1981). In the established attack, chlorpromazine can be used to treat behavioural disturbances and control pain. Hypertension may require treatment with propranolol and assisted ventilation is sometimes needed. Intravenous glucose reduces urinary excretion of porphyrin precursors and the use of intravenous laevulose and haematin has been recommended (Bonkowsky *et al.*, 1976; Watson, *et al.*, 1973; Brodie *et al.*, 1977).

The neurological complications of abetalipoproteinaemia can be prevented by the administration of large doses (100 mg/kg/day) of oral or parenteral vitamin E. The role of vitamin A in the treatment of this disorder is less clear (Muller, Lloyd and Bird, 1977, Muller, Lloyd and Wolff, 1983; Azizi *et al.*, 1978). Improvement and arrest of the neurological syndrome associated with Refsum's disease can be achieved by a low phytate diet (Steinberg *et al.*, 1970). If severe abrupt deterioration occurs, plasma exchange may be beneficial (Gibberd *et al.*, 1979).

Attempts at exogenous enzyme replacement in metachromatic leucodystrophy have failed (Austin, 1973), as have trials of low vitamin A or sulphur diets aimed at reducing sulphatide synthesis (Moser, Moser and McKhann, 1967; Melchior and Clausen, 1968). Enzyme replacement in Fabry's disease is being explored (Mapes *et al.*, 1970; Brady *et al.*, 1973). Carbamazepine can be effective in suppressing the often severe pain which occurs in this disorder.

In patients with the various types of HMSN, management is essentially supportive. It is worthwhile following patients regularly until the growth period has ceased in order to ensure that severe skeletal deformity does not develop. Both pes cavus and other foot deformities, and scoliosis, can be corrected surgically with benefit (Shapiro and Bresnan, 1982). Orthotic appliances or tenodesis may be required for severe foot-drop. Dyck (1982) has recommended the use of broad foot-wear with a heat-moulded insole bearing the patient's imprint inside the shoes to distribute body weight evenly. It is particularly important to prevent the development of severe kyphoscoliosis because of the risk of later respiratory complications. Thoracic braces followed by spinal fusion once the adolescent growth spurt has ceased may be necessary in some instances. Periods of bedrest should be minimized as they often enhance motor disability; this point should particularly be borne in mind if surgical procedures are undertaken. Excessive weight gain should be avoided in any patient with loss of functional motor ability due to neuropathy, and regular exercise is to be recommended. Swimming appears to be particularly beneficial in this respect as it does not demand particular feats of strength or coordination.

In HMSN, but to a much greater extent in HSN, prevention of plantar ulcers and their complications is of paramount importance. Patients should not walk barefoot, and should inspect their shoes for protrusions daily. Application of vaseline to the feet has protective value. The toenails need careful attention. Callus formation should not be removed with sharp implements but rubbed off gently after immersion in water. If ulcers do develop, weightbearing should cease until they have healed. Antibiotic therapy may be required if infection spreads beyond the ulcer. In the recessive form of HSN, it can be very difficult to prevent damage to the fingers and feet in young children (Dyck, 1982).

GENETIC COUNSELLING IN THE INHERITED NEUROPATHIES

As so few specific treatments are available for the genetically determined neuropathies, prevention is one of the mainstays of management. Genetic counselling is important in this respect; 'It is a basic human need to know what went wrong, whether it will happen again, and whether it can be prevented' (Baraitser, 1982). Genetic counselling should not, nevertheless, be undertaken lightly. There are frequently problems in diagnosis and the evaluation of genetic risks which are often best dealt with jointly by a neurologist and a clinical geneticist. An accurate neurological diagnosis is an essential requirement. The aim of counselling is to allow the individual at risk to make an informed reproductive decision. Genetic advice should be educational but not instructive.

In autosomal dominant disorders, the risk of developing the disease is 50% to each child of a patient. This applies to the amyloid neuropathies, the porphyrias, hereditary liability to pressure palsies, and the dominant forms of HMSN and HSN. Problems arise if gene carriers cannot be identified with certainty before they reproduce. This applies to the Portuguese type of amyloid neuropathy, although it is likely that clinical and neurophysiological abnormalities antedate the onset of symptoms. Asymptomatic adult patients with variegate porphyria excrete excess coproporphyrin and protoporphyrin in their faeces, and those with hereditary coproporphyria excrete coproporphyrin III by the same route. In neither disorder is gene detection by means of these tests fully reliable, but the frequency of gene carriers who cannot be detected after puberty is low (Mustajoki, 1978). Heterozygotes for acute intermittent porphyria can usually be identified by the demonstration of reduced uroporphyrinogen-I-synthetase activity. There is some overlap between gene carriers and normal controls (Tishler, Knighton and Schumaker, 1976). Identification of these individuals is important from the therapeutic as well as the genetic point of view.

In HMSN it is useful to distinguish between types I and II, as this affects recurrence risks to sibs and offspring of single cases as well as aiding the interpretation of neurophysiological findings in relatives. If the pedigree is clearly autosomal dominant, it is important to stress that the course and severity of both types of HMSN are very variable. Less than 10% of patients are severely disabled. In counselling asymptomatic children of sibs of patients with type I HMSN, the available evidence suggests that motor nerve conduction velocity is reduced in early childhood, regardless of the presence or absence of symptoms (Dyck, Lambert and Mulder, 1963). A clinically and electrophysiologically normal individual of childbearing age can therefore be reassured that the risks of transmission to offspring are negligible. The situation is more difficult in HMSN type II because of the later onset and more subtle nerve conduction changes. It has been suggested that the probability of a clinically and electrophysiologically normal at risk person aged 25 or over developing the disease is less than 20% (Thomas and Harding, 1983).

The recent demonstration of linkage of the locus for dominant HMSN type I to the Duffy blood group locus on chromosome 1 raises the possibility of antenatal diagnosis (Bird, Ott and Giblett, 1982; Guiloff *et al.*, 1982). This would not be completely reliable in view of the relatively low lod scores obtained, and not all families are likely to be informative for segregation of the Duffy locus.

Autosomal recessive inheritance cannot be assumed in either type of HMSN unless both parents are clinically and electrophysiologically normal. If more than one individual in a sibship is affected, and the parents are normal, the risk of HMSN developing in the patient's further sibs is 1 in 4. Risks to the patient's offspring or any other relatives are negligible unless cousin marriage is contemplated. The identification and genetic counselling of single or sporadic cases of HMSN are difficult; some empirical risk estimates have been formulated by Thomas and Harding (1983).

As has been mentioned, subsequent sibs of a patient with any neuropathy of autosomal recessive inheritance have a 25% chance of being affected. This applies to the metachromatic leucodystrophies, Krabbe's disease, Refsum's disease, xeroderma pigmentosum, abetalipoproteinaemia, ataxia telangiectasia, the Cockayne syndrome, giant axonal neuropathy, and the Riley-Day syndrome, as well as the recessive forms of HSN and HMSN. Unfortunately, many of these disorders do not give rise to symptoms until younger sibs have already been born, which makes prevention impossible. Antenatal diagnosis is possible in metachromatic leucodystrophy, Krabbe's disease, and xeroderma pigmentosum, and potentially possible in ataxia telangiectasia.

Fabry's disease, adrenoleucodystrophy, adrenomyeloneuropathy and X-linked bulbospinal neuronopathy are of X-linked recessive inheritance. Generally speaking in this context, half the sons of carrier females are affected and half their daughters are carriers. None of the sons of male patients are affected, but all their daughters are carriers. Isolated affected males can give rise to problems in risk estimates to relatives because of the possibility of fresh mutation. This situation is best handled by a clinical geneticist. In Fabry's disease female carriers can be identified biochemically and antenatal diagnosis of affected males is possible (Brady *et al.*, 1971). Carriers for adrenoleucodystrophy are detectable from assay of the C22:C26 fatty acid ratio in skin fibroblast cultures (Moser *et al.*, 1980; O'Neill, Moser and Saxena, 1981), but as yet antenatal diagnosis has not been attempted.

References

Aguayo, A. J., Nair, C. P. V. and Bray, G. M. (1971) Peripheral nerve abnormalities in the Riley-Day syndrome: findings in a sural nerve biopsy. *Archives of Neurology (Chicago)*, **24**, 106–116

Allan, W. (1939) Relation of hereditary pattern to clinical severity as illustrated by peroneal atrophy. *Archives of Internal Medicine*, **63**, 1123–1131

Anderson, R. M., Dennett, X., Hopkins, I. J. and Shield, L. K. (1973) Hypertrophic interstitial polyneuropathy in infancy. *Journal of Pediatrics*, **82**, 619–624

Andrade, C. (1952) A peculiar form of peripheral neuropathy: familial atypical generalized amyloidosis with special involvement of the peripheral nerves. *Brain*, **75**, 408–427

Araki, S., Mawatari, S., Ohta, M., Nakajima, A. and Kuroiwa, Y. (1968) Polyneuritic amyloidosis in a Japanese family. *Archives of Neurology (Chicago)*, **18**, 593–602

Arbuse, D. I., Cantor, M. B. and Barenberg, P. A. (1949) Congenital indifference to pain. *Journal of Pediatrics*, **35**, 221–226

Asbury, A. K., Gale, M. K., Cox, S. C., Baringer, J. R. and Berg, B. O. (1972) Giant axonal neuropathy: a unique case with segmental neurofilamentous masses. *Acta Neuropathologica (Berlin)*, **20**, 237–247

Austin, J. H. (1965) Metachromatic leukodystrophy. In *Medical Aspects of Mental Retardation*, edited by C. O. Carter, p. 768. Springfield: Thomas

Austin, J. H. (1973) Studies in metachromatic leukodystrophy. XI. Therapeutic considerations. In *Enzyme Therapy in Genetics*, edited by D. Bergsma, R. J. Desnick, P. W. Bernlohr and W. Krivit, p. 125. Baltimore: Williams and Wilkins

Austin, J. H., Armstrong, D., Fouch, S. *et al.* (1968) Metachromatic leukodystrophy. *Archives of Neurology (Chicago)*, **18**, 225–240

Azizi, E., Zaidman, J. L., Eschchar, J. and Szeinberg, A. (1978) Abetalipo-proteinaemia treated with parenteral and oral vitamins A and E, and with medium chain triglycerides. *Acta Paediatrica Scandinavica*, **67**, 797–801

Baraitser, M. (1982) *The Genetics of Neurological Disorders*. Oxford: Oxford University Press

Baxter, D. W. and Olszewski, J. (1960) Congenital universal insensitivity to pain. *Brain*, **83**, 381–393

Behse, F., Buchthal, F., Carlsen, F. and Knappeis, G. G. (1972) Hereditary liability to pressure palsies: electrophysiological and histopathological aspects. *Brain*, **95**, 777–797

Bell, J. (1935) On the peroneal type of progressive muscular atrophy. *Treasury of Human Inheritance*, **4**, part VI

Berg, B. O., Rosenberg, S. H. and Asbury, A. K. (1972) Giant axonal neuropathy. *Pediatrics*, **49**, 894–899

Bird, T. D., Cederbaum, S., Valpey, R. W. and Stahl, W. L. (1978) Familial degeneration of the basal ganglia with acanthocytosis: a clinical, neuropathological and neurochemical study. *Annals of Neurology*, **3**, 253–258

Bird, T. D., Ott, J. and Giblett, E. R. (1982) Evidence for linkage of Charcot-Marie-Tooth neuropathy to the Duffy locus on chromosome 1. *American Journal of Human Genetics*, **34**, 388–394

Bird, T. D. and Shaw, C. M. (1978) Progressive myoclonus and epilepsy with dentatorubral degeneration. *Journal of Neurology, Neurosurgery and Psychiatry*, **41**, 140–149

Bischoff, A. (1975) Neuropathy in leukodystrophies. In *Peripheral Neuropathy*, edited by P. J. Dyck, P. K. Thomas and E. H. Lambert, pp. 891–913. Philadelphia: W. B. Saunders

Bischoff, A., Fierz, U., Regli, F. and Ulrich, J. (1968) Peripherneurologische Störungen bie der Fabryschen Krankheit (Angiokeratoma corporis diffusum universale). Klinischelektronenmikrosopische Befunde bei einen Fall. *Klinische Wochenschrift*, **46**, 666–671

Bischoff, A. and Ulrich, J. (1969) Peripheral neuropathy in globoid cell leukodystrophy (Krabbe's disease); ultrastructural and histochemical findings. *Brain*, **92**, 861–870

Blume, R. S. and Wolff, S. M. (1972) The Chediak-Higashi syndrome: studies in four patients and a review of the literature. *Medicine (Baltimore)*, **51**, 247–280

Bonkowsky, H. L., Magnussen, C. R., Collins, A. R., Doherty, J. M., Hess, R. A. and Tschudy, D. P. (1976). Comparative effects of glycerol and dextrose on porphyrin precursor excretion in acute intermittent porphyria. *Metabolism*, **25**, 405–415

Bosch, E. P. and Hart, M. N. (1978) Late adult-onset metachromatic leukodystrophy. *Archives of Neurology (Chicago)*, **35**, 475–477

Boyd, D. A. and Nie, L. W. (1949) Congenital universal indifference to pain. *Archives of Neurology and Psychiatry*, **61**, 402–412

Boysen, G., Galassi, G., Kamieniecka, Z., Schlaeger, J. and Trojaborg, W. (1979) Familial amyloidosis with cranial neuropathy and corneal lattice dystrophy. *Journal of Neurology, Neurosurgery and Psychiatry*, **42**, 1020–1030

Bradley, W. G., Madrid, R., Thrush, D. C. and Campbell, M. J. (1975) Recurrent brachial plexus neuropathy. *Brain*, **98**, 381–398

Brady, R. O., Tallman, J. F., Johnson, W. G. and Gal, A. E. (1973) Replacement therapy for inherited enzyme deficiency: use of purified ceramidetrihexosidase in Fabry's disease. *New England Journal of Medicine*, **289**, 9–14

Brady, R. O., Uhlendorf, B. W. and Jacobson, C. B. (1971) Fabry's disease: antenatal detection. *Science*, **172**, 174–175

Brodie, M. J. (1981) Drug actions and interactions in metabolic disorders. *Medicine International*, **1**, 397–398

Brodie, M. J., Moore, M. R., Thompson, G. G. and Golberg, A. (1977) The treatment of acute porphyria with laevulose. *Clinical Science and Molecular Medicine*, **53**, 365–371

Buchthal, F. and Behse, F. (1977) Peroneal muscular atrophy and related disorders. I. Clinical manifestations as related to biopsy findings, nerve conduction and electromyography. *Brain*, **100**, 41–66

Byrne, E., Thomas, P. K. and Zilkha, K. J. (1982) Familial extrapyramidal disease with peripheral neuropathy. *Journal of Neurology, Neurosurgery and Psychiatry*, **45**, 372–374

Carpenter, S., Karpati, G., Andermann, F. and Gold, R. (1974) Giant axonal neuropathy. A clinically and morphologically distinct neurological disease. *Archives of Neurology (Chicago)*, **31**, 312–316

Cavanagh, N. P. C., Eames, R. A., Galvin, R. J., Brett, E. M. and Kelly, R. E. (1979) Hereditary sensory neuropathy with spastic paraplegia. *Brain*, **102**, 79–94

Church, A. (1906) The neuritic type of progressive muscular atrophy. A case with marked heredity. *Journal of Nervous and Mental Disease*, **33**, 447–453

Coimbra, A. and Andrade, C. (1971) Familial amyloid polyneuropathy: an electron microscope study of the peripheral nerve in five cases. II. Nerve fibre changes. *Brain*, **94**, 207–212

Crome, L., Hanefeld, F., Patrick, D. and Wilson, J. (1973) Late onset globoid cell leucodystrophy. *Brain*, **96**, 841–848

Davis, C. J. F., Bradley, W. G. and Madrid, R. (1978) The peroneal muscular atrophy syndrome (clinical, genetic, electrophysiological and nerve biopsy studies). *Journal de génétique Humaine*, **26**, 311–349

Dayan, A. D. (1967) Peripheral neuropathy of metachromatic leucodystrophy: observations on segmental demyelination and remyelination and the intracellular distribution of sulphatide. *Journal of Neurology, Neurosurgery and Psychiatry*, **30**, 311–318

Dearborn, G. V. (1932) Case of congenital pure general analgesia. *Journal of Nervous and Mental Disease*, **75**, 612–615

Denny-Brown, D. (1951) Hereditary sensory radicular neuropathy. *Journal of Neurology, Neurosurgery and Psychiatry*, **14**, 237–242

Dubois, G., Harzer, K. and Baumann, N. (1977) Very low arylsulfatase A and cerebroside sulfatase activities in leukocytes of healthy members of metachromatic leukodystrophy family. *American Journal of Human Genetics*, **29**, 191–194

Dulaney, J. T. and Moser, H. W. (1978) Sulfatide lipidosis: metachromatic leukodystrophy. In *The Metabolic Basis of Inherited Disease*, edited by J. B. Stanbury, J. B. Wyngaarden and D. S. Fredrickson, pp. 770–809. New York: McGraw Hill

Dunn, H. G. (1973) Nerve conduction studies in children with Friedreich's ataxia and ataxia-telangiectasia. *Developmental Medicine and Child Neurology*, **15**, 324–337

Dunn, H. G., Lake, B. D., Dolman, C. L. and Wilson, J. (1969) The neuropathy of Krabbe's infantile cerebral sclerosis (globoid cell leucodystrophy). *Brain*, **92**, 329–344

Duvoisin, R. C., Chokroverty, S., Nicklas, W., Lepore, F. and Sage, J. (1983) The clinical expression of glutamate dehydrogenase deficiency. *Neurology (Cleveland)*, **33** (in press)

Dyck, P. J. (1982) Advice for patients and their families with inherited neuropathy. In *International Conference on Peripheral Neuropathies*, edited by S. Refsum, C. L. Bolis and A. Portera Sanchez, pp. 123–129. Amsterdam: Excerpta Medica

Dyck, P. J. (1983) Neuronal atrophy affecting peripheral sensory neurons. In *Peripheral Neuropathy*, edited by P. J. Dyck, P. K. Thomas, E. H. Lambert and R. Bunge, 2nd edition. Philadelphia: W. B. Saunders (in press)

Dyck, P. J., Ellefson, R. D., Lais, A. C., Smith, R. C., Taylor, W. F. and Van Dyke, R. A. (1970) Histologic and lipid studies of sural nerve in inherited hypertrophic neuropathy: preliminary report of a lipid abnormality in nerve and liver in Dejerine-Sottas disease. *Mayo Clinic Proceedings*, **45**, 286–327

Dyck, P. J., Ellefson, R. D., Yao, J. K. and Herbert, P. N. (1978) Adult onset of Tangier disease. 1. Morphometric and pathological studies suggesting delayed degradation of neutral lipids after fiber degeneration. *Journal of Neuropathology and Experimental Neurology*, **37**, 119–137

Dyck, P. J. and Lambert, E. H. (1968a) Lower motor and primary sensory neuron diseases with peroneal muscular atrophy. II. Neurologic, genetic and electrophysiologic findings in hereditary polyneuropathy. *Archives of Neurology (Chicago)*, **18**, 603–618

Dyck, P. J. and Lambert, E. H. (1968b) Lower motor and primary sensory neuron diseases with peroneal muscular atrophy. I. Neurologic, genetic and electrophysiologic findings in various neuronal degenerations. *Archives of Neurology (Chicago)*, **18**, 619–625

Dyck, P. J., Lambert, E. H. and Mulder, D. W. (1963) Charcot-Marie-Tooth disease: nerve conduction and clinical studies of a large kinship. *Neurology (Minneapolis)*, **13**, 1–11

Dyck, P. J., Lambert, E. H. and Nichols, P. C. (1972) Quantitative measurement of sensation related to compound action potential and number and sizes of myelinated and unmyelinated fibers of sural nerve in health, Friedreich's ataxia, hereditary sensory neuropathy and tabes dorsalis. In *Handbook of Electroencephalography and Clinical Neurophysiology*, edited by W. A. Cobb, pp. 83–118. Amsterdam: Elsevier

Dyck, P. J., Lambert, E. H., Sanders, K. and O'Brien, P. C. (1971) Severe hypomyelination and marked abnormality of conduction in Dejerine-Sottas hypertrophic neuropathy: myelin thickness and compound action potential of sural nerve *in vitro*. *Mayo Clinic Proceedings*, **46**, 432–436

Dyck, P. J., Mellinger, J. F., Reagan, T. J. *et al.* (1983) Not 'indifference to pain' but varieties of hereditary sensory and autonomic neuropathy. *Brain*, **106**, 373–390

Dyck, P. J., Oviatt, K. F. and Lambert, E. H. (1981) Intensive evaluation of referred unclassified neuropathies yields improved diagnosis. *Annals of Neurology*, **10**, 222–226

Earl, C. J., Fullerton, P. M., Wakefield, G. S. and Schutta, H. S. (1964) Hereditary neuropathy with liability to pressure palsies. *Quarterly Journal of Medicine*, **33**, 481–498

Elder, G. H., Evans, J. O., Thomas, N. *et al.* (1976) The primary enzyme defect in hereditary coproporphyria. *Lancet*, **2**, 1217–1219

Estes, J. W., Morley, T. J., Levine, I. M. and Emerson, C. P. (1967) A new hereditary acanthocytosis syndrome. *American Journal of Medicine*, **42**, 868–881

Fullerton, P. M. (1964) Peripheral nerve conduction in metachromatic leucodystrophy (sulphatide lipidosis). *Journal of Neurology, Neurosurgery and Psychiatry*, **27**, 100–105

Geiger, L. R., Mancall, E. L., Penn, A. S. and Tucker, S. H. (1974) Familial neuralgic amyotrophy: report of three families with review of the literature. *Brain*, **97**, 87–102

Gibberd, F. B., Billimoria, J. D., Page, N. G. R. and Retsas, S. (1979) Heredopathia atactica polyneuritiformis (Refsum's disease) treated by diet and plasma-exchange. *Lancet*, **1**, 575–578

Goebel, H. H., Veit, S. and Dyck, P. J. (1980) Confirmation of virtual unmyelinated fiber absence in hereditary sensory neuropathy type IV. *Journal of Neuropathology and Experimental Neurology*, **39**, 670–675

Goodman, W. N., Cooper, W. C., Kessler, G. B., Fischer, M. S. and Garner, M. B. (1969) Ataxia telangiectasia, a report of two cases in siblings presenting a picture of progressive spinal muscular atrophy. *Bulletin of the Los Angeles Neurological Association*, **34**, 1–22

Gordon, N. (1978) The insidious presentation of the juvenile form of metachromatic leucodystrophy. *Postgraduate Medical Journal*, **54**, 335–337

Griffin, J. W., Goren, E., Schaumburg, H., Engel, W. K. and Loriaux, L. (1977) Adrenomyeloneuropathy: a probable variant of adrenoleukodystrophy. 1. Clinical and endocrinologic aspects. *Neurology (Minneapolis)*, **12**, 1107–1113

Guiloff, R. J., Thomas, P. K., Contreras, M., Armitage, S., Schwarz, G. and Sedgwick, E. M. (1982) Evidence of linkage of type I hereditary motor and sensory neuropathy with the Duffy locus on chromosome 1. *Annals of Human Genetics*, **46**, 25–27

Guzzetta, F., Ferrière, G. and Lyon, G. (1982) Congenital hypomyelination polyneuropathy: pathological findings compared with polyneuropathies starting later in life. *Brain*, **105**, 395–416

Haas, L. F., Austad, W. L. and Bergin, J. D. (1974) Tangier disease. *Brain*, **97**, 351–354

Hagberg, B. (1963) Clinical symptoms, signs and tests in metachromatic leucodystrophy. In *Brain Lipids and Lipoproteins and the Leucodystrophies*, edited by J. Folch-Pi and H. J. Bauer, pp. 134–146. Amsterdam: Elsevier

Hagberg, B. and Lyon, G. (1981) Pooled European series of hereditary peripheral neuropathies in infancy and childhood. A 'correspondence workshop' report of the European Federation of Child Neurology Societies (EFCNS). *Neuropediatrics*, **12**, 9–17

Hahn, A. F., Gordon, B. A., Feleki, V., Hinton, G. G. and Gilbert, J. J. (1982) A variant form of metachromatic leukodystrophy without arylsulphatase deficiency. *Annals of Neurology*, **12**, 33–36

Hahn, A. F., Gordon, B. A., Gilbert, J. J. and Hinton, G. G. (1981) The AB-variant of metachromatic leukodystrophy (postulated activator protein deficiency). Light and electron microscopic findings in a sural nerve biopsy. *Acta Neuropathologica (Berlin)*, **55**, 281–287

Harding, A. E. (1981) Friedreich's ataxia: a clinical and genetic study of 90 families with an analysis of early diagnostic criteria and intrafamilial clustering of clinical features. *Brain*, **104**, 589–620

Harding, A. E. and Thomas, P. K. (1980a) The clinical features of hereditary motor and sensory neuropathy types I and II. *Brain*, **103**, 259–280

Harding, A. E. and Thomas, P. K. (1980b) Distal spinal muscular atrophy: a report on 34 cases and a review of the literature. *Journal of the Neurological Sciences*, **45**, 337–348

Harding, A. E. and Thomas, P. K. (1980c) Autosomal recessive forms of hereditary motor and sensory neuropathy (Types I and II). *Journal of Neurology, Neurosurgery and Psychiatry*, **43**, 669–678

Harding, A. E. and Thomas, P. K. (1980d) Genetic aspects of hereditary motor and sensory neuropathy (Types I and II). *Journal of Medical Genetics*, **17**, 329–336

Harding, A. E. and Thomas, P. K. (1984) Peroneal muscular atrophy with pyramidal features. *Journal of Neurology, Neurosurgery and Psychiatry* (in press)

Harding, A. E., Thomas, P. K., Baraitser, M., Bradbury, P. G., Morgan-Hughes, J. A. and Ponsford, J. R. (1982) X-linked recessive bulbospinal neuronopathy: a report of ten cases. *Journal of Neurology, Neurosurgery and Psychiatry*, **45**, 1012–1019

Herbert, P. N., Gotto, A. M. and Fredrickson, D. S. (1978) Familial lipoprotein deficiency (abetalipoproteinemia, hypobetalipoproteinemia and Tangier disease). In *The Metabolic Basis of Inherited Disease*, edited by J. B. Stanbury, J. B. Wyngaarden and D. S. Fredrickson, pp. 545–588. New York: McGraw Hill

Herndon, J. H., Steinberg, D. and Uhlendorf, B. W. (1969) Refsum's disease. Defective oxidation of phytanic acid in tissue cultures derived from homozygotes and heterozygotes. *New England Journal of Medicine*, **281**, 1034–1038

Herringham, W. P. (1889) Muscular atrophy of the peroneal type affecting many members of a family. *Brain*, **11**, 230–236

Hicks, E. P. (1922) Hereditary perforating ulcer of the foot. *Lancet*, **1**, 319–321

Hierons, R. (1957) Changes in the nervous system of acute porphyria. *Brain*, **80**, 176–192

Humberstone, P. M. (1972) Nerve conduction studies in Charcot-Marie-Tooth disease. *Acta Neurologica Scandinavica*, **48**, 176–190

Iwashita, H., Inoue, N., Araki, S. and Kuroiwa, Y. (1970) Optic atrophy, neural deafness and distal neurogenic amyotrophy. Report of a family with two affected siblings. *Archives of Neurology (Chicago)*, **22**, 357–364

Jacob, J. C., Andermann, F. and Robb, J. P. (1961) Heredofamilial mononeuritis multiplex with brachial predilection. *Brain*, **83**, 113–137

Johnson, R. H. and Spalding, J. M. K. (1964) Progressive sensory neuropathy in children. *Journal of Neurology, Neurosurgery and Psychiatry*, **27**, 125–130

Johnston, A. W., Frost, F., Spaeth, G. L. and Renwick, J. H. (1968) Linkage relationships of the angiokeratoma (Fabry) locus. *Annals of Human Genetics*, **32**, 369–374

Jones, M. A., Nigro, M. A. and Barre, P. S. (1979) Familial 'giant axonal neuropathy'. *Journal of Neuropathology and Experimental Neurology*, **38**, 324

Kahlke, W. (1964) Refsum-Syndrom. Lipoidchemische Untersuchungen bei 9 Fällen. *Klinische Wochenschrift*, **42**, 1011–1016

Kennedy, W. R., Alter, M. and Sung, J. H. (1968) Progressive proximal spinal and bulbar muscular atrophy of late onset. *Neurology (Minneapolis)*, **18**, 671–680

Kennedy, W. R., Sung, J. H. and Berry, J. F. (1977) A case of congenital hypomyelination neuropathy. Clinical, morphological and chemical studies. *Archives of Neurology (Chicago)*, **34**, 337–345

Killian, J. M. and Kloepfer, H. W. (1979) Homozygous expression of a dominant mutant gene for Charcot-Marie-Tooth neuropathy. *Annals of Neurology*, **5**, 515–522

Kint, J. A. (1970) Fabry's disease, alpha-galactosidase deficiency. *Science*, **167**, 1268–1269

Kirkham, T. H., Guitton, D. and Coupland, S. G. (1980) Giant axonal neuropathy: visual and oculomotor deficits. *Canadian Journal of Neurological Science*, **7**, 177–184

Kocen, R. S., King, R. H. M., Thomas, P. K. and Haas, L. F. (1973) Nerve biopsy findings in two cases of Tangier disease. *Acta Neuropathologica (Berlin)*, **26**, 317–327

Kocen, R. S., Lloyd, J. K., Laselles, P. T., Fosbrooke, A. S. and Williams, D. (1967) Familial α-lipoprotein deficiency (Tangier disease) with neurological abnormalities. *Lancet*, **1**, 1341–1345

Kocen, R. S. and Thomas, P. K. (1970) Peripheral nerve involvement in Fabry's disease. *Archives of Neurology (Chicago)*, **22**, 81–88

Koenig, R. H. and Spiro, A. J. (1970) Hereditary spastic paraparesis with sensory neuropathy. *Developmental Medicine and Child Neurology*, **12**, 576–581

Langenbeck, U., Dunker, P., Heipertz, R. and Pilz, H. (1977) Inheritance of metachromatic leukodystrophy. *American Journal of Human Genetics*, **29**, 639–640

Lapresle, J. and Salisachs, P. (1973) Onion bulbs in a nerve biopsy specimen from an original case of Roussy-Lévy disease. *Archives of Neurology (Chicago)*, **29**, 346–348

Lewis, R. A., Grunnet, M. L. and Zimmerman, A. W. (1982) Peripheral nerve demyelination in Cockayne's syndrome. *Muscle and Nerve*, **5**, 557

Liu, H. M. (1970) Ultrastructure of globoid leukodystrophy (Krabbe's disease) with reference to the origin of the globoid cells. *Journal of Neuropathology and Experimental Neurology*, **29**, 441–462

Lockman, J. A., Kennedy, W. R. and White, J. G. (1967) The Chediak-Higashi syndrome: electrophysiological and electron microscopic observations on the peripheral neuropathy. *Journal of Pediatrics*, **70**, 942–951

Low, P. A., Burke, W. J. and McLeod, J. G. (1978) Congenital sensory neuropathy with selective loss of small myelinated nerve fibers. *Annals of Neurology*, **3**, 179–182

Lyon, G. (1969) Ultrastructure study of a nerve biopsy from a case of early infantile chronic neuropathy. *Acta Neuropathologica (Berlin)*, **13**, 131–142

Mahloudji, M., Brunt, P. W. and McKusick, V. A. (1970) Clinical neurological aspects of familial dysautonomia. *Journal of the Neurological Sciences*, **11**, 383–395

Mahloudji, M., Teasdall, R. D., Adamkiewicz, J. J., Hartmann, W. H., Lambird, P. A. and McKusick, V. A. (1969) The genetic amyloidoses, with particular reference to hereditary neuropathic amyloidosis type II (Indiana or Rukavina type). *Medicine (Baltimore)*, **48**, 1–37

Mapes, C. A., Anderson, R. L., Sweeley, C. C., Desnick, R. J. and Krivit, W. (1970) Enzyme replacement in Fabry's disease, an inborn error of metabolism. *Science*, **169**, 987–989

Massion-Verniory, L., Dumont, E. and Potvin, A. M. (1946) Rétinite pigmentaire familiale compliqué d'une amyotrophie neurale. *Revue Neurologique (Paris)*, **78**, 561–571

McLeod, J. G. (1971) An electrophysiological and pathological study of peripheral nerves in Friedreich's ataxia. *Journal of the Neurological Sciences*, **12**, 333–349

McLeod, J. G. and Evans, W. A. (1981) Peripheral neuropathy in spinocerebellar degenerations. *Muscle and Nerve*, **4**, 51–61

McLeod, J. G., Low, P. A. and Morgan, J. A. (1978) Charcot-Marie-Tooth disease with Leber optic atrophy. *Neurology (Minneapolis)*, **28**, 179–184

McMurray, G. A. (1950) Experimental study of a case with insensitivity to pain. *Archives of Neurology and Psychiatry*, **64**, 650–667

Meier, C. and Moll, C. (1982) Hereditary neuropathy with liability to pressure palsies. Report of two families and review of the literature. *Journal of Neurology*, **228**, 73–96

Melchior, J. C. and Clausen, J. (1968) Metachromatic leucodystrophy in early childhood. Treatment with a diet deficient in vitamin A. *Acta Paediatrica Scandinavica*, **37**, 2–8

Meretoja, J. and Teppo, L. (1971) Histopathological findings of familial amyloidosis with cranial neuropathy as principal manifestation. Report of three cases. *Acta Pathologica Microbiologica Scandinavica*, **79**, 432–440

Miller, R. G., Davis, C. J. F., Illingworth, D. R. and Bradley, W. G. (1980) The neuropathy of abetalipoproteinaemia. *Neurology (Minneapolis)*, **30**, 1286–1291

Moosa, A. and Dubowitz, V. (1970) Peripheral neuropathy in Cockayne's syndrome. *Archives of Disease in Childhood*, **45**, 674–677

Moser, H. W., Moser, A. B., Kawamura, N. *et al.* (1980). Adrenoleukodystrophy: elevated C26 fatty acid in cultured skin fibroblasts. *Annals of Neurology*, **7**, 542–549

Moser, H. W., Moser, A. B. and McKhann, G. M. (1967) The dynamics of a lipidosis: turnover of sulfatide, steroid sulfate and polysaccharide sulfate in metachromatic leukodystrophy. *Archives of Neurology (Chicago)*, **17**, 494–511

Moser, H., Sugita, M., Harbison, M. D. and Williams, S. R. (1972) Liver glycolipids, steroid sulfates and steroid sulfatases in a form of metachromatic leucodystrophy associated with multiple sulfatase deficiency. In *Sphingolipids, Sphingolipidoses and Applied Disorders*, edited by B. Volk and S. Aronson, p. 429. New York; Plenum Press

Muller, D. P. R., Lloyd, J. K. and Bird, A. C. (1977) Long-term management of abetalipoproteinaemia. Possible role of vitamin E. *Archives of Disease in Childhood*, **52**, 209–214

Murray, T. J. (1973) Congenital sensory neuropathy. *Brain*, **96**, 387–394

Mustajoki, P. (1978) Variegate porphyria. *Annals of Internal Medicine*, **89**, 238–244

Mustajoki, P. (1980) Variegate porphyria. *Quarterly Journal of Medicine*, **49**, 191–203

Nordborg, C., Conradi, N., Sourander, P. and Westerberg, B. (1981) A new type of non-progressive sensory neuropathy in children with atypical dysautonomia. *Acta Neuropathologica (Berlin)*, **55**, 135–141

Norman, R. M., Urich, H., and Tingey, A. H. (1960) Metachromatic leucodystrophy: a form of lipidosis. *Brain*, **83**, 369–380

Nukuda, H., Pollock, M. and Haas, L. F. (1982) The clinical spectrum of type II hereditary sensory neuropathy. *Brain*, **105**, 647–665

O'Brien, J. S. (1964) A molecular defect of myelination. *Biochemical and Biophysical Research Communications*, **15**, 484–486

Ohnishi, A. and Dyck, P. J. (1974) Loss of small peripheral sensory neurons in Fabry disease. Histologic and morphometric evaluation of cutaneous nerves, spinal ganglia and posterior columns. *Archives of Neurology (Chicago)*, **31**, 120–127

Ohnishi, A., Sato, Y., Nagara, H. *et al.* (1981) Neurogenic muscular atrophy and low density of large myelinated fibres of sural nerve of chorea-acanthocytosis. *Journal of Neurology, Neurosurgery and Psychiatry*, **44**, 645–648

Ohta, M., Ellefson, R. D., Lambert, E. H. and Dyck, P. J. (1973) Hereditary sensory neuropathy type II. Clinical, electrophysiologic, histologic and biochemical studies of a Quebec kinship. *Archives of Neurology (Chicago)*, **29**, 23–37

O'Neill, B. P., Moser, H. W. and Saxena, K. M. (1981) Familial X-linked Addison disease as an expression of adrenoleukodystrophy (ALD): elevated C26 fatty acid in cultured skin fibroblasts. *Neurology (Minneapolis)*, **32**, 543–547

Opitz, J. M., Stiles, F. C., Wise, D. *et al.* (1965) The genetics of angiokeratoma corporis diffusum (Fabry's disease) and its linkage relations with the Xg locus. *American Journal of Human Genetics*, **17**, 325–374

Ouvrier, R. A., McLeod, J. G., Morgan, G. J., Wise, G. A. and Conchin, T. E. (1981) Hereditary motor and sensory neuropathy of neuronal type with onset in early childhood. *Journal of the Neurological Sciences*, **51**, 181–197

Pearson, J., Budzilovich, G. and Finegold, M. J. (1971) Sensory, motor and autonomic dysfunction: the nervous system in familial dysautonomia. *Neurology (Minneapolis)*, **21**, 486–493

Percy, A. K., Kaback, M. M. and Herndon, R. M. (1977) Metachromatic leukodystrophy: comparison of early and late onset forms. *Neurology (Minneapolis)*, **27**, 933–941

Pilz, H. (1972) Late adult metachromatic leukodystrophy. *Archives of Neurology (Chicago)*, **27**, 87–90

Pilz, H., Duensing, I., Heipertz, R. *et al.* (1977) Adult metachromatic leukodystrophy. *European Neurology*, **15**, 301–307

Pinksy, L. and DiGeorge, A. M. (1966) Congenital familial sensory neuropathy with anhidrosis. *Journal of Pediatrics*, **68**, 1–13

Pollock, M., Nukada, H., Frith, R. W., Simcock, J. P. and Allpress, S. (1983) Peripheral neuropathy in Tangier disease. *Brain* (in press)

Powers, J. M. and Schaumburg, H. H. (1974) Adrenoleukodystrophy: similar ultrastructural changes in adrenal cortical cells and Schwann cells. *Archives of Neurology (Chicago)*, **30**, 406–408

Rampini, S., Isler, W., Baerlocher, K., Bischoff, A., Ulrich, J. and Plüss, H. (1970) Die Kombination von metakromatischer Leukodystrophie und Mukopolysaccharidose als selbständiges Krankheitsbild (Mukosulfatidose). *Helvetica Paediatrica Acta*, **25**, 436–461

Refsum, S., Stokke, O., Eldjarn, L. and Fardeau, M. (1975) Heredopathia atactica polyneuritiformis (Refsum's disease). In *Peripheral Neuropathy*, edited by P. J. Dyck, P. K. Thomas and E. H. Lambert, pp. 868–890. Philadelphia: W. B. Saunders

Richterich, R., Rosen, S. and Rossi, E. (1965) Refsum's disease (heredopathia atactica polyneuritiformis): an inborn error of lipid metabolism with storage of 3, 7, 11, 15-tetramethyl hexadecanoic acid. Formal genetics. *Humangenetik*, **1**, 333–336

Robbins, J. H., Kraemer, K. H., Lutzner, M. A., Festoff, B. W. and Coon, H. G. (1974) Xeroderma pigmentosum. An inherited disease with sun sensitivity, multiple cutaneous neoplasms and abnormal DNA repair. *Annals of Internal Medicine*, **80**, 221–248

Rosenberg, R. N. and Chutorian, A. (1967) Familial opticoacoustic nerve degeneration and polyneuropathy. *Neurology (Minneapolis)*, **17**, 827–832

Rukavina, J. G., Block, W. D., Jackson, C. E., Falls, H. F., Carey, J. H. and Curtis, A. C. (1956) Primary systemic amyloidosis: a review and an experimental, genetic and clinical study of cases with particular emphasis on the familial form. *Medicine (Baltimore)*, **35**, 239–334

Salisachs, P. (1974) Wide spectrum of motor conduction velocity in Charcot-Marie-Tooth disease. An anatomico-physiological interpretation. *Journal of the Neurological Sciences*, **23**, 25–31

Salisachs, P. (1982) Ataxia and other data reviewed in Charcot-Marie-Tooth and Refsum's disease. *Journal of Neurology, Neurosurgery and Psychiatry*, **45**, 1085–1091

Satya-Murti, S., Cacace, A. T. and Hanson, P. A. (1979) Abnormal auditory evoked potentials in hereditary motor-sensory neuropathy. *Annals of Neurology*, **5**, 445–459

Schaumburg, H. H., Powers, J. M., Raine, C. S., Suzuki, K. and Richardson, E. P. Jr. (1975) Adrenoleukodystrophy: a clinical and pathological study of 17 cases. *Archives of Neurology (Chicago)*, **32**, 577–591

Schilder, P. and Stengel, E. (1931) Asymbolia for pain. *Archives of Neurology and Psychiatry*, **25**, 598–600

Schutta, H. S., Pratt, R. T. C., Metz, H., Evans, K. A. and Carter, C. O. (1966) A family study of the late infantile and juvenile forms of metachromatic leucodystrophy. *Journal of Medical Genetics*, **3**, 86–91

Serratrice, G., Gastaut, J. L. and Dubois-Gambarelli, D. (1973) Amyotrophie neurogène périphérique au cours du syndrome de Marinesco-Sjögren. *Revue Neurologique (Paris)*, **128**, 432–441

Shapiro, F. and Bresnan, M. J. (1982) Orthopedic management of childhood neuromuscular disease. Part II: Peripheral neuropathies, Friedreich's ataxia, and arthrogryposis multiplex congenita. *Journal of Bone and Joint Surgery*, **64A**, 949–953

Skre, H. (1974) Genetic and clinical aspects of Charcot-Marie-Tooth disease. *Clinical Genetics*, **6**, 98–118

Sluga, E. (1974) *Polyneuropathien. Typen und Differenzierung. Ergebnisse bioptischer Untersuchungen.* Berlin: Springer-Verlag

Steinberg, D., Mize, C. E., Herndon, J. H. Jr, Fales, H. M., Engel, W. K. and Vroom, F. Q. (1970) Phytanic acid in patients with Refsum's syndrome and response to dietary treatment. *Archives of Internal Medicine*, **125**, 75–87

Strand, L. J., Felsher, B. W., Redeker, A. G. and Marver, H. S. (1970) Enzymatic abnormalities in heme biosynthesis in intermittent acute porphyria. Decreased hepatic conversion of porphobilinogen to porphyrins and an increase in δ-aminolevulinic acid synthetase activity. *Proceedings of the National Academy of Sciences USA*, **67**, 1315–1320

Swanson, A. G., Buchan, G. C. and Alvord, E. C. Jr (1965) Anatomic changes in congenital insensitivity to pain. *Archives of Neurology*, **12**, 12–18

Taylor, A. M. R., Harnden, D. G., Arlett, C. F. *et al.* (1975) Ataxia telangiectasia: a human mutation with abnormal radiation sensitivity. *Nature*, **258**, 427–429

Thomas, P. K., Calne, D. B. and Stewart, G. (1974) Hereditary motor and sensory polyneuropathy (peroneal muscular atrophy). *Annals of Human Genetics*, **38**, 111–153

Thomas, P. K. and Harding, A. E. (1983) Peripheral neuropathies. In *The Principles and Practice of Medical Genetics*, edited by A. E. H. Emery and D. L. Rimoin, pp. 296–312. Edinburgh: Churchill Livingstone

Thomas, P. K., King, R. H. M., Kocen, R. S. and Brett, E. M. (1977) Comparative ultrastructural observations on peripheral nerve abnormalities in the late infantile, juvenile and late onset forms of metachromatic leukodystrophy. *Acta Neuropathologica (Berlin)*, **39**, 237–245

Thrush, D. C., Holt, I. G., Bradley, W. G., Campbell, M. J. and Walton, J. N. (1974) Neurological manifestations of xeroderma pigmentosum in two siblings. *Journal of the Neurological Sciences*, **22**, 91–104

Tishler, P. V., Knighton, D. J. and Schumaker, H. M. (1976) Screening test for intermittent acute porphyria. *Lancet*, **1**, 303–305 van Allen, M. W., Frohlich, J. A. and Davis, J. R. (1969) Inherited predisposition to generalized amyloidosis: clinical and pathological study of a family with neuropathy, nephropathy and peptic ulcer. *Neurology (Minneapolis)*, **19**, 10–25

Vassella, F., Emrich, H. M., Kraus-Ruppert, R., Aufdermaur, F. and Tönz, O. (1968) Congenital sensory neuropathy with anhidrosis. *Archives of Disease in Childhood*, **43**, 124–130

Watson, C., Dhar, G. J., Bossenmaier, I., Cardinal, R. and Petryka, Z. J. (1973) Effect of hematin in acute porphyria relapse. *Annals of Internal Medicine*, **79**, 80–83

Wetterberg, L. (1967) *A Neuropsychiatric and Genetical Investigation of Acute Intermittent Porphyria.* Stockholm: Svenska Bökförlaget

Wilson, J., Lake, B. D. and Dunn, H. G. (1970) Krabbe's leukodystrophy. Some clinical, genetic and pathogenetic considerations. *Journal of the Neurogical Sciences*, **10**, 541–561

Woratz, G. (1964) Neurale Muskelatrophie mit dominantem X-chromosomalem Erbgang. *Abhandlungen der Deutschen Akademie der Wissenschaften zu Berlin Klasse für medizinische Wissenschaften*, **2**, 1–99

Yao, J. K. and Dyck, P. J. (1981) Lipid abnormalities in hereditary neuropathy. Part 4. Endoneurial and liver lipids of HMSN-III (Dejerine-Sottas disease). *Journal of the Neurological Sciences*, **52**, 179–190

Yao, J. K., Herbert, P. N., Fredrickson, D. S. *et al.* (1978) Biochemical studies in a patient with Tangier syndrome. *Journal of Neuropathology and Experimental Neurology*, **37**, 138–154

Yudell, A., Gomez, M. R., Lambert, E. H. and Dockerty, M. B. (1967) The neuropathy of sulfatide lipidosis (metachromatic leukodystrophy). *Neurology (Minneapolis)*, **17**, 103–111

Ziegler, D. K., Schimke, R. N., Kepes, J. J. and Rose, D. L. (1972) Late onset ataxia, rigidity and peripheral neuropathy. *Archives of Neurology (Chicago)*, **27**, 52–66

10
Nerve compression and entrapment
R. W. Gilliatt and M. J. G. Harrison

INTRODUCTION

The terms compression and constriction are not synonymous, and entrapment means something different again.

Compression is the correct term when sustained pressure is applied to a localized region of nerve, either through the skin (as in Saturday-night palsy) or from a source within the tissues (such as a haematoma adjacent to the nerve). In both cases there is a pressure differential between one part of the nerve and another. Pressure which is uniformly distributed throughout the body does not cause nerve dysfunction, so that a deep-sea diver can work safely at pressures which would cause nerve demyelination or degeneration if these were applied locally to a portion of a nerve (Gilliatt, 1981).

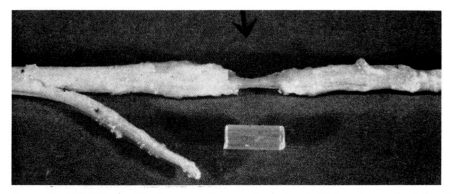

Figure 10.1 Rabbit popliteal nerve after prolonged constriction by a short length of siliconized rubber tubing (shown in foreground). The tube was placed round the nerve in young animals and left in place for 9 months so that gradual constriction occurred during growth. Demyelination sufficient to cause slowing of conduction occurred at the site of constriction, but there was no muscle weakness or evidence of Wallerian degeneration. (From Aguayo, Nair and Midgley, 1971)

Constriction indicates that a reduction in calibre is imposed on a nerve by adjacent tissues. If this happens gradually it may not be possible to demonstrate a rise in pressure. The non-neural elements of the nerve trunk are capable of adapting to the constriction by a decrease in volume so that the cross-sectional area of a constricted region can be substantially reduced without a functional deficit (*Figure 10.1*). Beyond a certain point, however, there is increasing damage to nerve fibres.

Entrapment implies constriction or mechanical distortion of a nerve by a fibrous band or within a fibrous or fibro-osseous tunnel. In such cases angulation and stretching may be as important as compression or constriction; the insult to the nerve may be repetitive or sustained, according to circumstances. In spite of this variation in the mechanism of nerve damage the term *entrapment* is a useful one in that it implies that the lesions occur at particular sites where surgical intervention is required to release the entrapped nerves (Kopell and Thompson, 1963; Nakano, 1978b).

AETIOLOGICAL FACTORS

Many individual nerves are anatomically vulnerable either to external pressure and/or to entrapment. Some of them lie superficially between major limb bones and the skin, protected only by a small amount of subcutaneous fat. The weight of the limb, or of a sleeping, drugged, anaesthetized or comatose body may thus compress the nerve between bone and a hard external surface. The pressure may be focal and protracted if the patient sleeps heavily after taking alcohol or a hypnotic, or is not regularly moved when nursed in a drowsy or comatose state, or is paralysed (e.g. a stroke victim). Repetitive percussion or compression may have a cumulative effect. For example, the repeated wearing of a rucksack may tend to brachial plexus damage (Daube, 1969) or the ulnar nerve in the hand may be damaged in long-distance cycling (Noth, Dietz and Mauritz, 1980).

Most peripheral nerves at some point in their course run under a ligament or retinaculum, or pass through or under the often fibrous origin of a muscle. Others, like the ulnar nerve at the elbow, loop round an anatomical landmark that exposes them to stretch during limb movement. The use of intraneural recording electrodes brought to light the fact that nerves move in the long axis of the limb during limb movements. Thus a needle placed in the median nerve in the upper arm can be seen to sway as the wrist is passively flexed and extended, revealing that the nerve must normally slide inside the carpal tunnel. Limitation of movement at an entrapment site due to fibrosis and tethering of the nerve may have the effect of exaggerating the amount of stretching and angulation occurring at the edge of the lesion, and thus increase the nerve fibre damage. Congenital differences in anatomy may well play an important role in determining vulnerability. Thus patients with symptomatic entrapment of the median nerve at the wrist have been shown to have an anatomically smaller carpal space (Dekel and Coates, 1979). Neary, Ochoa and Gilliatt (1975) and Jefferson, Neary and Eames (1981) also showed that subclinical damage of peripheral nerves was common at the traditional sites of acquired entrapment, confirming the anatomical vulnerability of such points.

It should be added that in some forms of generalized neuropathy the liability to local pressure palsies is increased. In 'tomaculous' neuropathy, for example, there is a generalized abnormality of compact myelin but patients usually only develop symptoms as a result of pressure from an external force (Behse *et al.*, 1972; Madrid and Bradley, 1975). This force can be trivial compared with that required to produce a lesion in a normal nerve; in a personal case, for example, the patient noticed numbness of the thumb for several weeks after using a heavy pair of scissors to cut up some cloth. Diabetic neuropathy is another condition in which lesions at common entrapment sites occur more often than would be expected in the general population. In an electrophysiological study Mulder *et al.* (1961) found evidence of localized conduction delay in the carpal tunnel in 9 out of 103 unselected diabetic patients. Further examples of carpal tunnel compression and of ulnar nerve entrapment at the elbow in diabetic patients have been described by others (*see* Chapter 6). Local lesions at entrapment sites can also occasionally occur in other forms of polyneuropathy, including hereditary and inflammatory neuropathies and those associated with neoplasia and amyloidosis.

In an experimental study of the susceptibility of pathological nerve fibres to compression from an external source, Hopkins and Morgan-Hughes (1969) utilized the known fact that guinea pigs kept in cages with wire mesh flooring may, after many weeks, develop a plantar neuropathy. When these animals were given small systemic doses of diphtheria toxin, the plantar neuropathy developed relatively quickly, although the dose of toxin was insufficient to cause much change in other nerves not subject to compression. The authors then went on to show that a diphtheritic plantar neuropathy could also occur in animals kept in cages with solid floors covered with sawdust, and that the only way to prevent the lesion was to suspend the animals in canvas slings for several weeks after the administration of toxin, so that the hind feet did not touch the floor of the cage. From their results it seemed that diphtheria toxin impaired the capacity of Schwann cells to maintain compact myelin in the face of mild but recurrent nerve compression.

FEATURES OF ACUTE NERVE COMPRESSION

When an external compressive force acts on a limb for a short period, as in the genesis of Saturday-night palsy or tourniquet paralysis, there is good evidence that the nerve damage is due to mechanical distortion of nerve fibres and not to ischaemia. The evidence may be summarized as follows:

(1) The short duration of the compression. In experimental animals it is possible to produce persistent damage by a tourniquet inflated for a period as short as 1 hour (Fowler, Danta and Gilliatt, 1972). In human pressure palsies the duration of compression can be even shorter. A personal case may be cited in which the patient, an otherwise healthy woman aged 48, made a short journey in an overcrowded car, during which her grown-up daughter sat on her knee. On arrival the patient had unilateral footdrop which took several weeks to recover. The duration of the journey was not more than 25 minutes but

investigation showed no evidence of a special susceptibility to pressure palsies in this particular case.

(2) In acute compression of this type, the paralysis is typically due to local demyelination at the site of pressure, causing conduction block. This is good evidence against an ischaemic aetiology since ischaemia alone, for example that produced in experimental animals by ligation of the internal and external iliac arteries, is more likely to produce Wallerian-type degeneration than demyelination (Fowler and Gilliatt, 1981).

(3) The strongest evidence for direct mechanical damage to nerve fibres during this type of compression comes from animal experiments in which the compressive force has been shown to cause movement of axoplasm along the nerve fibres, with displacement of the nodes of Ranvier and consequent damage to paranodal myelin (*Figure 10.2*). Since the movement of axoplasm is in response

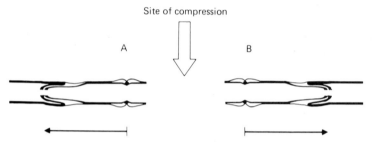

Figure 10.2 Schematic diagram of displacement of nodes of Ranvier by localized pressure, with stretching and invagination of paranodal myelin. There is no corresponding movement of the Schwann-cell junctions which indicate the original sites of the nodes (modified from Ochoa, Fowler and Gilliatt, 1972)

to a pressure gradient along the fibre between its compressed and uncompressed parts, the lesions in experimental tourniquet paralysis tend to occur under the edges of the compressing cuff; in the centre where there is no pressure gradient there is little if any movement of axoplasm and a corresponding absence of demyelination (Ochoa, Fowler and Gilliatt, 1972).

(4) It might be suggested that coincident ischaemia due to occlusion of neural vessels would make an acute compressive lesion worse, by rendering nerve fibres more susceptible to the effect of mechanical distortion. This possibility was tested directly in experimental animals by the use of a proximal cuff to arrest limb blood flow, combined with distal compression (Williams, Jefferson and Gilliatt, 1980). In this experimental situation, periods of limb ischaemia of 3–4 hours did not affect the outcome of local nerve compression for 1 hour, the resulting lesions being similar (in respect of the amount of demyelination and Wallerian-type degeneration) to those produced by a similar period of local compression in a limb with an intact blood supply.

For these reasons it is difficult to accept an ischaemic contribution to the nerve damage in the type of pressure palsy which occurs when a large external force acts on a small skin area for a short period. Some estimates of the force and pressure required to produce persistent conduction block have been made. In the baboon it seemed that a pressure in the region of 1.5 kg/cm^2 (147 kPa) on the skin would produce demyelinating conduction block in an underlying nerve whereas a pressure of 0.75 kg/cm^2 (74 kPa) would not (Gilliatt, 1975).

Attention should be drawn to two interesting features of acute pressure palsies in man. The first of these is the presence of wasting in patients after acute compression injury. The classical teaching (from the time of Erb) is that conduction block causes paralysis without wasting, and often with sparing of sensation. Why then should limb wasting sometimes be present? Animal experiments suggest that these are usually mixed lesions with conduction block in some fibres and complete degeneration in others (Rudge, Ochoa and Gilliatt, 1974). For this reason the presence of wasting and fibrillation in affected muscles should not be taken to indicate a bad prognosis if nerve stimulation shows that there are surviving motor axons distal to the site of injury. There is the additional complication that the inactivity of a muscle caused by blocking conduction in its motor nerve is itself associated with changes in the muscle membrane (increased extra-junctional acetylcholine sensitivity and the appearance of fibrillation) which may confuse the picture (Trojaborg, 1978; Gilliatt, Westgaard and Williams, 1978; Bray, Hubbard and Mills, 1979). With regard to sensory sparing, the main effect of acute compression is on large myelinated fibres and animal evidence does not suggest that motor fibres are more susceptible than afferent fibres of comparable size (Fowler, Danta and Gilliatt, 1972). The relative sparing of sensation in acute pressure palsies is more likely to be due to the sparing of small myelinated and non-myelinated afferents. For the same reason it is unusual for post-ganglionic sympathetic efferent fibres to be damaged during an episode of acute compression, although this has been described by Bolton and McFarlane (1978).

Another feature of acute compressive lesions to which particular attention should be drawn is the long delay which can elapse in severe cases before recovery commences. There are good examples in the literature of cases in which 2 or 3 months have elapsed before evidence of conduction through the blocked region has been detected (Rudge, 1974; Harrison, 1976; Trojaborg, 1977). An example is illustrated in *Figure 10.3*. Two factors in particular contribute to this delay. In the first place the time-course of recovery of the individual paranodal lesions is known to vary. Resumption of conduction through the whole length of a damaged nerve must wait until the last of these individual lesions has recovered; thus the length of the initial lesion and number of nodes of Ranvier affected are important factors. Animal experiments have confirmed this and have shown that with lesions of comparable severity (as judged by the amount of Wallerian degeneration) the demyelination caused by a narrow weighted cord across the nerve recovers more quickly than that in a long lesion caused by a broad compressing cuff (Rudge, Ochoa and Gilliatt, 1974). The other important factor affecting the rate of recovery is the nature of the myelin damage. After severe compression intracytoplasmic Schwann-cell oedema may cause myelin splitting or, if the adaxonal Schwann-cell cytoplasm is affected, distension of an otherwise intact myelin sheath. In some of the animal material studied by Ochoa, Fowler and Gilliatt (1972), such lesions appeared to persist for long periods of time before the distorted myelin was removed by macrophages, leading to a delayed demyelination/remyelination cycle.

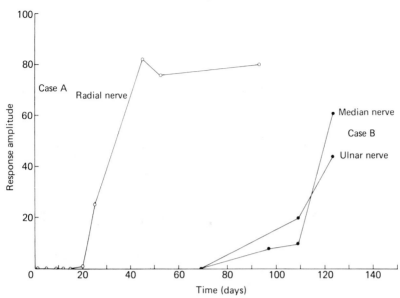

Figure 10.3 Recovery from conduction block after compression injury in man. Amplitude of muscle response on stimulation proximal to the block, expressed as a percentage of response on distal stimulation. Case A represents data for the radial nerve from case 19 of Trojaborg (1970) and the curves for case B are data for the median and ulnar nerves of the patient studied by Rudge (1974)

From the practical point of view it should be emphasized that the delayed recovery of conduction block is not in itself an indication for surgical exploration after a single compressive injury. If recurrent compression is thought to be occurring the problem is a very different one.

What has been said so far does not imply that all acute nerve pressure syndromes are due to mechanical distortion rather than to nerve ischaemia. When compression arises internally from haemorrhage into the nerve sheath or into adjacent structures, or as part of a muscle compartment syndrome, the pressure acting on the nerve is likely to be very much less than that associated with an external compressive force. For example, Hargens *et al.* (1979) have recently shown that when pressure in the anterior tibial compartment of dogs is increased experimentally by plasma infusion, degeneration in the deep peroneal nerve may be seen after pressures of 60–80 mmHg sustained for 8 hours. Ischaemia due to obliteration of intraneural blood vessels seems the likely cause of nerve damage in such a case.

Further study of nerve pathology in this model, including the use of teased fibres, would be helpful in resolving this question.

If, as seems likely, low pressures acting for relatively long periods produce ischaemic nerve damage in muscle compartment syndromes and in cases of nerve compression due to haemorrhage, the clinical implications are important. The likelihood of complete Wallerian degeneration or even of ischaemic necrosis would seem to be high, and early surgical treatment to be essential in order to prevent this.

Prolonged coma due to drugs or carbon monoxide provides a situation in which both 'high-pressure' and 'low-pressure' nerve injury may occur. The lesion shown in *Figure 10.4* was sustained by a man who was unconscious for approximately 24 hours after taking whisky and a barbiturate. When he was found, his left arm was lying across a table and it seems likely that the edge of this had caused the skin blisters running obliquely across the inner side of the arm above the elbow.

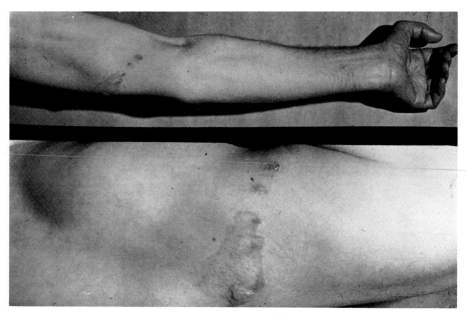

Figure 10.4 A line of skin blisters running obliquely across the ulnar side of the arm just above the elbow, thought to be due to contact with a table-edge during coma lasting approximately 24 hours. Complete median and ulnar lesions were present at this level. (Case report and photograph kindly provided by Dr Eric Nieman)

Although blisters of this kind were at one time called 'barbiturate blisters' and were thought to represent some skin reaction to the drug which had been ingested, they are now known to be due to pressure. In this particular case, they indicated the site of underlying nerve damage, and neurological examination revealed complete median and ulnar nerve lesions at this level. The sharply defined skin blistering makes it likely that a relatively large compressive force acting on a small area had caused direct mechanical damage to nerve fibres in this particular patient.

There are others, however, in which skin blistering involves a larger area, as in the following example (for which we are indebted to Dr C. J. Earl).

A 59-year-old woman had taken an overdose of barbiturates and was unconscious on the floor for 36 hours. During this time she was lying on her right side, with her right arm underneath her. On admission to hospital she was found to have a large blister on the anterior surface of the right forearm. A year later she still had a complete median nerve lesion at this level and a partial ulnar nerve lesion; the area of the skin which had been blistered was depressed and the underlying tissues were indurated. Surgery subsequently showed the median nerve passing into an area of dense fibrous tissue in which it was markedly constricted over several centimetres. In such a case it is impossible to distinguish between the direct effect of compression and the effect of prolonged ischaemia.

While prolonged compression may produce localized necrosis of part of a muscle (Howse and Seddon, 1966), it can also lead to a general rise in tissue pressure throughout a muscle compartment, with the risk of secondary ischaemic damage to both muscle and nerve. Examples have been described by Mubarak and Owen (1975) who emphasize that prompt fasciotomy is required to reduce the increased compartment pressure before it leads to irreversible changes in muscle and nerve.

FEATURES OF CHRONIC COMPRESSION/ENTRAPMENT

The mechanism of nerve damage in chronic compression is less well understood than in acute syndromes, but certain generalizations can be made.

(1) The high pressures which may act on nerve fibres during acute compression are unlikely to arise in chronic entrapment lesions, and displacement of the nodes of Ranvier leading to paranodal demyelination is not thought to be an important mechanism of nerve damage in such cases.

(2) While there is still uncertainty over the role of ischaemia, present evidence suggests that demyelination at an entrapment site results from the detachment of the terminal loops of the myelin lamellae from the axolemma at the nodes of Ranvier, followed by retraction of myelin along the internodes (*Figure 10.5*). The fact that the retraction of myelin appears to take place in opposite directions on the two sides of a lesion would favour local mechanical distortion of nerve fibres as the cause, rather than nerve ischaemia (Ochoa and Marotte, 1973).

(3) Demyelination leading to conduction block is, however, only one feature of the chronic entrapment lesion, and not necessarily the most important in relation to the patient's deficit or the likelihood of recovery. In ulnar lesions at the elbow conduction block in some fibres can persist for long periods (Miller and Olney, 1982), but such fibres constitute a minority and significant Wallerian degeneration is always present in addition to the conduction block. In a study of entrapped nerves at the time of operative decompression, Brown *et al.* (1976) found conduction block in only one-third of the ulnar nerves and one-quarter of the median nerves examined, although conduction delay at the site of the lesion was present in all. This was an important observation as it implies that in most cases the patient's deficit is likely to be due to Wallerian degeneration rather than demyelination.

Histological specimens of entrapped human nerves are rarely obtained, but the naturally occurring median nerve lesion in the guinea-pig has proved valuable in supplementing the small amount of information available from human studies. From both of these it is clear that considerable recovery can occur after

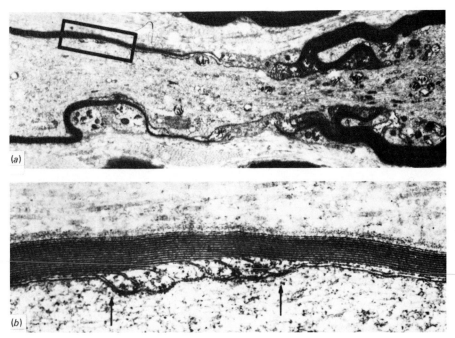

Figure 10.5 Guinea-pig median nerve at the proximal edge of a compression lesion at the wrist. (*a*) Low power electron micrograph of a node of Ranvier showing tapering of the paranodal myelin on the proximal side of the node (*left*) and purse-like folding of the myelin on the distal side of the node (*right*); ×7000. (*b*) Enlargement of the area enclosed in the rectangle in (*a*). The terminal loops (arrowed) of the inner myelin lamellae have become detached from the axon membrane at the node and have retracted some distance along the internode. (From Ochoa and Marotte, 1973)

The progressive thinning of the myelin sheath as the node is approached might seem in (*a*) to be a gradual process but it is clear from (*b*) that it occurs in a step-wise fashion as groups of lamellae lose their terminal attachment to the nodal axon membrane and subsequently shorten or retract along the internode

demyelination or Wallerian degeneration in untreated lesions (Marotte 1974; Neary and Eames, 1975). Thus, thinly remyelinated internodes indicative of previous paranodal or segmental demyelination are easily identified in teased fibre preparations; they are presumably responsible for the localized conduction delay which is such a characteristic feature. Evidence of regeneration comes from the presence in transverse sections of 'regeneration clusters' (Schröder, 1968; Thomas, 1968) in which several small thinly myelinated fibres appear to have arisen from sprouts within a single Schwann-tube (*Figure 10.6*). That some of these regenerating fibres can re-innervate distal muscles, even in untreated cases, seems likely from nerve conduction studies which sometimes reveal grossly reduced motor conduction velocity extending from the level of the lesion to the muscle itself. Motor latencies of more than 20 msec have been described in ulnar lesions at the elbow or in the hand when the ulnar nerve has been stimulated immediately proximal to the site of damage and muscle action potentials recorded from an affected hand muscle (Gilliatt and Thomas, 1960; Ebeling, Gilliatt and Thomas, 1960). Motor latencies of this order, particularly when associated with temporal dispersion of the muscle response, suggest regeneration, even when they are seen in untreated cases.

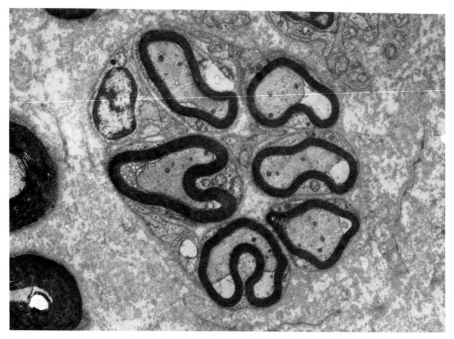

Figure 10.6 A regeneration cluster from the ulnar nerve distal to an untreated entrapment lesion at the elbow. Human post-mortem specimen (×7600). (From Neary and Eames, 1975)

A conspicuous feature of chronic entrapment is neuromatous thickening of the affected nerve. The nerve thickening may be proximal or (less commonly) distal to the actual site of entrapment, or it may extend diffusely through the region. From transverse sections of both animal and human specimens it seems that while there is some increase in epineurial connective tissue, the enlargement of the cross-sectional area of the nerve is due to the increased endoneurial area of individual fascicles, together with some increase in the thickness of the perineurial sheath (*Figure 10.7*). In the endoneurium itself there is oedema and increased deposition of collagen, with a decreased nerve fibre density. Renaut bodies are seen in greatly increased numbers at entrapment sites (Asbury, 1973; Jefferson, Neary and Eames, 1981). While their nature has been the source of some uncertainty in the past, it is now clear that they result from recurrent trauma or sustained compression (Ortman, Sahenk and Mendell, 1983).

The extent to which the endoneurial changes described above might impair the normal vascular perfusion of the endoneurium is uncertain. Experiments in which the endoneurial pressure has been measured directly by a micro-manometer have shown that in certain situations this can be increased to an extent which might be expected to cause capillary closure (Gelberman *et al.*, 1981; Rydevik, Lundborg and Bagge, 1981), but whether this is an important factor in the genesis of nerve damage is not yet clear. It is known that endoneurial swelling (*Figure 10.7*) can occur at an entrapment site in a patient without a clinical deficit and in the absence of significant nerve fibre damage (Neary, Ochoa and Gilliatt, 1975). In mild cases at least, there is no correlation between the endoneurial enlargement or increased perineurial sheath thickness and the nerve fibre damage itself.

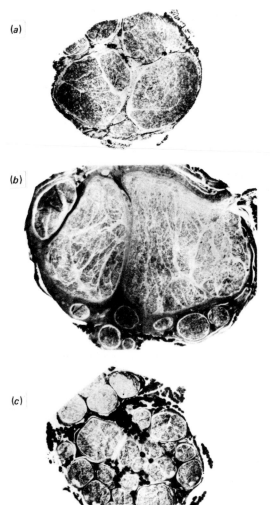

(a)

(b)

(c)

Figure 10.7 Transverse sections of the ulnar nerve of a 40-year-old man with subclinical entrapment at the elbow. (*a*) 6 cm proximal to the elbow; (*b*) in the ulnar groove; (*c*) 4 cm distal to the elbow. There is gross fascicular enlargement in (*b*), × 15 (From Neary *et al.*, 1975)

The continuity of individual fascicles through an entrapment neuroma should provide much better opportunities for successful regeneration following surgery than is the case when a nerve has been partly or completely divided, or when the fascicular architecture has been destroyed by infarction. It may therefore be asked

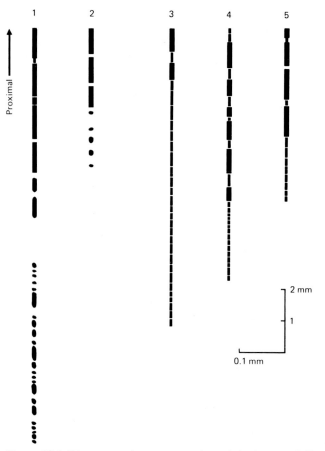

Figure 10.8 Diagrammatic representation of single teased fibres from the median nerve of the guinea-pig to show degenerative changes 2–3 cm proximal to long-standing compression under the carpal ligament. Distal degeneration is present in fibres 1 and 2. This has been followed by regeneration in fibres 3–5. Paranodal demyelination is present proximal to the level of axonal degeneration. (Unpublished material reproduced by courtesy of Dr J. A. Jarratt)

why recovery is sometimes poor after what had seemed to be a satisfactory surgical procedure on an entrapped nerve. Answers to this question are necessarily speculative but the following factors may be relevant.

(1) After Wallerian degeneration has occurred at an entrapment site, atrophic changes develop in the axons proximal to this level which are followed by secondary demyelination (Anderson *et al.*, 1970; Dyck *et al.*, 1981), and dying-back (*Figure 10.8*). Ultimately these are likely to lead to anterior horn cell loss.

(2) Excessive fibrosis at the level of entrapment may produce such a severe degree of constriction that regenerating axons are unable to penetrate the constricted region. If, for example, a ligature is tied tightly round a peripheral nerve in an

experimental animal and left in place, there may be no regeneration except for a few fibres which circumvent the ligature by taking an aberrant course through superficial connective tissue, and which re-join the nerve fascicles below the level of the lesion (Krarup, Gilliatt and Jacobs, 1982). When the ligature is tied less tightly some regeneration through the constricted region is possible but this may occur after a substantial delay, relatively few motor axons finally reaching their target muscles.

(3) Even if fibrosis at the level of entrapment is insufficient to produce such severe constriction as in (2), it may result in slowly progressive atrophy of the distal axon. This process, first studied by Weiss and Hiscoe (1948) was subsequently described as 'axonocachexia' by Bauwens (1961). Recent work has show that this distal axonal atrophy may be followed by secondary demyelination and dying-back of affected axons (Baba *et al.*, 1982).

From the foregoing considerations it is clear that the pathological changes associated with entrapment involve the proximal and distal portions of the nerve as well as the entrapped region itself. While some of these changes are reversed by surgical decompression, there are others which are likely to persist. In this respect time is not necessarily on the side of the patient, and there are many clinical situations in which the early decompression of entrapped nerves is justified, not only in the hope of obtaining improvement, but also to preserve such function as remains.

INDIVIDUAL ENTRAPMENT SYNDROMES

Thoracic outlet syndrome

The eighth cervical and first thoracic roots commonly unite to form the lower trunk of the brachial plexus at the inner border of the first rib. If there is an extra rib on the seventh cervical vertebra or a band running from its transverse process to the scalene tubercle on the first rib, the C8/T1 roots or the lower trunk may be stretched over the abnormal structure. However, nerve injury is rare and X-rays of the thoracic outlet commonly reveal cervical ribs or abnormalities of transverse processes in asymptomatic individuals.

The patients who develop the neurological syndrome usually experience pain in the arm and hand; occasionally this is nocturnal and suggestive of the carpal tunnel syndrome (CTS). Distinction from the latter is made more difficult by the selective thenar wasting which is sometimes present (Gilliatt *et al.*, 1970). More severe cases show thinning of the medial border of the forearm (*Figure 10.9*) and of all the intrinsic hand muscles. Sensory change is usually detectable over the inner aspect of the forearm. It may extend along the medial border of the hand to the ring and little fingers, but the ring finger is not split as in an ulnar lesion, and the sensory deficit is more marked on the inner side of the forearm (T1 territory) than in the hand itself (C8 territory).

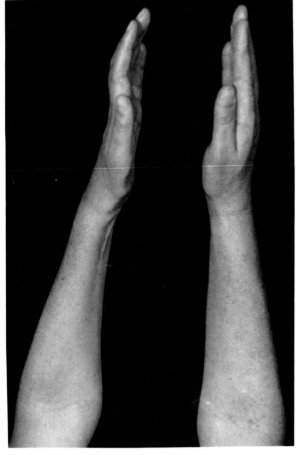

Figure 10.9 Wasting of left forearm and thenar muscles, with claw deformity of the hand (indicating interosseous/lumbrical weakness) in a patient with a rudimentary cervical rib and band. (From Gilliatt, 1979)

Prominence of the neurovascular bundle in the supraclavicular fossa, which can be confirmed by palpation, is present when there is a fully developed cervical rib but is not usually detectable with a rudimentary rib and band. There may be a bruit due to kinking of the subclavian artery over the rib or band. Some patients have vascular symptoms in the hands, with or without embolic phenomena in the digits, but these rarely seem to coincide with the neurological sequelae of a cervical rib.

Neurophysiological studies are needed to exclude the carpal tunnel syndrome or an ulnar neuritis at the elbow. To this end a comparison of the ulnar sensory action potential (SAP), F5 to wrist, with that recorded from F5 to elbow is valuable (Gilliatt *et al.*, 1978). If the ulnar SAP is small due to a cervical rib causing axonal loss in the sensory fibres of C8, then the response at the elbow preserves its usual relative amplitude. If there is an ulnar nerve lesion at the elbow there will be a discrepant reduction or absence of the response at the elbow. Partial denervation in both median and ulnar supplied hand muscles may be demonstrable and not explicable by any distal delay in either median and ulnar nerve conduction. The F wave in the affected hand muscles may be delayed when compared with the asymptomatic side (*Figure 10.10*).

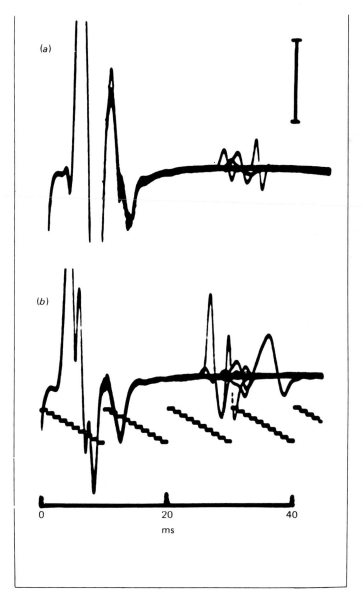

Figure 10.10 F waves recorded from abductor digiti minimi with ulnar nerve stimulation at the wrist, in a patient with a rudimentary cervical rib and band, to show improvement after operation.Twenty superimposed traces (*a*) before and (*b*) 3 months after removal of the band, by which time F-wave amplitude had increased and latency decreased. (From Wulff and Gilliatt, 1979)

When wasting, weakness and sensory loss are accompanied by signs of denervation and a reduced ulnar SAP, there is no controversy about the indication to explore the region of the cervical rib, even if only a minor radiological abnormality is present. The neurological signs often appear on the side of lesser X-ray changes, due to the fact that the sharp edge of a fibrous band is more likely to cause neurological symptoms than a fully developed bony rib (*Figure 10.11*). Successful decompression relieves pain and paraesthesiae and arrests progression, but wasting usually persists. The management of patients with pain in the arm which is thought to be due to a cervical rib or band but which is not accompanied by wasting or weakness of typical distribution is more controversial. The problem is

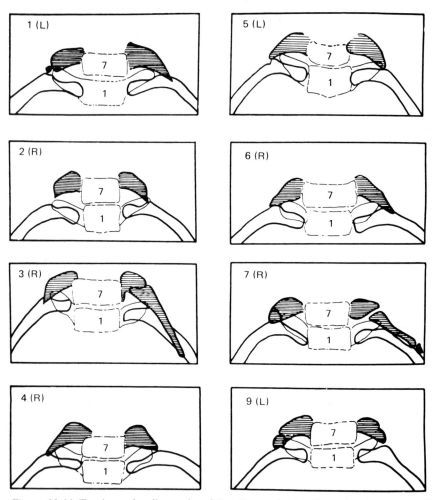

Figure 10.11 Tracings of radiographs of 8 patients with hand wasting due to a rudimentary cervical rib and band. The side of the muscle wasting in each case is indicated in brackets next to the case number. It can be seen that in two cases (3 and 7) there was a large cervical rib on one side and a long C7 transverse process on the other; in each case the hand wasting was on the side of the latter. (From Gilliatt *et al.*, 1970)

magnified when X-rays fail to reveal a bony abnormality. In some clinics surgical removal of the first rib via the axilla is the treatment of choice (Urschel and Razzuk, 1972; Roos, 1976); in others this operation is rarely performed. Some of the difficulties which prevent the development of an agreed treatment policy for such cases are discussed elsewhere (Gilliatt, 1984).

Long thoracic nerve

Isolated weakness of the serratus anterior with winging of one scapula is more common than any other single nerve lesion around the shoulder (Kaplan, 1980). The nerve may be damaged by radical breast surgery or by the wearing of heavy backpacks, but the aetiology is frequently mysterious. Some cases are thought to be variants of neuralgic amyotrophy (brachial plexus neuropathy) in which pain around the shoulder is followed by denervation in the territory of roots or peripheral nerves or combinations of both. If there are associated changes, for example if there is evidence of sensory loss in the territory of the circumflex nerve, then a lesion of the long thoracic nerve can reasonably be attributed to this cause. The prognosis is uncertain, some patients taking at least a year before re-innervation is seen.

Suprascapular nerve

This nerve is rarely damaged by external pressure, but is occasionally affected by a ganglion. The nerve may be entrapped in the suprascapular notch, when there is weakness of both the supraspinatus and infraspinatus, or at the lateral border of the spine of the scapula, when only the infraspinatus is wasted and/or weak (Ganzhorn *et al.*, 1980; Aiello *et al.*, 1982). Wasting of spinati muscles is often difficult to detect with confidence, especially in the aged, and a flat contour without demonstrable weakness should not be accepted as proof of abnormality. Most patients with proven denervation of the spinati will have a C5/6 root lesion or plexus damage with appropriate changes in arm muscles and reflexes. It may be possible to show a prolonged latency to the spinati from stimulation at Erb's point when the suprascapular nerve is damaged (Aiello *et al.*, 1982).

Pain in the region of the shoulder after stretching the adducted arms across the chest, and in the familiar frozen shoulder, may be partly due to involvement of the suprascapular nerve, but this is a controversial point.

Dorsal scapular nerve

Doubt surrounds the entity of entrapment of this nerve which innervates the rhomboids (Nakano, 1978b). There is unilateral weakness of the rhomboids with partial winging of the scapula and weak retraction of the shoulder blades. Posterior displacement of the elbow when the hand is placed on the hip is similarly weak.

Tenderness over the nerve at the level of the scalene muscle is said to be confirmatory. Rest and local anesthetic injections can be helpful. Again there is little hard proof of the existence of an entrapment syndrome.

Notalgia paraesthetica

Burning, pruritus and paraesthesiae develop over an area the size of the palm of a hand at the medial magin of the scapula (Pleet and Massey, 1978). Examination reveals some reduction in pinprick over the same area. It is suggested that this is the territory of the dorsal branches of roots T2–6 and further that these branches are vulnerable as they make a 90° turn on passing through the multifidus spinae. Nonetheless, the aetiology is uncertain. The prognosis appears benign and no intervention is warranted.

Musculocutaneous nerve

Lesions of this nerve are rarely recognized. It supplies the biceps and brachialis and is responsible for sensation over the radial side of the forearm. A cervical 5/6 root lesion is partly mimicked but there is no weakness of spinati, deltoid or brachioradialis and the brachioradialis reflex is normal. Nor is there sensory change in the thumb and index as with C6 root problems. The cause is usually obvious external trauma, or a hyperextension injury of the forearm (Trojaborg, 1976).

Axillary (circumflex) nerve

This may be damaged by fractures and dislocation around the shoulder, and by deep intramuscular injections in the deltoid but, rarely, may develop without a history of trauma. There is isolated weakness of the deltoid, and a small area of sensory change over the lateral aspect of the upper arm. As Seddon has emphasized, simple testing of abduction of the shoulder may be misleading due to the action of the supraspinatus which occasionally permits a full range of movement. Usually abduction is limited to 155° with the arm a little anterior to the coronal plane (Seddon, 1975).

Radial nerve

The nerve is most vulnerable in the upper arm at the level of the spiral groove, usually below the take-off of the motor branch to the triceps muscle. Whilst blunt trauma and fracture of the humerus may cause radial nerve palsies, the commonest cause is external pressure as in a 'Saturday-night' paralysis. The sleeping patient, often affected by alcohol, compresses the nerve between the humerus and the back of a chair, waking with a fully developed radial nerve lesion. A comparable disturbance may occur if an arm hangs over the edge of the operating table during general anaesthesia. A deep intramuscular injection in the upper arm may similarly produce an iatrogenic radial nerve palsy.

Clinically there is a wrist and finger drop (*Figure 10.12*) with weakness of the brachioradialis in most instances. The brachioradialis reflex is lost. A sensory disturbance over the back of the base of the thumb is inconstant.

The position of the hand affected by a wrist drop produces an apparent weakness of grip and abduction of the digits, sometimes leading the inexperienced to diagnose additional weakness in the median and ulnar territories. It is important that these functions are only tested after passive correction of the wrist position.

Electrical studies can be helpful in predicting recovery. If pressure changes in the upper arm are restricted to the appearance of a conduction block due to local

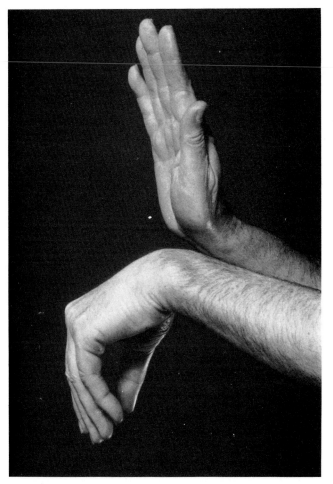

Figure 10.12 Wrist drop due to a 'Saturday-night' pressure palsy of the left radial nerve. The radial sensory action potential recorded in the forearm remained intact, and recovery occurred over the course of approximately 8 weeks

demyelination, the radial SAP in the forearm will be preserved, sampling of the brachioradialis and common extensor origin reveal no denervation, and stimulation at the spiral groove elicits a much smaller muscle action potential from the extensor group than does a stimulus at the lateral epicondyle. Such a demonstration of conduction block enables one to predict a spontaneous resolution of symptoms usually within 6–8 weeks. If the SAP is reduced after 6–10 days and there is denervation of the radial supplied muscles, then Wallerian degeneration can be inferred and recovery predicted to await upon regeneration. Mixed findings, for example retention of the SAP but some fibrillation potentials, are commonly encountered (Trojaborg, 1970). A cockup splint may enable the patient to make good use of the hand during the interim.

Posterior interosseous nerve

The posterior interosseous nerve arises from the radial nerve at the elbow, and passes through the supinator, an opening between the tip of the lateral epicondyle and the medial aspect of the epicondyle (Spinner, 1968). If the elbow is extended with pronation of the palmar flexed wrist the supinator is tightened across the nerve. Hyperextension and repeated pronation and supination of the forearm may therefore provoke symptoms. Synovial bulging from the elbow joint in rheumatoid arthritis, bursitis and ganglia are all rarer causes of the posterior interosseous nerve syndrome. The nerve branches into two, one branch supplying the extensor carpi ulnaris and extensor communis, the other the extensor pollicis longus, abductor longus and extensor indicis.

The patient complains of a deep ache in the forearm, perhaps after unaccustomed use of something like a screwdriver, and develops weakness of finger extension with relative sparing of the radial wrist extensors (Goldman *et al.*, 1969). Radial deviation may thus occur during attempted extension of the wrist. The weakness may be confined to extension of the thumb and index finger, or occasionally to more lateral digits, according to which branch is maximally affected.

If spontaneous recovery does not occur in 6–8 weeks of rest, exploration may be indicated.

Median nerve at elbow (Pronator syndrome: anterior interosseous nerve)

The median nerve may be damaged at the elbow by external trauma including supracondylar fractures, and iatrogenically with catheterization of the brachial artery or even venepuncture in the antecubital fossa (Winer and Harrison, 1982). Entrapment is thought to occur at three sites. In about 1% of subjects the median nerve lies behind a supracondylar process of the humerus, a caudally directed process 5 cm above the medial epicondyle. A fibrous band may pass from this spur to the medial epicondyle (ligament of Struthers) representing a possible site of compression. The nerve is also vulnerable behind the bicipital aponeurosis, and again as it enters the forearm, passing between two heads of the pronator teres in

80% of individuals. Entrapment at this site by hypertrophy of the pronator teres, by tendinous bands or a taut arch gives rise to the 'pronator' syndrome (Morris and Peters, 1976; Nigst and Dick, 1979).

Patients with the pronator syndrome complain of an ache in the forearm. Pain may be aggravated by forceful pronation of the arm with the fingers flexed. Writing is often painful, and paraesthesiae felt over the median supplied fingers and palm. Acute symptoms may be provoked by carrying a heavy load on the forearm. Examination may reveal tenderness and a Tinel sign over the pronator teres. Thenar atrophy is commonly present with weakness of the abductor pollicis brevis and opponens pollicis as well as of the muscles supplied by the anterior interosseous branch (flexor pollicis longus and flexor digitorum profundus to the index finger). Sensory change is detected over the median supplied digits and palm. Location of the lesion by nerve conduction studies is difficult, though slowing may be detected between the elbow and wrist. Usually, however, there are signs of denervation without major conduction disturbance, suggesting that acute local damage rather than chronic entrapment is responsible for the nerve lesion.

The symptoms may remit spontaneously with avoidance of repetitive forearm use, particularly of supination and pronation with flexed fingers. Infiltration of the pronator teres with local steroid has its advocates as has surgical decompression if no improvement occurs in 2–3 months.

Anterior interosseous nerve

The anterior interosseous nerve arises as a branch of the median nerve approximately 5–8 cm distal to the lateral epicondyle. It is therefore vulnerable following fractures at or about the elbow, and during open reduction of forearm fractures (Spinner, 1970). Some cases of damage are due to direct trauma but the majority are attributed to entrapment. The nerve may be compressed by a tendinous origin of the deep head of the pronator teres and this may be the explanation for the development of symptoms after the repeated use of the forearm. The nerve supplies the flexor digitorum profundus, flexor pollicis longus and the pronator quadratus. It has no cutaneous sensory branch (but supplies some sensory fibres to the joints of the carpus). The symptoms consist of deep aching in the forearm and loss of pinch grip. The patient is unable to make an 'O' between the tip of the index and thumb due to loss of flexion of the tips of these two digits (*Figure 10.13*). Hyperextension of the distal interphalangeal joints causes the point of contact of the index on the thumb to be more proximally displaced than normal. Weakness of the pronator quadratus can be detected by testing pronation with the elbow fully flexed (to eliminate the effect of pronator teres). There is no sensory loss. The Martin Gruber anastomosis commonly involves the anterior interosseous nerve and the ulnar nerve so a lesion of the former may also produce weakness of the ulnar supplied small hand muscles.

Recovery may occur spontaneously but, if there is no sign of improvement in 2–3 months, exploration is usually advised though proof of its necessity has never been formally obtained. The differential diagnosis includes rupture of the long flexor

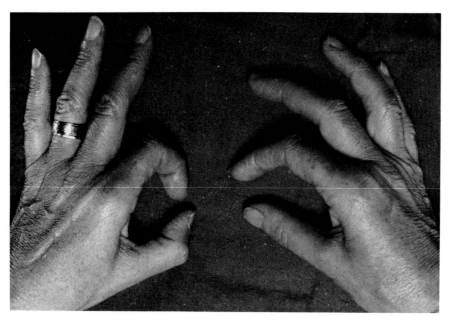

Figure 10.13 Anterior interosseous nerve lesion. This 46-year-old woman developed sudden weakness of the thumb and index finger of the right hand. She was unable to make an 'O' on the right due to paralysis of flexion of the tip of both digits. As no recovery could be detected after 3 months, the forearm was explored. No abnormality was detected. Six months later the patient's weakness remained unchanged

tendon of the thumb or index (e.g. rheumatoid arthritis) which can be difficult when it is appreciated that cases of anterior interosseous palsy have been reported in which weakness is confined to the thumb. Electromyography may be necessary to make the distinction. Abnormalities may be confined to the demonstration of denervation in the deep forearm flexors and pronatus quadratus, with delay in conduction to the latter muscle.

Median nerve at the wrist (Carpal tunnel syndrome)

For many years the condition of burning pins and needles at night in the fingers of middle-aged females was known as the acro-paraesthesia syndrome. It is interesting that the cause of this syndrome was not appreciated until McArdle (1949) proposed that the symptoms could be due to compression of the median nerve in the carpal tunnel. Recent pathological studies have confirmed this explanation and have also shown that subclinical abnormalities are common in asymptomatic subjects. Thus, Neary, Ochoa and Gilliatt (1975) showed an increase in the connective tissue elements in the median nerve with some endoneurial oedema at the point where it passes under the transverse retinaculum. Teased fibre preparations on these asymptomatic cases show some of the changes seen in experimental mechanical nerve compression.

The carpal tunnel has been shown to be anatomically smaller in symptomatic cases (Dekel and Coates, 1979) and it seems likely that an anatomical predisposition exists, which probably helps to explain the female predominance (3:1). Other circumstances or conditions which alter the dimensions of the tunnel can provoke or aggravate symptoms. Thus acromegaly, myxoedema, amyloidosis, rheumatoid arthritis and tenosynovitis may all cause a pressure rise in the narrowing of the tunnel. Venous engorgement of the hand, for example after the creation of an arteriovenous shunt at the wrist for renal dialysis, can also provoke median nerve symptoms, as can local trauma or osteoarthritic deformity of the wrist. Lymphoedema after breast surgery is another cause and needs to be distinguished from coexistent brachial plexus infiltration or radiation fibrosis of the nerve. Flexion and extension movements at the wrist may cause further nerve damage (Gelberman *et al.*, 1981). This may explain aggravation of symptoms during such tasks as wringing out wet clothes and knitting, and is the basis of Phalen's test (*see below*).

The nocturnal exacerbation of symptoms may be due to ischaema since it is mimicked by placing a cuff above arterial pressure on the symptomatic arm and relieved by hanging the arm out of the bed (Fullerton, 1963). It is also possible that venous engorgement, vasodilation or fluid retention also cause changes in sleep. Finally, some patients sleep with their wrists fully flexed. Fluid retention may explain an increase in symptoms during pregnancy.

The symptoms are well exemplified by case 1 from the influential early clinical paper by Kremer *et al.* (1953):

'A right-handed housewife aged 49 had had symptoms for two years in both hands before she was seen. She would be wakened in the early hours of the morning by burning tingling in the thumb, index and middle and to a lesser extent, ring fingers of both hands, the right being more severely affected. This would be accompanied by a numb swollen feeling in the fingers and by a deep ache passing up the forearm on the inner aspect and into the upper arm almost to the shoulder. This would last up to an hour, during which time she would try to rid herself of the pain, by shaking the hands or getting out of bed and walking about. Her own impression was that nothing made much difference to the pain, and that it would ease spontaneously after a certain time. The attacks were always at their worst at night but could appear in the day. When this happened the tingling in the thumb and neighbouring fingers would precede numbness by as much as ten minutes. The precipitating factors for diurnal attacks were knitting, sewing, wringing washing or writing. Just before she was seen, the attacks were so severe that she was afraid to go to bed and suffered greatly from insomnia.'

Many patients are less precise than this. Difficulties arise particularly with patients who insist that paraesthesiae affect all digits. Kremer *et al.* (1953) found that patients, when asked to observe their attacks of nocturnal symptoms more closely, would often correct their earlier impressions and usually report back that in fact the little finger was strikingly spared. Pain, though maximal in the thenar eminence or palm, is also felt deep in the forearm and even in the upper part of the arm, raising the differential diagnosis of a cervical root lesion. Paraesthesiae are restricted to the fingers, however, unlike those with root irritation, and there is no effect of neck positioning on the symptoms; nor is there neck pain. Both conditions may coexist and it has been suggested that root damage may make symptoms from early carpal tunnel compression more likely or more prominent (double crush hypothesis).

Other symptoms often suggest a rheumatological condition, with complaints of flexed stiff fingers on waking, and of swollen fingers. These resolve with decompression of the nerve, however. There are cases with associated trigger fingers, tennis elbows and frozen shoulders suggesting a more widespread disorder of soft tissues. A carpal tunnel syndrome may prove to be the first presentation of rheumatoid arthritis.

A diffuse neuropathy may underlie an increased vulnerability of the median nerve to local compressive damage (Earl *et al.*, 1964) and personal cases have subsequently been found to be suffering from diabetic neuropathy, lymphomatous neuropathy and hypertrophic (presumably hereditary) neuropathy. Therefore, symptoms of more diffuse neuropathy should be sought in the history.

Examination may reveal some softness or flattening of the lateral aspect of the thenar eminence (*Figure 10.14*) with weakness of abduction of the thumb at 90° to the plane of the hand. Some abduction by the long abductor and extensor is avoided by testing in this position. Wasting of the thenar eminence is common in old age and care needs to be taken in interpreting the appearance of the hand in the elderly. This is also true in the presence of rheumatoid arthritis when disuse atrophy occurs about the deformed and often subluxed joints. Median nerve entrapment due to the synovial thickening may coexist and sensory changes and electrical studies make the distinction. Severe atrophy and weakness may be seen without a history of pain or sensory change, whilst in other patients severe pain and painful paraesthesiae have brought the patient to medical attention and no motor changes are apparent. The reason for these two types of presentation is not clear though it may be that direct compression causes atrophy due to axonal loss, whilst the nocturnal painful paraesthesiae are more common when ischaemia plays an important role (Fullerton, 1963).

Sensory testing often reveals little, but there may be diminished appreciation of light touch and pinprick over the median-supplied 3½ digits. The index finger is often more affected than the thumb. The sensory changes are often restricted to the pulp of the digit and may only be detected as an elevation of two point threshold when compared with that in the little finger or in a truly asymptomatic contralateral index. Symptoms may be aggravated by 30–60 s of forced flexion (Phalen's test) or forced extension (sometimes called a reversed Phalen's test). Phalen (1970) found the test positive in 76.7% of 200 surgically confirmed cases. Others have found it less reliable. He also found a positive Tinel sign at the wrist in two-thirds of his cases; personal experience suggests that the incidence is lower than this.

It is often stated that electrical tests are not needed to make the diagnosis. Whilst this is sometimes true it is always prudent to confirm the diagnosis before surgery. Failure of symptoms to be relieved after decompression is usually due to an incorrect diagnosis that might have been avoided by nerve conduction studies, though sometimes it is due to inadequate surgery (*see below*).

EMG studies may demonstrate fasciculation in abductor pollicis brevis and electrical signs of denervation, with normal findings in ulnar supplied muscles and forearm flexor groups, though such extensive muscle sampling is surely unnecessary if conduction studies demonstrate abnormalities confined to the median nerve at the wrist.

The distal motor latency may be prolonged as proof of local slowing at the wrist (Simpson, 1956; Buchthal, Rosenfalck and Trojaborg, 1974). Motor conduction velocity from the elbow to the wrist will be normal in mild cases. When the distal abnormality is severe, mild or moderate proximal slowing is found. Marked slowing in the forearm should raise suspicions that the lesion is not distal, unless the

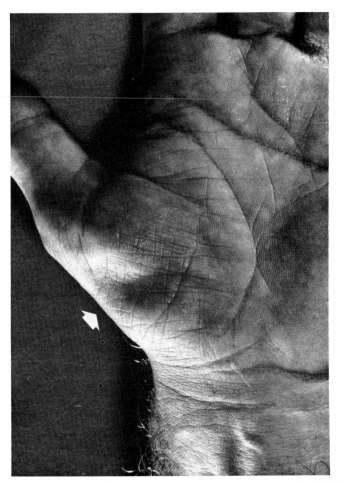

Figure 10.14 Selective wasting of the abductor pollicis brevis. The muscle was electrically silent, and no sensory action potential could be recorded at the wrist with stimulation of the index finger. The abnormality in the median nerve could not therefore be localized by the nerve conduction studies and division of the flexor retinaculum at the wrist was advised on clinical criteria. Severe median nerve compression in the carpal tunnel was confirmed at surgery.

distal delay is still disproportionately greater or the muscle sampling has revealed that one is studying only one or two surviving fibres. In some cases threshold stimulation elicits a late response even though the latency for supramaximal shocks is within the normal range.

Sensory testing is more valuable since normal motor latencies can be found despite compression. The 'classical' finding is of a small and late sensory action potential (SAP) at the wrist during stimulation of the index (Buchthal, Rosenfalck and Trojaborg, 1974; Kimura, 1979). Comparison with the ulnar or radial SAP is essential to exclude a generalized abnormality as a cause of the reduced median SAP. A direct comparison with the ulnar SAP may be helpful to detect reduction in the median SAP even though its amplitude remains within normal range (Loong and Seah, 1971). Normally the median SAP is greater than the ulnar. A median SAP equal to or smaller than the ulnar SAP, even though over $9\mu V$, may thus be a sign of abnormality. Similarly a discrepancy of 1.5 ms in the latency implies median nerve compression, as does a difference of 1 ms between the symptomatic and asymptomatic hands. The difference between the median and ulnar SAP latency may be conveniently tested by stimulation of the ring finger and recording over both median and ulnar nerves. An increase in the yield of abnormalities can also be achieved by stimulating motor and sensory fibres in the palm. This enables calculation of conduction directly across the wrist. Palmar stimulation can be painful however and this test is not universally applied. Another way to localize the restricted changes is to record the digital SAP which may be normal when the finger to wrist SAP is relatively small.

Rarely, conduction studies reveal no definite abnormality but help to exclude rival diagnoses. Treatment must then proceed on the basis of clinical evidence (*Figure 10.14*).

Rest is undoubtedly effective. This is commonly obvious to the patient who reports relief of symptoms while on holiday or in hospital. Unilateral carpal tunnel decompression sometimes 'cures' both hands due to the enforced rest. Fullerton (1963) showed improvement after splinting of the wrist and it is clear that this simple device relieves nocturnal pain. It may be enough to relieve symptoms in late pregnancy, a further spontaneous improvement occurring after delivery. Local steroid injections may also relieve symptoms, the effect often being only temporary. If there is muscle atrophy, if clearcut conduction abnormalities have been obtained or pain is severe, surgery is normally advised. An early sequential trial showed the superiority of surgery over immobilization (Garland et al., 1964). The point of compression has been located by careful pre-operative electro-physiological studies and coincides with the point of greatest narrowing of the tunnel in many cases. The critical point is usually 2–4 cm distal to the distal wrist crease. Occasionally, however, the site of damage is proximal to the wrist crease and in 50% the change appears more diffuse (Brown et al., 1976). It is clear from these remarks that the whole tunnel must be decompressed. This is best achieved by open decompression through a curved longitudinal incision. Cases of failed surgery with confirmed electrical abnormality have usually in personal experience had blind surgery through a small transverse wrist incision, with incomplete decompression.

Pain is usually relieved at once, as are painful paraesthesiae. Intraneural recordings confirm that conduction may recover in some fibres at the time of decompression (Hougell and Mattsson, 1971). Weakness may recover rapidly except when accompanied by atrophy. Electrical abnormalities may take 18 months to return to normal, a fact which must be recalled when assessing cases of 'failed' surgery; this can create difficulties if there has been no pre-operative study (Goodman and Gilliatt, 1961).

Ulnar nerve lesions

The ulnar nerve in the axilla is vulnerable to pressure from the use of crutches, and occasionally to a Saturday-night paralysis from pressure between the back of a chair and the humerus (Harrison, 1976). However, the commonest site by far for a lesion is at the elbow. Richards (1945) described four common possible lesions – distal fractures of the humerus; delayed damage long after a fracture due to deformity (tardy ulnar palsy) (Shelden, 1921); recurrent dislocation of the nerve; osteoarthritis of the elbow.

External trauma at the elbow commonly occurs during general anaesthesia for major surgery (Miller and Camp, 1979) or during bed rest for disabling medical illnesses (e.g. in the intensive care unit). It also follows the use of unpadded elbow crutches. At surgery, the risk of a pressure lesion is greater if the elbow is flexed, or pronated though extended. A narrow ulnar groove or a hypermobile nerve which easily dislocates out of the groove is thought to increase the nerve's vulnerability, as does diabetes or a hereditary neuropathy. In practice, constriction of the nerve by the aponeurosis of the flexor carpi ulnaris in the cubital tunnel predominates as the mechanism for an ulnar neuropathy, rather than those related to acute pressure (Wadsworth and Williams, 1973; Wadsworth, 1977).

Intraneural pressure is also increased by simple changes of posture, for example when the arm is flexed above the head (Pechan and Julis, 1975), a position sometimes adopted in sleep. One personal case of bilateral ulnar nerve lesions at the elbow proved to be due to the woman sleeping with an arm around each of her two pet poodles!

The patients complain of painful paraesthesiae in the ulnar side of the hand, the little and ring fingers. The pain is often said to be worse in cold weather. Flexion of the elbow or habitual pressure on it may increase paraesthesiae. Weakness of the hand develops followed by guttering of the back of the hand as wasting of the interossei develops.

Examination may reveal a deformity of the elbow (*Figure 10.15*) in cases of tardy ulnar paralysis, many years after a fracture or with the development of osteoarthritis of the joint. Extension is limited and the carrying angle increased. The nerve may be palpably thickened above or in the ulnar groove. Wasting may be obvious in the hypothenar eminence, though this may be more palpable than visible; it is more readily detected in the first dorsal interosseous (*Figure 10.16*). The inner aspect of the forearm may look thinner if the flexor carpi ulnaris or flexor digitorum profundus are affected. Weakness of the interossei and hypothenar eminence is obvious in abduction and adduction of individual digits. The loss of

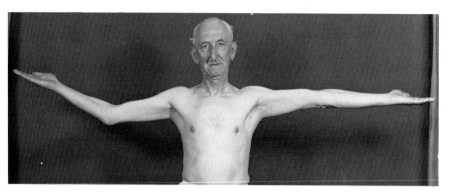

Figure 10.15 Limitation of extension of the right elbow resulting from an old fracture in a patient who developed an ulnar neuropathy many years after the original injury. The results of nerve conduction studies in this patient are given by Simpson (1956)

lumbricals to the fourth and fifth fingers with preserved long extensor muscles leads to the hyperextension deformity at the metacarpo-phalangeal joints with flexion at the interphalangeal joints. Loss of adduction of the little finger leads to another abnormal posture of the hand with a tendency of the little finger to drift away from the rest of the hand, although this is more frequently seen with lesions of the deep palmar branch.

Attempts to adduct the thumb to the index, for example when holding a sheet of paper horizontally with the thumb above the page and the rest of the hand below, reveal a trick movement. The long flexors of the thumb are used and pronounced flexion of the interphalangeal joint of the thumb is obvious (Froment's sign). The metacarpal arch may be obviously flat and the patient is unable to make the hand into a cone shape. The middle finger cannot be swayed from side to side in the plane of the extended fingers. Powerful extension of the fingers may provoke some flexion at the wrist. During abduction of the little finger there is normally a dimpling of the hypothenar eminence due to contraction of the palmaris brevis. In an ulnar palsy this dimpling is lost. If there is weakness of the flexors of the distal phalanges of the fourth and fifth digits, the patient may also have difficulty playing musical instruments, e.g. the flute or the high notes of the violin if the left hand is affected. Weakness of the flexor digitorum profundus to the fourth and fifth fingers and of the flexor carpi ulnaris may or may not be obvious even when the nerve is injured at the elbow above the branches to the forearm muscles. When present their weakness helps to locate the lesion at least as high as the elbow. If not, the lesion may yet be at the ulnar groove. The relative immunity of fibres to these two muscles probably lies in their deep position in the groove and the origin of the branch to flexor carpi ulnaris in many individuals above the cubital aponeurosis.

Sensory change is found over the little finger and the adjacent side of the ring finger. The ulnar border of the hand may also show diminished pinprick and light touch sensibility but no change will be found above the wrist crease (in contrast to T1 root lesions which involve the ulnar border of the forearm). Two point discrimination on the pads of the fingers is often the most sensitive test for ulnar (or

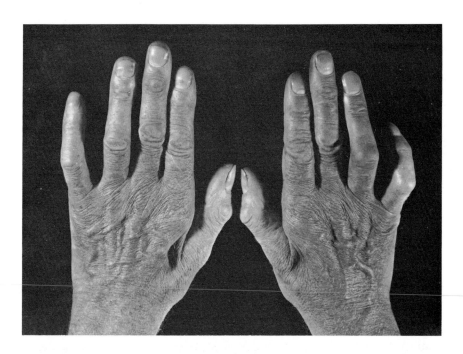

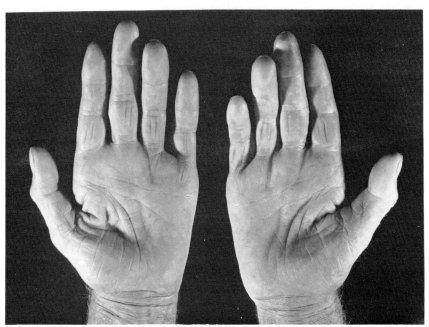

Figure 10.16 Selective wasting of the ulnar-supplied hand muscles due to bilateral lesions at the elbow associated with generalised osteoarthritis in a 56-year-old man. The sparing of the median-supplied first and second lumbrical muscles results in a claw deformity limited to the ring and little fingers

median) territory impairment. It is often possible to demonstrate a difference between the ulnar and median supplied halves of the ring finger by this method.

The diagnostic neurophysiological approach depends to some extent on the circumstances (Payan, 1969). When there has been obvious axonal damage with marked wasting, the ulnar SAP will be lost and the nerve action potential (NAP) small or absent (wrist to elbow). Conduction velocity measurements hold out the best chance of localizing the lesion by defining a discrepancy in velocity between the axilla to elbow segment, and the elbow to wrist, or demonstrating disproportionate slowing across the elbow segment (Eisen, 1974). If there has been severe fibre loss the nerve may even be inexcitable – then the presence of signs of denervation in the ulnar supplied forearm muscles may at least indicate that the lesion is not at the wrist. When there is no wasting and the symptoms are of short duration, one may only be dealing with local demyelination at the site of mechanical trauma. The ulnar SAP at the wrist may be of normal amplitude reflecting the lack of Wallerian change in sensory fibres. It is then valuable to compare the amplitude of the response recordable at the elbow with that at the wrist during stimulation of the little finger, a low ratio suggesting conduction block at the elbow. Similarly the NAP (wrist to elbow) volley may be reduced, delayed and dispersed, when compared with that on the asymptomatic side. Finally, the muscle action potential should be recorded by surface electrodes from abductor digiti minimi while the nerve is stimulated at wrist, below elbow, above elbow and in the axilla. A decrement of over 20% when comparing the response above the elbow with that below the elbow or at the wrist implies a degree of local conduction block. A small response from the wrist implies loss of motor units and a degree of axonal loss.

When there is little or no wasting and the electrical studies confirm that the lesion is presumably one of conduction block, rest, protection of the elbow, and a wait-and-see policy are indicated. This is particularly true after a history of acute trauma when spontaneous recovery, given these precautions, can be anticipated. When there is fibre loss and the electrical changes support the view that there is a significant degree of Wallerian change, the situation is a little different. If there has been acute trauma (e.g. during anaesthesia) there is no need to explore the nerve unless arthritis of the joint suggests regeneration will be impeded. The prognosis for recovery is less certain, however. If the changes have appeared insidiously, cubital tunnel compression should be assumed and the patient offered surgery. Prolonged symptoms represent an adverse prognostic factor for successful decompression so patients should be encouraged to submit to surgery within a year of symptoms. Two procedures have their advocates – decompression of the tunnel (Miller and Hummel, 1980) and transposition into a mechanically less vulnerable anterior site (Harrison and Nurick, 1970). The latter procedure is preferred if the joint is abnormal, or if the nerve dislocates. If there is clear-cut local change with, for example, pseudoneuroma formation at the upper edge of a tight aponeurosis, a simple decompression is sufficient (MacNicol, 1979).

Postoperatively, pain and painful paraesthesiae are relieved and function in the hand improves though some wasting and weakness may remain. Failure of a local decompression should be considered an indication for transposition. Failure of transposition may be due to nerve entrapment in the muscle bed (Harrison and Nurick, 1970).

Ulnar nerve at the wrist

Damage to the ulnar nerve at the wrist is far less common. The nerve may however be affected by open injuries at the wrist (putting a hand through a glass window or slashing of the wrists in a suicide attempt), recurrent trauma (Noth, Dietz and Mauritz, 1980) and, rarely, by a ganglion. There is weakness of the ulnar intrinsic muscles and sensory change but no involvement of the flexor digitorum profundus or flexor carpi ulnaris; this aggravates clawing of the fourth and fifth digits. The lack of involvement of the long flexors is, however, unreliable in locating the lesion at the wrist rather than the elbow. There is usually an obvious visible or palpable abnormality at the wrist and nerve conduction studies demonstrate prolonged distal latencies to both abductor digiti minimi (ADM) and the first dorsal interosseous with preserved conduction more proximally. The ulnar SAP will be reduced and/or delayed.

In Guyton's canal the nerve runs between the pisiform bone and the hook of the hamate (Shea and McClain, 1969). A lesion here – a ganglion (Brooks, 1952) or repetitive occupational trauma – may spare sensation but affect all the ulnar intrinsic muscles. Again latencies to both the first dorsal interosseous and the hypothenar muscles will be prolonged but the SAP normal. The differential bedside diagnosis includes motor neurone disease when there is insidious wasting of the intrinsic hand muscles with no sensory loss. Sparing of the median supplied abductor pollicis brevis (APB) and the conduction studies should leave little doubt of ulnar nerve involvement.

At its exit from Guyton's canal the deep branch of the ulnar nerve crosses the palm to innervate the interossei. Visible wasting of the first dorsal interosseous may be the presenting feature of damage to the nerve in the palm. The cause is usually by occupational trauma (Noth, Dietz and Mauritz, 1980). A personal case concerned a greengrocer who took delivery of boxes of oranges by catching them at two lower corners in the palm of each hand as they were allowed to slide down a chute into his basement store. Bilateral wasting of the web space between the thumb and index finger developed over a few months and examination revealed characteristic weakness of all the interossei and of adductor pollicis, with hypothenar sparing.

The distal latency to the first dorsal interosseous will be prolonged, that to ADM and the SAP normal (Ebeling, Gilliatt and Thomas, 1960). If there is a clear-cut history of trauma its avoidance may suffice to allow recovery; if a ganglion is palpable, exploration is advisable. This applies to lesions at the wrist or in the canal. Subluxation of carpal bones in rheumatoid arthritis may cause deep ulnar branch lesions with a risk that the wasting of interossei be attributed to disuse.

Cheiralgia paraesthetica

Pressure on the superficial branch of the radial nerve may produce sensory disturbance over the dorsum of the lateral aspect of the wrist and of the first two fingers. The nerve is vulnerable at the wrist and its damage has been recorded following the wearing of a tight watch strap, wrist bands and handcuffs (Massey and Pleet, 1978).

Digital nerves

Isolated lesions of individual digital nerves are rare and usually due to obvious trauma to the palm or to a finger. Pallis (1966) drew attention to the frequency of a digital neuropathy in patients with rheumatoid arthritis, usually in individuals with nodules and evidence of vascular complications. A true digital entrapment neuropathy has also been postulated (Wartenberg, 1954; Kopell and Thompson, 1963).

Numbness may affect one side of a finger or asymmetrically affect the terminal phalanx. In rheumatoid cases the symptoms usually develop insidiously and subside spontaneously after some months.

Recording digital sensory action potentials, as described by Casey and Le Quesne (1972), or the finger to wrist SAPs from separate digits can be confirmatory. Thus, in a personal case, the digit to wrist potentials from the thumb and middle finger were 25–27 μV while that from the index, which was the site of a unilateral digital nerve lesion, was 13 μV.

Abdominal cutaneous nerves

Entrapment of cutaneous nerves in the abdominal wall may give rise to abdominal pain with tenderness at the rectus margin where the nerve turns through an acute angle. Applegate (1972) has suggested that this is a not infrequent cause of abdominal pain. Injections of local anaesthetic are both diagnostic and therapeutic.

Proximal lesions of the sciatic nerve

The nerve is subject to stretch and direct trauma at hip surgery, during prolonged recumbency especially after weight loss, and to intramuscular injections placed too medially in the gluteal muscles. Some believe that the nerve may be entrapped under the pyriformis muscle (Solheim, Siewers and Paus, 1981) but, as in some of the other situations discussed, the argument rests on the interpretation of local tenderness and the response to local injections of anaesthetic materials. These phenomena may, however, be seen distal to root lesions and thus are not proof of local irritation. There is weakness of the hamstrings and of all muscle groups below the knee, commonly producing a flail foot. Sensory change is detected laterally below the knee, over the dorsum and sole of the foot and a distal area of the calf. Nerve conduction studies are usually needed to exclude root lesions, and slow conduction in the sciatic nerve may be detectable (Yap and Hirota, 1967).

Common peroneal nerve

The nerve is superficial behind the head and neck of the fibula and may be compressed against the fibula by external forces. Sitting cross-legged may be enough especially after weight loss has removed the protective subcutaneous fat. One personally studied case lost 38 kg under medical advice after sustaining a myocardial infarct, but reappeared in the clinic wth bilateral footdrop due to pressure palsies localized behind the head of the fibula. Rarer causes include surgery for popliteal aneurysm, Baker's cysts (Nakano, 1978a), ganglia (Stack, Bianco and McCarty, 1965) and prolonged squatting. Ganglia tend to affect the deep branch and spare the peronei (Seddon, 1975). A painless footdrop may develop (*Figure 10.17*) or, more usually, there is pain and numbness over the lower outer aspect of the leg and dorsum of the foot together with weakness of dorsiflexion and eversion of the foot. In some individuals the peronei are either relatively spared or particularly involved. An isolated lesion of the deep branch causes footdrop but with sensory change limited to the web space between the first two toes. A rarer isolated disturbance of the superficial sensory branch where it emerges from the fascia causes sensory disturbance over the lateral side of the leg and top of the foot but no weakness (Bannerjee and Koons, 1981). It may follow an inversion injury or the wearing of high lace-up boots as used by skaters.

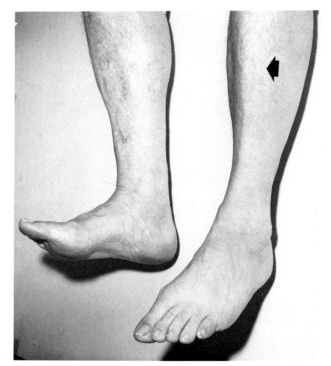

Figure 10.17 Left-sided foot drop with some wasting of the anterior tibial compartment due to acute pressure on the common peroneal nerve at the head of the fibula. Incomplete recovery occurred over the followng 12 months

The differential diagnosis includes sciatic nerve lesions in which calf muscles and inversion of the foot may be affected, but it should be realized that, in many individuals, the common peroneal and tibial branches of the sciatic nerve are anatomically distinct within the trunk of the sciatic nerve high in the thigh. A lesion in the thigh may then cause an isolated deficit corresponding to the common peroneal nerve alone. The other differential diagnostic problem concerns L5 root lesions. In theory, weakness due to the root lesion will predominantly affect the extensor hallucis longus, and also affect hip abduction and hamstrings, and may reduce the ankle jerk and/or medial hamstring reflex. In practice, L5 root lesions may spare more proximal muscles and the ankle jerk may be preserved. In these difficult cases electrical testing may be essential. A local conduction block may be demonstrated across the head of the fibula recording from extensor digitorum brevis. When the muscle is wasted or congenitally small this technique may fail. The distal motor latencies to the tibialis anterior on each side from the popliteal fossa may be the only way of demonstrating a local lesion. If there has been axonal loss the peroneal NAP recorded over the 12 cm above the lateral malleolus may be lost. If there is a local block at the knee the NAP recorded there by subcutaneous needle electrodes during stimulation at the ankle may be detectable at the neck of the fibula but not in the popliteal fossa. It may be useful to sample S1 muscles such as the medial gastrocnemius and record the ankle jerk latency to further exclude root lesions.

If acute trauma can be traced as a cause of the footdrop conservative measures are appropriate. These will need to include some form of footdrop appliance if there has been axonal loss and recovery must await regeneration. When the lesion develops insidiously and/or is aggravated by exercise, exploration may be necessary to determine if there is some unexpected local abnormality, such as a ganglion. If there is a palpable lesion on the nerve it should be explored (Berry and Richardson, 1976). However, spontaneous progressive lesions are unusual and most cases are due to acute trauma.

Posterior tibial nerve

This may occasionally be affected, for example by a Baker's cyst in the popliteal fossa, but lesions usually result from fractures of the lower leg or trauma to the calf. Wasting and weakness of plantar flexion of the foot and of long flexors of the toes are accompanied by denervation of small foot muscles. A flat foot with hyperextended metatarso-phalangeal joints results with numbness over the sole of the foot.

Femoral nerve

Femoral nerve lesions are encountered with some frequency. Haemorrhage into the psoas sheath (in haemophilia or due to anticoagulant drugs) may cause a rapidly evolving femoral nerve paralysis. The haematoma may be shown on CT scans

(Simeone *et al.*, 1977). Frequently, the nerve lesion is permanent. Rarely, operations cause an iatrogenic femoral neuropathy but the majority of clinical cases are idiopathic or occur in diabetic subjects when the pathogenesis is likely to be ischaemic. In diabetics the differential diagnosis is between an isolated femoral neuropathy (Calverley and Mulder, 1960) and diabetic amyotrophy (Casey and Harrison, 1972), in which the weakness involves other proximal muscles. The other distinction to be made is between femoral neuropathy and an L3/4 root lesion. In the cases of a femoral nerve lesion, wasting and weakness of the quadriceps are accompanied by loss of the knee jerk and sensory change over the anterior thigh and medial aspect of the lower leg. An L3/4 lesion additionally causes weakness of adduction of the thigh and particularly inversion of the foot, and there may be a history of associated back pain. When the femoral nerve is affected proximally as with a haematoma of the psoas sheath, there may also be some weakness of hip flexion (*Figures 10.18* and *10.19*).

A femoral nerve conduction study may be helpful. Latencies to two sites, one proximal and one distal in rectus femoris, may be compared from the groin (Gassell, 1963), though the authors prefer to stimulate at the inguinal ligament and in Hunter's canal while recording in vastus medialis.

Ilio-inguinal nerve

This is virtually always an iatrogenic problem (Winer and Harrison, 1982) although entrapment has been described (Kopell, Thompson and Postel, 1962; Mumenthaler *et al.*, 1965). Damage to the nerve causes some weakness of the lower fibres of the internal oblique muscle of the abdominal wall, sensory changes over the root of the scrotum, an area of the upper thigh medially, and the skin over the inguinal ligament. Exploration of the site of the previous surgery may be necessary to relieve pain.

Genitofemoral nerve

This, too, is vulnerable at the time of appendectomy (Nakano, 1978b). A small area of sensory change and sometimes pain may develop over the femoral triangle. The nerve may supply the cremaster so there may be loss of the cremasteric reflex unilaterally. Genitofemoral neuropathy can also be caused by the wearing of skin-tight jeans (O'Brien, 1979).

Obturator nerve

Rarely pelvic fractures, genitourinary operations or an obturator hernia catch this nerve in its foramen. The muscles of the adductor group are weak, the adductor jerk is lost and there is sensory change over the inner side of the thigh. In the case of an obturator hernia, pain and paraesthesiae over the inner side of the thigh may be increased by any manoeuvre that raises intra-abdominal pressure, e.g. coughing.

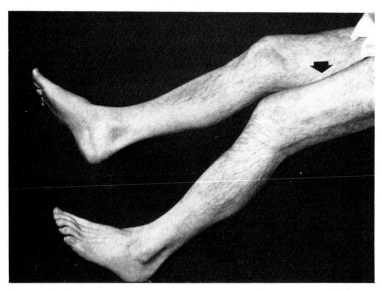

Figure 10.18 Femoral nerve lesion. The seated patient is attempting to extend both legs. Weakness on the left is associated with some wasting of the quadriceps (arrowed). The knee jerk was lost. Although this lesion may develop from a retroperitoneal haematoma, this patient was found to be diabetic. With institution of diabetic treatment he made a complete recovery

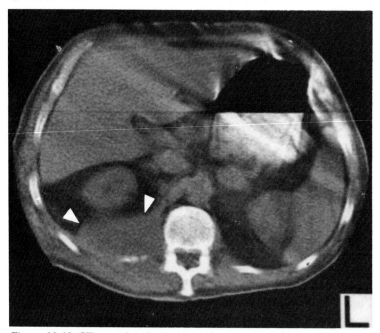

Figure 10.19 CT scan showing isodense mass in the right paravertebral gutter due to a psoas sheath haematoma (arrows). The right kidney is displaced forwards. The stomach contains gastrograffin and a fluid level. (Scan kindly supplied by Dr W. Lees)

This may superficially suggest a lumbar root lesion. Intrapelvic section of the nerve is recommended if there is severe pain, since exploration in the obturator foramen may damage the artery (Nakano, 1978b).

Meralgia paraesthetica

Damage to the lateral cutaneous nerve of the thigh is always thought to be due to pressure at the anterior superior iliac spine (Jefferson and Eames, 1979) not along its intrapelvic course, although it lies behind the caecum and could theoretically be affected by pelvic cancer. Pressure in the groin can be simply measured in the sitting position by a sphygmomanometer (Deal and Canoso, 1982). In normal subjects this rarely exceeds 35 mmHg. Pressures over 60 mmHg are common in obese individuals and in the presence of ascites. Lesions of this nerve are commonly held to be due to obesity. Clinical experience suggests that stretch may also play a part in patients of normal weight. Standing to attention may cause symptoms, as may the development of a pelvic tilt as in some muscular dystrophies. External compression may result from the wearing of corsets ('corset neuralgia'), trusses, sabre belts, or tight jeans.

The patients complain of painful pins and needles and a sense of numbness over the anterolateral aspect of the thigh. The affected area can often be covered by the patient's hand and spreads from 3 cm above the knee to 2 cm below the groin. The patient may sit forward to rub his thigh and this becomes a mild habit. The examination reveals no muscle wasting or weakness, making a femoral nerve or lumbar root lesion unlikely, and the characteristic territory shows some mild sensory change. The syndrome is often detected when the patient is examined for some other problem and appears most often in adults aged 20–60 years and more commonly in males (Stevens, 1957).

There is a good chance (2:1) of spontaneous recovery if the history is short. If weight loss does not help and painful paraesthesiae are unduly bothersome to the patient, steroid injections or exploration of the nerve medial to the anterior superior iliac spine may be necessary.

Gonyalgia paraesthetica

Damage to the infrapatellar branch of the saphenous nerve may produce a restricted area of numbness and paraesthesiae in the skin over the patella (Wartenberg, 1954). The symptoms usually develop insidiously without a history of acute trauma though resting the knee joint against a car door on long tours can be responsible. Sharp pain may be felt in the same territory on stretch. No treatment is necessary for what is a minor complaint; only reassurance that it is not due to some more significant disorder.

Tarsal tunnel syndrome

The posterior tibial nerve enters the plantar compartment of the foot under a retinaculum analogous to the carpal tunnel. Compression at this site may occur after fractures or dislocation of the ankle or in the presence of post-traumatic oedema around the ankle. Venous engorgement may also compress the nerve in the tunnel, as may tenosynovitis.

The patients complain of numbness, pain and paraesthesiae in the sole of the foot. Inversion of the foot may increase the pain as may venous occlusion by a cuff around the lower leg. Nocturnal pain is quite common, as in the carpal tunnel syndrome, and the patients may obtain relief by hanging the leg out of bed (Kopell and Thompson, 1960).

Examination may reveal wasting or weakness of the abductor hallucis with sensory loss over the distal part of the sole of the foot over the heads of the metatarsals and toes. There may be a Tinel sign at the ankle below and behind the medial malleolus.

Electrical studies may reveal denervation of the abductor hallucis and a prolonged distal latency to abductor hallucis or abductor digiti quinti or both (Fu, Delisa and Kraft, 1980). An asymmetry of over 1 ms in the motor latency when compared with the asymptomatic side is considered abnormal as is an absolute latency of 7.0 ms or more. Abnormalities may only be detected in 50% of cases, however. The medial plantar SAP recorded behind the medial malleolus during stimulation of the big toe may be lost and is abnormal in perhaps 90% of instances (Oh *et al.*, 1979).

Lam (1967) reported that three out of ten of his patients also had carpal tunnel syndromes and the possibility of other nerve compression syndromes should be considered. Normally decompression will be necessary except in those with temporary swelling of the foot.

References

Aguayo, A., Nair, C. P. V. and Midgley, R. (1971) Experimental progressive compression neuropathy in the rabbit. *Archives of Neurology*, **24**, 358–364

Aiello, I., Serra, G., Traina, G. C. and Tugnoli, V. (1982) Entrapment of the suprascapular nerve at the spinoglenoid notch. *Annals of Neurology*, **12**, 314–316

Anderson, M. H., Fullerton, P. M., Gilliatt, R.W. and Hern, J. E. C. (1970) Changes in the forearm associated with median nerve compression at the wrist in the guinea-pig. *Journal of Neurology, Neurosurgery and Psychiatry*, **33**, 70–79

Applegate, W. V. (1972) Abdominal cutaneous nerve entrapment syndrome. *Surgery*, **71**, 118–124

Asbury, A. K. (1973) Renaut bodies – a forgotten endoneurial structure. *Journal of Neuropathology and Experimental Neurology*, **32**, 334–343

Baba, M., Fowler, C. J., Jacobs, J. M. and Gilliatt, R. W. (1982) Changes in peripheral nerve fibres distal to a constriction. *Journal of the Neurological Sciences*, **54**, 197–208

Banerjee, T. and Koons, D. D. (1981) Superficial peroneal nerve entrapment. *Journal of Neurosurgery*, **55**, 991–992

Bauwens, P. (1961) Electrodiagnosis revisited: Tenth John Stanley Coulter Memorial Lecture. *Archives of Physical Medicine and Rehabilitation*, **42**, 6–18

Behse, F., Buchthal, F., Carlsen, F. and Knappeis, G. G. (1972) Hereditary neuropathy with liability to pressure palsies: electrophysiological and histopathological aspects. *Brain*, **95**, 777–794

Berry, H. and Richardson, P. M. (1976) Common peroneal nerve palsy: a clinical and electrophysiological study. *Journal of Neurology, Neurosurgery and Psychiatry*, **39**, 1162–1171

Bolton, C. F. and McFarlane, R. M. (1978) Human pneumatic tourniquet paralysis. *Neurology (Minneapolis)*, **28**, 787–793

Bray, J. J., Hubbard, J. I. and Mills, R. G. (1979) The trophic influence of tetrodotoxin-inactive nerves on normal and reinnervated rat skeletal muscles. *Journal of Physiology*, **297**, 479–491

Brooks, D. M. (1952) Nerve compression by simple ganglia. *Journal of Bone and Joint Surgery*, **34B**, 391–400

Brown, W. F., Ferguson, G. G., Jones, M. W. and Yates, S. K. (1976) The location of conduction abnormalities in human entrapment neuropathies. *Canadian Journal of Neurological Sciences*, **3**, 111–122

Buchthal, F., Rosenfalck, A. and Trojaborg, W. (1974) Electrophysiological findings in entrapment of the median nerve at wrist and elbow. *Journal of Neurology, Neurosurgery and Psychiatry*, **37**, 340–360

Calverley, J. R. and Mulder, D. W. (1960) Femoral neuropathy. *Neurology (Minneapolis)*, **10**, 963–967

Casey, E. B. and Harrison, M. J. G. (1972) Diabetic amyotrophy. *British Medical Journal*, **1**, 656–659

Casey, E. B. and Le Quesne, P. M. (1972) Digital nerve action potentials in healthy subjects and in carpal tunnel and diabetic patients. *Journal of Neurology, Neurosurgery and Psychiatry*, **35**, 612–623

Daube, J. R. (1969) Rucksack paralysis. *Journal of the American Medical Association*, **208**, 2447–2452

Deal, C. L. and Canoso, J. J. (1982) Meralgia paresthetica and large abdomens. *Annals of Internal Medicine*, **96**, 787–788

Dekel, S. and Coates, R. (1979) Primary carpal stenosis as a cause of 'idiopathic' carpal tunnel syndrome. *Lancet*, **2**, 1024

Dyck, P. J., Lais, A. C., Karnes, J. L. *et al.* (1981) Permanent axotomy: a model of axonal atrophy and secondary segmental demyelination and remyelination. *Annals of Neurology*, **9**, 575–583

Earl, C. J., Fullerton, P. M., Wakefield, G. S. and Schutta, H. S. (1964) Hereditary neuropathy, with liability to pressure palsies. *Quarterly Journal of Medicine*, **33**, 481–498

Ebeling, P., Gilliatt, R. W. and Thomas, P. K. (1960) A clinical and electrical study of ulnar nerve lesions in the hand. *Journal of Neurology, Neurosurgery and Psychiatry*, **23**, 1–9

Eisen, A. (1974) Early diagnosis of nerve palsy. *Neurology*, **24**, 256–262

Fowler, T. J., Danta, G. and Gilliatt, R. W. (1972) Recovery of nerve conduction after a pneumatic tourniquet: observations on the hind-limb of the baboon. *Journal of Neurology, Neurosurgery and Psychiatry*, **35**, 638–647

Fowler, C. J. and Gilliatt, R. W. (1981) Conduction velocity and conduction block after experimental ischaemic nerve injury. *Journal of the Neurological Sciences*, **52**, 221–238

Fu, R., Delisa, J. A. and Kraft, G. H. (1980) Motor nerve latencies through the tarsal tunnel in normal adult subjects: standard determinations corrected for temperature and distance. *Archives of Physical Medicine and Rehabilitation*, **61**, 243–248

Fullerton, P. M. (1963) The effect of ischaemia on nerve conduction in the carpal tunnel syndrome. *Journal of Neurology, Neurosurgery and Psychiatry*, **26**, 385–397

Ganzhorn, R. W., Hocker, J. T., Horowitz, M. and Switzer, H. E. (1981) Suprascapular nerve entrapment. *Journal of Bone and Joint Surgery*, **63A**, 492–494

Garland, H., Langworth, E. P., Taverner, D. and Clark, J. M. P. (1964) Surgical treatment for the carpal tunnel syndrome. *Lancet*, **1**, 1129–1130

Gassell, M. M. (1963) A study of femoral nerve conduction time. *Archives of Neurology (Chicago)*, **9**, 607–614

Gelberman, R. H., Hergenroeder, P. T., Hargens, A. R., Lundborg, G. N. and Akeson, W. H. (1981) The carpal tunnel syndrome. A study of carpal canal pressures. *Journal of Bone and Joint Surgery*, **63A**, 380–383

Gilliatt, R. W. (1975) Peripheral nerve compression and entrapment. In *Eleventh Symposium on Advanced Medicine: Proceedings of a Conference held at the Royal College of Physicians of London, 1975*, edited by A. F. Lant, pp. 144–163. Tunbridge Wells: Pitman Medical

Gilliatt, R. W. (1979) The classical neurological syndrome associated with a cervical rib and band. In *Pain in the Shoulder and Arm*, edited by J. M. Greep, H. A. J. Lemmens, D. B. Roos and H. C. Urschel, pp. 173–183. The Hague: Martinus Nijhoff Publishers

Gilliatt, R. W. (1981) Physical injury to peripheral nerves – physiologic and electrodiagnostic aspects. *Mayo Clinic Proceedings*, **56**, 361–370

Gilliatt, R. W. (1984) Thoracic outlet syndromes. In *Peripheral Neuropathy*, 2nd Edition, edited by P. J. Dyck, E. H. Lambert, P. K. Thomas and R. Bunge. Philadelphia: W. B. Saunders (in press)

Gilliatt, R. W., Le Quesne, P. M., Logue, V. and Sumner, A. J. (1970) Wasting of the hand associated with a cervical rib or band. *Journal of Neurology, Neurosurgery and Psychiatry*, **33**, 615–624

Gilliatt, R. W. and Thomas, P. K. (1960) Changes in nerve conduction with ulnar lesions at the elbow. *Journal of Neurology, Neurosurgery and Psychiatry*, **23**, 312–320

Gilliatt, R. W., Westgaard, R. H. and Williams, I. R. (1978) Extrajunctional acetylcholine sensitivity of inactive muscle fibres in the baboon during prolonged nerve pressure block. *Journal of Physiology*, **280**, 499–514

Gilliatt, R. W., Willison, R. G., Dietz, V. and Williams, I. R. (1978) Peripheral nerve conduction in patients with a cervical rib and band. *Annals of Neurology*, **4**, 124–129

Goldman, S., Honet, J. C., Sobel, R. and Goldstein, A. S. (1969) Posterior interosseous nerve palsy in the absence of trauma. *Archives of Neurology (Chicago)*, **21**, 435–441

Goodman, H. V. and Gilliatt, R. W. (1961) The effect of treatment on median nerve conduction in patients with carpal tunnel syndrome. *Annals of Physical Medicine*, **6**, 137–155

Hargens, A. R., Romine, J. S., Sipe, J. C., Evans, K. L., Mubarak, S. J. and Akeson, W. H. (1979) Peripheral nerve-conduction block by high muscle-compartment pressure. *Journal of Bone and Joint Surgery*, **61A**, 192–200

Harrison, M. J. G. (1976) Pressure palsy of the ulnar nerve with prolonged conduction block. *Journal of Neurology, Neurosurgery and Psychiatry*, **39**, 96–99

Harrison, M. J. G. and Nurick, S. (1970) Results of anterior transposition of the ulnar nerve for ulnar neuritis. *British Medical Journal*, **1**, 27–29

Hopkins, A. P. and Morgan-Hughes, J. A. (1969) The effect of local pressure in diphtheritic neuropathy. *Journal of Neurology, Neurosurgery and Psychiatry*, **32**, 614–623

Hougell, A. and Mattsson, H. S. (1971) Neurographic studies before, after and during operation for median nerve compression in the carpal tunnel. *Scandinavian Journal of Plastic and Reconstructive Surgery*, **5**, 103–109

Howse, A. J. G. and Seddon, H. (1966) Ischaemic contracture of muscle associated with carbon monoxide and barbiturate poisoning. *British Medical Journal*, **1**, 192–195

Jefferson, D. and Eames, R. A. (1979) Subclinical entrapment of the lateral femoral cutaneous nerve: an autopsy study. *Muscle and Nerve*, **2**, 145–154

Jefferson, D., Neary, D. and Eames, R. A. (1981) Renaut body distribution at sites of human peripheral nerve entrapment. *Journal of the Neurological Sciences*, **49**, 19–29

Kaplan, P. E. (1980) Electrodiagnostic confirmation of long thoracic nerve palsy. *Journal of Neurology, Neurosurgery and Psychiatry*, **43**, 50–52

Kimura, J. (1979) The carpal tunnel syndrome. *Brain*, **102**, 619–635

Kopell, H. P. and Thompson, W. A. L. (1960) Peripheral entrapment neuropathies of the lower extremity. *New England Journal of Medicine*, **262**, 56–60

Kopell, H. P. and Thompson, W. A. L. (1963) *Peripheral Entrapment Neuropathies*. Baltimore: Williams and Wilkins

Kopell, H. P., Thompson, W. A. L. and Postel, A. H. (1962) Entrapment neuropathy of the ilioinguinal nerve. *New England Journal of Medicine*, **266**, 16–19

Krarup, C., Gilliatt, R. W. and Jacobs, J. M. (1982) Conduction in constricted and aberrant regenerating fibres. In *Abstracts of Fifth International Congress on Neuromuscular Diseases*, Marseilles

Kremer, M., Gilliatt, R. W., Golding, J. S. R. and Wilson, J. G. (1953) Acroparaesthesiae in the carpal tunnel syndrome. *Lancet*, **2**, 590–595

Lam, S. J. S., (1967) Tarsal tunnel syndrome. *Journal of Bone and Joint Surgery*, **49B**, 87–92

Loong, S. C. and Seah, C. S. (1971) Comparison of median and ulnar sensory nerve action potentials in the diagnosis of the carpal tunnel syndrome. *Journal of Neurology, Neurosurgery and Psychiatry*, **32**, 750–754

MacNicol, M. F. (1979) The results of operation for ulnar neuritis. *Journal of Bone and Joint Surgery*, **61B**, 159–164

Madrid, R. and Bradley, W. G. (1975) The pathology of neuropathies with focal thickening of the myelin sheath (tomaculous neuropathy): studies on the formation of the abnormal myelin sheath. *Journal of the Neurological Sciences*, **25**, 415–448

Marotte, L. R. (1974) An electron microscope study of chronic median nerve compression in the guinea-pig. *Acta Neuropathologica (Berlin)*, **27**, 69–82

Massey, E. W. and Pleet, A. B. (1978) Handcuffs and cheiralgia paresthetica. *Neurology*, **28**, 1312–1313

McArdle, M. J. (1949) quoted by Kremer *et al.* (1953)

Miller, R. G. and Camp, P. E. (1979) Postoperative ulnar neuropathy. *Journal of the American Medical Association*, **242**, 1636–1639

Miller, R. G. and Hummel, E. E. (1980) The cubital tunnel syndrome: treatment with simple decompression. *Annals of Neurology*, **7**, 567–569

Miller, R. G. and Olney, R. K. (1982) Persistent conduction block in compression neuropathy. Special Lambert Symposium, Mayo Clinic. *Muscle and Nerve*, **5**, S154–156

Morris, H. H. and Peters, B. H. (1976) Pronator syndrome: clinical and electrophysiological features in seven cases. *Journal of Neurology, Neurosurgery and Psychiatry*, **39**, 461–464

Mubarak, S. and Owen, C. A. (1975) Compartmental syndrome and its relation to the crush syndrome; a spectrum of disease: a review of 11 cases of prolonged limb compression. *Clinical Orthopaedics*, **113**, 81–89

Mulder, D. W., Lambert, E. H., Bastron, J. A. and Sprague, R. G. (1961) The neuropathies associated with diabetes mellitus. *Neurology*, **11**, 275–284

Mumenthaler, A., Mumenthaler, M., Luciani, G. and Kramer, J. (1965) Das Ilioinguinalis Syndrom. *Deutsche medizinische Wochenschrift*, **90**, 1073–1078

Nakano, K. K. (1978a) Entrapment neuropathy from Baker's cyst. *Journal of the American Medical Association*, **239**, 135

Nakano, K. K. (1978b) The entrapment neuropathies. *Muscle and Nerve*, **1**, 264–279

Neary, D. and Eames, R. A. (1975) The pathology of ulnar nerve compression in man. *Neuropathology and Applied Neurobiology*, **1**, 69–88

Neary, D., Ochoa, J. and Gilliatt, R. W. (1975) Sub-clinical entrapment neuropathy in man. *Journal of the Neurological Sciences*, **24**, 283–298

Nigst, H. and Dick, W. (1979) Syndromes of compression of the median nerve in the proximal forearm (pronator teres syndrome; anterior interosseous nerve syndrome). *Archives of Orthopaedic and Traumatic Surgery*, **93**, 307–312

Noth, J., Dietz, V. and Mauritz, K. H. (1980) Cyclist's palsy: neurological and EMG study in 4 cases with distal ulnar lesions. *Journal of the Neurological Sciences*, **47**, 111–116

O'Brien, M. D. (1979) Genitofemoral neuropathy. *British Medical Journal*, **1**, 1052

Ochoa, J., Fowler, T. J. and Gilliatt, R. W. (1972) Anatomical changes in peripheral nerves compressed by pneumatic tourniquet. *Journal of Anatomy*, **113**, 433–455

Ochoa, J. and Marotte, L. R. (1973) The nature of the nerve lesion caused by chronic entrapment in the guinea-pig. *Journal of the Neurological Sciences*, **19**, 491–495

Oh, S. J., Sarala, P. K., Kuba, T. and Elmore, R. S. (1979) Tarsal tunnel syndrome: electrophysiological study. *Annals of Neurology*, **5**, 327–330

Ortman, J. A., Sahenk, Z. and Mendell, J. R. (1983) The experimental production of Renaut bodies in response to mechanical stress. *Journal of the Neurological Sciences* (in press)

Pallis, C. A. (1966) The neuropathies of rheumatoid arthritis. *Journal of Royal College of Physicians of London*, **1**, 19–28

Payan, J. (1969) Electrophysiological localization of ulnar nerve lesions. *Journal of Neurology, Neurosurgery and Psychiatry* **32**, 208–220

Pechan, J. and Julis, I. (1975) The pressure measurement in the ulnar nerve: a contribution to the pathophysiology of the cubital tunnel syndrome. *Journal of Biomechanics*, **8**, 75–79

Phalen, G. S. (1970) Reflections on 21 years' experience with the carpal tunnel syndrome. *Journal of the American Medical Association*, **212**, 1365–1367

Pleet, A. B. and Massey, E. W. (1978) Notalgia paresthetica. *Neurology*, **28**, 1310–1311

Richards, R. L. (1945) Traumatic ulnar neuritis. *Edinburgh Medical Journal*, **52**, 14–21

Roos, D. B. (1976) Congenital anomalies associated with thoracic outlet syndrome. *American Journal of Surgery*, **132**, 771–778

Rudge, P. (1974) Tourniquet paralysis with prolonged conduction block: an electrophysiological study. *Journal of Bone and Joint Surgery*, **56B**, 716–720

Rudge, P., Ochoa, J. and Gilliatt, R. W. (1974) Acute peripheral nerve compression in the baboon. *Journal of the Neurological Sciences*, **23**, 403–420

Rydevik, B., Lundborg, G. and Bagge, U. (1981) Effects of graded compression on intraneural blood flow. *Journal of Hand Surgery*, **6**, 3–12

Schröder, J. M. (1968) Die Hyperneurotisation Bungnerscher Bander bei der experimentellen Isoniazid-Neuropathie: Phasenkontrast und elektronenmikroskopische Untersuchungen. *Virchows Archiv Abteilung B. Zellpathologie*, 131–156

Seddon, H. (1975) *Surgical Disorders of Peripheral Nerves*, 2nd Edn. Edinburgh: Churchill Livingstone

Shea, J. D. and McClain, E. J. (1969) Ulnar nerve compression syndromes at and below the wrist. *Journal of Bone and Joint Surgery*, **51A**, 1095–1103

Shelden, W. D. (1921) Tardy paralysis of the ulnar nerve. *Medical Clinics of North America*, **5**, 499–509

Simeone, J. F., Robinson, F., Rothman, S. L. G. and Jaffe, C. C. (1977) Computerized tomographic demonstration of a retroperitoneal hematoma causing femoral neuropathy. *Journal of Neurosurgery*, **47**, 946–948

Simpson, J. A. (1956) Electrical signs in the diagnosis of carpal tunnel and related syndromes. *Journal of Neurology, Neurosurgery and Psychiatry*, **19**, 275–280

Singh, N., Behse, F. and Buchthal, F. (1974) Electrophysiological study of peroneal palsy. *Journal of Neurology, Neurosurgery and Psychiatry*, **37**, 1202–1213

Solheim, L. F., Siewers, P. and Paus, B. (1981) The piriformis muscle syndrome. *Acta Orthopaedica Scandinavica*, **52**, 73–75

Spinner, M. (1968) The arcade of Frohse and its relationship to posterior interosseous nerve paralysis. *Journal of Bone and Joint Surgery*, **50B**, 809–812

Spinner, M. (1970) The anterior interosseous nerve syndrome. *Journal of Bone and Joint Surgery*, **52A**, 84–94

Stack, R. E., Bianco, A. J. and MacCarty, C. S. (1964) Compression of the common peroneal nerve by ganglion cysts. *ournal of Bone and Joint Surgery*, **47A**, 773–778

Stevens, H. (1957) Meralgia parasthetica. *Archives of Neurology and Psychiatry*, **77**, 557–574

Thomas, P. K. (1968) The effect of repeated regenerative activity on the structure of peripheral nerve. In *Research in Muscular Dystrophy*, edited by Research Committee Muscular Dystrophy Group, pp. 413–416. London: Pitman Medical

Trojaborg, W. (1970) Rate of recovery in motor and sensory fibres of the radial nerve: clinical and electrophysiological aspects. *Journal of Neurology, Neurosurgery and Psychiatry*, **33**, 625–638

Trojaborg, W. (1976) Motor and sensory conduction in the musculocutaneous nerve. *Journal of Neurology, Neurosurgery and Psychiatry*, **39**, 890–899

Trojaborg, W. (1977) Prolonged conduction block with axonal degeneration: an electrophysiological study. *Journal of Neurology, Neurosurgery and Psychiatry*, **4**, 50–57

Trojaborg, W. (1978) Early electrophysiologic changes in conduction block. *Muscle and Nerve*, **1**, 400–403

Urschel, H. C. and Razzuk, M. A. (1972) Management of the thoracic-outlet syndrome. *New England Journal of Medicine*, **286**, 1140–1143

Wadsworth, T. G. The external compression syndrome of the ulnar nerve at the cubital tunnel. *Clinical Orthopaedics and Related Research*, **124**, 189–204

Wadsworth, T. G. and Williams, J. R. (1973) Cubital tunnel external compression syndrome. *British Medical Journal*, **1**, 662–666

Wartenberg, R. (1954) Digitalgia paresthetica and gonyalgia paresthetica. *Neurology*, **4**, 106–115

Weiss, P. and Hiscoe, H. B. (1948) Experiments on the mechanism of nerve growth. *Journal of Experimental Zoology*, **107**, 315–395

Williams, I. R., Jefferson, D. and Gilliatt, R. W. (1980) Acute nerve compression during limb ischaemia. *Journal of the Neurological Sciences*, **46**, 199–207

Winer, J. B. and Harrison, M. J. G. (1982) Iatrogenic nerve injuries. *Postgraduate Medical Journal*, **58**, 142–145

Wulff, C. H. and Gilliatt, R. W. (1979) F waves in patients with hand wasting caused by a cervical rib and band. *Muscle and Nerve*, **2**, 452–457

Yap, C. B. and Hirota, T. (1967) Sciatic nerve motor conduction velocity study. *Journal of Neurology, Neurosurgery and Psychiatry*, **30**, 233–239

11
Geographical patterns of neuropathy: India

Noshir H. Wadia

INTRODUCTION

This common neurological disorder affects Indians probably as much as anybody else. The same aetiological agents operate, but there is some difference in their frequency distribution. This chapter attempts to highlight this difference, and draw attention to the relevant Indian literature. No acceptable incidence or prevalence study has been carried out for India as a whole; however, a recent report from North-West India gives some information (Kaur *et al.*, 1982). This clinical study supported by laboratory data, electromyography and sural nerve biopsy examination was restricted to patients admitted to a teaching hospital in the capital city of Chandigarh. In 3 years 570 cases were seen and constituted 8.5/1000 hospital admissions. Patients with diabetic neuropathy (65.6%) and leprosy (14.4%) formed the majority. The remaining 114 patients were classified as in *Table 11.1*. Whilst useful as the only serious effort to document data it cannot truly reflect the total picture of this disease in India as the authors themselves mention. Thus, the incidence of Guillain-Barré syndrome is disproportionately high as the majority of these patients have to be hospitalized, whilst the role of malnutrition is probably underplayed. The milder case, the outpatient, and the vast rural population remain unrepresented. Although an unusually large number of patients with leprosy were hospitalized, the true incidence of leprosy can only be gauged in the outpatient department and by population survey. Finally, this report shows that in India diabetes is a major cause of peripheral neuropathy as elsewhere. *Table 11.1* also gives some comparative information of a simultaneous collaborative study from a teaching hospital in Madras in the South-east of India (Arjundas, unpublished observations, 1983).

LEPROSY

Endemic in India since 1400 BC, this commonest peripheral neuropathy (neuritis) is believed to affect 3.2 million Indians (Noordeen, 1980) though this is probably an underestimate. Unfortunately, not enough has changed since Charles Morehead

Table 11.1 Inpatient cases of peripheral neuropathy over 3 years
(1977–1979)

	Chandigarh* (114)	Madras† (77)
Guillain-Barré syndrome	53	37
Vaccine/sera	3	1
Arsenic	13	0
Alcohol	3	1
Organophosphorus compounds	1	1
INH	0	2
Varnish	0	1
Unidentified toxins	0	3
Malnutrition	2	5
Polyarteritis nodosa	3	0
Rheumatoid arthritis	0	2
Malignancy	3	3
Uraemia	1	0
Porphyria	4	0
Diphtheria	1	0
Peroneal muscular atrophy	5	0
Refsum's disease	0	1
Compressive (carpal tunnel syndrome)	0	4
Degeneration	0	2
Neurofibroma	0	1
Undetermined	22	13

* Modified from Kaur *et al.*, 1982
† Arjundas (unpublished observations)

(1860) wrote that 391 cases of leprosy were admitted to a special ward at the Sir Jamsetjee Jeejeebhoy (JJ) Hospital between 1848 and 1853. Today, the overall prevalence rate is 6/1000 population in South and East India, and 2/1000 in the North and North-west.

Leprosy spreads between humans with no alternate host. Prolonged close skin contact was once believed to be the only mode of transmission of *Mycobacterium leprae*, but today inhalation of infected droplets from nasal discharge of patients and the role of arthropods, especially flies, as carriers is increasingly recognized.

Depending on the host response to infection, leprosy presents in a variety of identifiable types. The classification is based on clinical, histological and bacteriological observations and the lepromin test. It indicates in turn the infectiousness of the patient, the prognosis and the duration of treatment required. Tuberculoid leprosy (TT) with a strong cell-mediated immune response is at one end of the spectrum, while lepromatous leprosy (LL) with no cell-mediated immunity and vigorous humoral antibody response occupies the other end. Graded borderline cases, borderline tuberculoid (BT), borderline (BB) and borderline lepromatous (BL) lie in between. Even finer shades and an 'indeterminate type' which cannot be classified early have been described. Dastur (1976) mentions that borderline tuberculoid variety predominates in India, and the non-lepromatous types considered together constitute about 80% of the leprosy cases.

Fite (1943) stated that 'all leprosy is neural leprosy', the difference is only in the degree and type of infection of the peripheral nervous system which extends from the dermal branches to the posterior root and sympathetic ganglia. Antia (1974) sums up the evidence for this succinctly, mentioning that biopsy from even the first small skin patch shows involvement of the cutaneous nerves as the earliest histological evidence of leprosy. Multiple tissue biopsies from 50 patient-volunteers at different stages of the disease showed that the earliest, heaviest and the most persistent bacillary invasion was in the nerves.

Types of leprosy

Tuberculoid leprosy

In tuberculoid leprosy, *M. leprae* enters the nerve (especially the Schwann cells) but the patient's hyperergic state prevents the bacilli from multiplying by producing an intense tissue reaction. A dermal nerve biopsy shows epithelioid reaction, giant cell formation and a tuberculoid granuloma (*Figure 11.1*). The patient often presents with numbness, loss of sensation, pain or tingling in the distribution of a single, or sometimes two or three randomly affected, nerves (mononeuritis multiplex). Wasting and weakness of muscles always follows. The infected nerve trunk is tender and thickened, especially in its cooler superficial parts (the ulnar at the elbow and the lateral popliteal at the knee), and even a painful swelling from a leprous abscess can be palpated.

Because there is nerve destruction due to a vigorous cell-mediated immune response, late detection leads to permanent disability such as claw-hand, foot-drop,

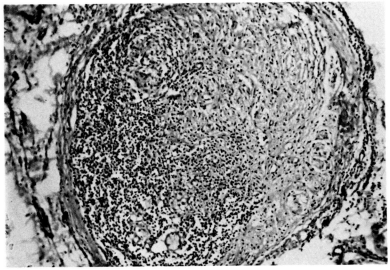

Figure 11.1 Tuberculoid leprosy. Section through a single nerve fascicle showing a granuloma composed of ephitheloid cells, giant cells and a peripheral rim of histiocytes. Haemotoxylin and eosin ×110 (Courtesy Dr R. Mani, Department of Pathology, Jaslok Hospital and Research Centre)

or trophic ulcer. Such a patient is likely to come first to a neurologist or internist, because he may not have an easily detectable dermal lesion, or may have one or two scattered erythematous or coppery, dry, raised patches which may go unnoticed unless looked for. These patches are not always anaesthetic or depilated.

Alternatively, a patient with tuberculoid leprosy may present to a general practitioner with a single dermal lesion. Failure to palpate carefully with the finger tips for a uniformly thickened cutaneous nerve, which almost invariably leaves the lesion, will lead to a costly misdiagnosis. The radial and ulnar cutaneous nerves at the wrist, the medial cutaneous nerve of the forearm, the superficial peroneal, the sural and the greater auricular nerves become easily palpable and even visible (*Figure 11.2*). As the small nerve fibres are affected first, fine examination for early

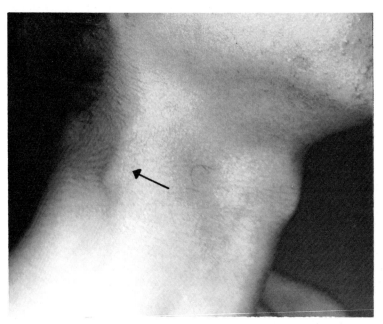

Figure 11.2 Tuberculoid leprosy. Lateral view of the neck of a patient showing visible enlargement (arrow) of the greater auricular nerve (Courtesy Dr N. H. Antia, Foundation for Medical Research)

impairment of temperature and pain sensitivity in the dermal patch should be performed. There is usually also absence of sweating. Biopsy of a nerve, skin or nasal mucosa in this variety usually reveals few or no leprae bacilli, the lepromin test is strongly positive and the patient essentially non-infectious.

Lepromatous leprosy

The anergic state of the patient in lepromatous leprosy permits a bacillaemia with spread of bacilli to many organs, the peripheral nervous system being most affected. Massive invasion of the Schwann cells by bacilli occurs but, in the absence of tissue reaction, very little early nerve damage occurs. There are, therefore, few or no neurological signs at the onset of the disease and the patient almost invariably presents to a dermatologist with a variety of obvious dermal lesions and the neurologist sees the late misdiagnosed case. Stuffiness of the nose, blood-stained nasal discharge and ankle oedema are early diagnostic indicators of lepromatous leprosy (Jopling, 1978). With advance of the disease and delayed treatment multiple, often symmetrical, peripheral neuropathy appears, so that classical glove and stocking anaesthesia, distal weakness and wasting, and even absent ankle reflexes may be found at a later stage. There is a uniform smooth thickening of nerves without much tenderness in the coolest subcutaneous parts. The diagnosis is easy, as the skin lesions are always present. Biopsy or smear of the skin, cutaneous nerves, or nasal mucosa will show tissue teeming with bacteria (*Figure 11.3*). The lepromin test is negative and the patient is highly infectious even at an early stage.

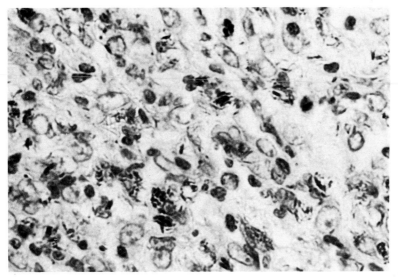

Figure 11.3 Lepromatous leprosy. Section through an intradermal nerve totally replaced by an infiltrate of foamy histiocytes teeming with *M. leprae*. Fite faraco ×800 (Courtesy Dr S. S. Pandya, Ackworth Hospital)

Untreated patients show the facial, nasal and other disfiguration so classical of this disease, whilst early diagnosis and treatment gives excellent results. In a proportion of patients, mostly those responding well to antibacillary treatment, an acute generalized systemic lepra reaction (type 2), due to deposition of immune complexes, occurs. This causes an acute painful neuritis which has to be recognized and treated vigorously as it can lead to permanent nerve damage and consequent deformities.

Borderline leprosy

Between these polar types various shades of borderline leprosy have been described, with graded change in clinical, bacteriological and histological examination and the lepromin test. The infectivity and treatment of such patients would accordingly vary. Considerable up and down grading occurs in these varieties, whilst the polar leprosy remains stable. Of interest to neurologists is the fact that in some of these borderline cases a prolonged polyneuritic (mononeuritis multiplex) phase occurs before skin lesions appear, leading to misdiagnosis unless the peripheral nerves, which are smoothly enlarged, are carefully palpated. Since this variety is immunologically unstable, severe widespread nerve destruction may occur, especially during acute episodes of cell-mediated hypersensitivity (lepra reaction, type 1) in patients responding well to treatment. Acute painful swelling of nerves and even an abscess may develop, causing pain and dysaesthesiae in their distribution. Wrist and foot drop or facial palsy with permanent sequelae are seen unless efficiently treated.

Differential diagnosis

Keeping the points made earlier in mind, the differential diagnosis has to be made from other varieties of peripheral neuropathy, especially sensory neuropathy and radiculopathy, syringomyelia and, at times, chronic anterior horn cell disease. In the absence of sensory loss, leprosy should not be diagnosed. Proximal muscle wasting and weakness and generalized loss of deep reflexes are very uncommon, and pyramidal tract signs are never seen in leprosy.

Prognosis

The prognosis depends on early diagnosis and sustained treatment. Examination of family contacts even by lay but trained health visitors yields great dividends. Electromyography has also helped in revealing subclinical neuropathy in contacts (Shetty *et al.*, 1977).

Treatment

When dapsone was first used in India by Cochrane in the 1940s, a great impact on the cure and spread of leprosy was expected. Unfortunately, primary and secondary drug resistance soon overtook this major advance (Pearson, 1981). Irregular insufficient monotherapy was blamed, and it was difficult to convince patients to take the drug for years. Bacterial persistence in tissues was noted over 10–12 years in patients treated with dapsone alone. With all this in mind and with the advent of other antileprosy drugs, WHO (1976) recommended two-drug therapy, especially for all active multibacillary cases. The latest recommendations for therapy come from a new WHO study group (WHO, 1982; *Lancet*, 1982) after review of the main antileprosy drugs (dapsone, rifampicin, clofazimine, ethionamide and prothionamide). It recommends for paucibacillary cases (T, BT) rifampicin 600 mg once a month with dapsone 100 mg daily. The treatment is for 6 months only. For multibacillary cases (LL, BL, BB) three drugs are advised:

rifampicin 600 mg monthly, dapsone 100 mg daily and clofazimine 300 mg monthly and 50 mg daily. Additionally, ethionamide or prothionamide 500 mg monthly may be given for certain patients. This treatment must be given for at least 2 years, and ideally until the slit-skin smears for *M. leprae* are negative. Close supervision must be kept on both groups during treatment, and for at least 4 years in paucibacillary and 8 years in multibacillary cases. This regimen has not yet been universally established and therapy has to be tailored to local and even individual needs and circumstances. There are those who hold the view that for abundant precaution dapsone should be continued for many years. Yet, the expectations of this shortened therapy are better compliance and greater impact on prevention and spread of the disease. The cost of treatment will also be lower and most patients, even in developing countries, can afford rifampicin once a month. Lepra reactions require quick attention. Corticosteroids should be used in type 1 reaction and anti-inflammatory drugs in type 2. If the latter reaction is severe, corticosteroids, clofazimine or thalidomide are indicated. Equally important as drug therapy are measures to prevent deformities and disfigurement. Health measures and efforts to detect and treat early cases must continue. The search for an effective antileprosy vaccine is still being actively pursued.

MALNUTRITION AND GASTROINTESTINAL MALABSORPTION

It is well recognized that malnutrition still prevails widely in India, but the extent of its effect on the peripheral nervous system has not been satisfactorily documented. Wadia (1979) mentions that an 11-year (1966–1977) search through Indian medical journals failed to reveal a comprehensive report on nutritional disorders of the nervous system, though some random observations were available. It is well known that peripheral neuropathy can occur through deprivation or malabsorption in the gut of vitamin B, but often in an individual case it is difficult to decide which of the two is more important. Strict vegetarianism, food fads, alcoholism, chronic infection such as pulmonary tuberculosis and multiple pregnancies contribute their share. The general experience has been that with exceptions (beriberi due to thiamine deficiency and selective vitamin B_{12} deficiency due to malabsorption) nutritional neuropathy can rarely be defined in terms of a single vitamin deficiency. Additionally, the disorder is not always strictly localized to the peripheral nervous system, but may have predominant features arising from central nervous system disease such as myelopathy, encephalopathy, etc.

Reviewing only Indian reports the following observations seem pertinent:

(1) Vitamin B complex deficiency

With the exception of pellagra, which is predominant in certain districts in India like Hyderabad and Udaipur, there are no identifiable areas where large scale vitamin B deficiency disorder now prevails (Wadia, 1979). Even though thiamine-dependent, mild peripheral neuropathy with distal paraesthesiae alone is still seen by physicians in practice, classical beriberi or Wernicke-Korsakoff syndrome are rarely seen or reported. According to Pallis and Lewis (1974a), those with experience of thiamine deficiency in areas where it is endemic see patients at a stage when they have anorexia, nausea, impaired gastrointestinal mobility, vague muscle pains, paraesthesiae and heaviness of legs, personality change, altered behaviour and hypotension. These patients probably respond quickly to specific or blunderbuss therapy without ever reaching a stage of overt peripheral neuropathy. The truth about what happens to the vast numbers beyond the pale of such medical attention is not recorded.

A 3-year prospective study of 67 consecutive malnourished patients admitted for neurological symptoms to a teaching hospital in Bombay found that 28 patients had peripheral sensory neuropathy (Wadia and Swami, 1970). All complained of intolerable acral burning and tingling paraesthesiae and essentially 'glove and stocking' sensory loss could be demonstrated in 27. The lower limbs were more affected. Vibration sense was lost at the ankles in 5 patients, and the deep reflexes were absent in only 9. Proximal limb girdle weakness, especially severe in the lower limbs, without much wasting was observed in some patients. Additionally, 6 had optic neuropathy and 3 had organic psychosis. Interestingly, 23 of the 28 were chronic alcoholics. Signs of malnutrition were evident elsewhere in the body, and all of them had classical dermal pellagra. Rapid regression of the skin lesions occurred in all patients with only a modest hospital diet without vitamin B supplement. In 18 the peripheral neuropathy also similarly subsided. In the remainder injectable niacin alone only worsened the paraesthesiae, while injectable thiamine alone in 6, and vitamin B complex in 3 gave rapid relief. This study demonstrated that:

(1) Although the skin changes were probably due to niacin deficiency, the peripheral neuropathy was caused by thiamine or multivitamin B deficiency
(2) Alcoholism played a significant role in urban 'nutritional' peripheral neuropathy, a facsimile of the West

This study was extended to the laboratory from 1970–1975. Fifty-nine new patients similar to those described above were seen. In this series (Dastur *et al.*, 1972, 1976) 100% were alcoholics, and only 66% had dermal pellagra. It confirmed the fact that a syndrome of dermal pellagra and sensory peripheral neuropathy most often in alcoholics was the commonest urban pattern of malnutrition. They found that, except for vitamin B_{12}, the concentration of all other B vitamins (thiamine, riboflavin, nicotinic acid, pantothenic acid, total and pyridoxal fraction of vitamin B_6) was 'highly significantly' lowered in the blood of these patients compared with controls. This reduction was even greater in the CSF. With the clinical improvement on the usual hospital diet there was a moderate increase in the blood levels of all vitamins, so that it was difficult to identify the individual vitamin B responsible for the clinical syndrome.

Electromyography revealed remarkable disorder of sensory nerve conduction by way of delayed latencies or total absence of conduction, especially in the lower limbs. The motor conduction velocities were less often and less severely reduced.

Sural nerve biopsies (Dastur *et al.*, 1977b) showed depletion of the large fibres with a unimodal distribution or shift of the normal bimodality to the left. It is interesting that the myelinated fibre count varied from very low to normal, and it varied between different funiculi of the same nerve. The overall impression was reduction in the fibre count as a whole. Degenerating and regenerating fibres were encountered, suggesting an active neuropathy. Electronmicroscopy revealed myelin degeneration and also degeneration of unmyelinated fibres with proliferation of their Schwann cells. Teased fibre preparations showed axon degeneration in various stages in the vast majority. Only a few also showed concurrent segmental demyelination even of the same fibre.

By contrast, peripheral neuropathy formed only a small part of the neurological manifestations of classical pellagra in the more rural populations (Shah and Singh, 1967; Shah, Singh and Jain, 1971; Gopalan, 1969), and there was some doubt whether it was due to the nicotinic acid deficiency itself or due to the accompanying deficiency of other B vitamins, especially thiamine.

(2) Malnutrition and tropical sprue (Vitamin B_{12} deficiency)

Clinically obvious peripheral neuropathy is not seen commonly with tropical sprue. Stefanini (1948), describing his observations amongst a thousand Italian prisoners of war suffering from tropical sprue in India, mentioned that 17% complained of acral paraesthesiae. Iyer *et al.* (1973) found only one out of 24 patients with tropical sprue who had obvious peripheral neuropathy, though 6 had acral paraesthesiae and a third had electrodiagnostic evidence of mild subclinical peripheral neuropathy. A definite correlation between the peripheral neuropathy and a megaloblastic bone marrow was established. Serum vitamin B_{12} levels were significantly reduced in half of these patients, but the serum folate was normal. Rao *et al.* (1981) also found only one patient out of 20 with clinically evident peripheral neuropathy, though 60% had paraesthesiae and 40% had motor nerve conduction abnormalities. Sensory conduction was not studied. Eighteen sural nerve biopsies revealed loss of myelinated fibres in 50% and segmental demyelination of varying degree in 88%. No correlation was observed between serum B_{12} or folate levels and subclinical neuropathy as established by biopsy or electrodiagnosis.

Earlier Jeejeebhoy, Wadia and Desai (1967), making a careful study of 12 patients presenting with features resembling subacute combined degeneration with mild to moderate sensory neuropathy, found conclusive evidence that eight had vitamin B_{12} deficiency, quickly responsive to appropriate therapy. Investigations revealed malabsorption in every case, although overt symptoms were absent. They stressed the importance of investigating for asymptomatic sprue in cases of neuromyelopathy. The other four patients with a somewhat similar neurological syndrome and latent sprue had no vitamin B_{12} deficiency, leaving open the possibility of other factors including other B vitamins (which they did not estimate) playing a part in the causation of this type of neuromyelopathy. Peripheral neuropathy due to vitamin B_{12} deficiency is mainly due to malabsorption. Undernutrition even in India plays a much smaller role and Addisonian pernicious anaemia is rare among Indians.

(3) Protein-calorie malnutrition

Although protein-calorie malnutrition is rampant amongst underprivileged Indian children, evidence of peripheral neuropathy directly related to it is not forthcoming. Sachdev, Taori and Pereira (1971) reported muscle wasting and weakness with a waddling gait, hypotonia and hyporeflexia in a high proportion of these children. No sensory disturbance was noted. Reduction in motor nerve conduction velocity, small motor units and, less commonly, fibrillation potentials were found. Three muscle biopsies showed small atrophic fibres in groups. On this evidence they considered that this disorder was due to a motor peripheral neuropathy or anterior horn cell disease, mentioning that it may have been caused by the commonly accompanying vitamin B complex deficiency rather than the protein-calorie malnutrition.

Dastur *et al.* (1977a) studying children with protein-calorie malnutrition found on quantitative histology of their sural nerve biopsy that (1) there was a retardation or suppression of development of the larger myelinated fibres, the severity depending on the degree of malnutrition regardless of age; (2) there was no difference in the mean nerve fibre density compared with controls, although there was a greater variation in the myelinated fibre density (counts both above and below the normal range were encountered). They did not detect any peripheral neuropathy in these children nor did they suggest a greater possibility of it occuring with sustained malnutrition alone or with additional toxic or metabolic factors.

ARSENICAL NEUROPATHY

Arsenical neuropathy has been well described in the Western literature. The only reason for including it here is to draw attention to the unusual source of intoxication and its common recognition in North-west India since the 1950s (Chuttani, Chawla and Sharma, 1967). Chuttani and Chopra (1979) mentioned that the main source of arsenic was in pills and powders administered by practitioners of indigenous medicine, and when added to tincture of ginger for potentiating action of alcohol or to opium to enhance its effect for addicts. Opium addicts are known to develop chronic peripheral neuropathy when they consume 0.039–0.4 mg of arsenic in 100 g of opium. Individual susceptibility, the daily dose and the period over which the opium is consumed seem to be the deciding factors.

Data gathered over 10 years at the postgraduate Institute of Medicine, Chandigarh, mentions 24 out of 205 patients investigated for peripheral neuropathy from 1970–1976, and 11 out of 570 patients from 1977–1979, as suffering from arsenic intoxication.

As chronic repeated low-dose intoxication with arsenic is more common in India, a relatively lower incidence of gastrointestinal disturbance such as vomiting, anorexia and diarrhoea has been reported. Pigmentation, palmar erythema, hyperkeratosis of palms and soles with exfoliation occur in nearly 50% of Indian patients. The peripheral neuropathy can be acute or chronically progressive. It is usually of the symmetrical, sensorimotor type and results from peripheral axonal degeneration. Electromyography demonstrates denervation with mild to moderate slowing of motor nerve conduction and marked abnormality of the sensory action potentials. Initially it may be difficult to distinguish it from alcoholic peripheral neuropathy, and that complicating malnutrition, especially pellagra, where dermal lesions and diarrhoea can also occur. The diagnosis is still more difficult when the addiction is for both alcohol and opium laced with arsenic. On the other hand, as a fair proportion of patients may not have both the dermal and gastrointestinal symptoms the cause of the neuropathy may remain undetected. However, once suspected, diagnosis is easily confirmed by high levels of arsenic in the blood, urine, hair or nails. BAL, D-penicillamine and symptomatic treatment are usually prescribed.

CLIOQUINOL

Clioquinol has been and is consumed as an anti-diarrhoeal drug since 1934, especially in the developing countries. Tsubaki, Honma and Hoshi (1971) first implicated this drug in the causation of a mysterious disease which had afflicted nearly 10 000 Japanese since 1955. The disease was redesignated as subacute myelo-opticoneuropathy (SMON), because the main damage was believed to be in the spinal cord, optic and peripheral nerves. The evidence for peripheral neuropathy was largely on the clinical grounds of distal ascending dysasthesiae, with objective sensory impairment, sensory ataxia and absent ankle jerks in the majority. The electrophysiological and pathological evidence (Miyakawa *et al.*, 1970; Sobue *et al.*, 1971) in support of this was not strong, but was acceptable enough to be recorded in standard monographs (Pallis and Lewis, 1974b; Le Quesne, 1975). Although occasional cases were described elsewhere from the Western world, SMON seemed to be essentially a Japanese malady.

As a very conservative estimate had indicated that 480 million tablets of clioquinol were sold in India in 1971 (Wadia, 1973) a search for SMON was initiated in Bombay city. As a result it was established (Wadia, 1973; 1977) that:

(1) There was considerable validity in the assertion that clioquinol caused SMON in Japan
(2) SMON was uncommon in India, even if some cases were being missed. Only 9 patients were diagnosed as SMON with varying degree of confidence
(3) The peripheral neuropathy component was not seen in Indian patients. In 8 out of 9 patients, the ankle jerks were present, the motor and sensory nerve conduction velocities were normal, and there was no distal denervation.

There has since been more questioning whether peripheral neuropathy results from clioquinol intoxication. The earlier Japanese reports on formalin-fixed tissue of peripheral degeneration have not been supported by more recent sophisticated animal studies (Schaumburg and Spencer, 1980) which showed the peripheral nervous system to be normal. Baumgartner *et al.* (1979) commented that in the absence of unequivocal evidence of peripheral neuropathy by electromyography and nerve conduction study, or muscle and nerve biopsy, the absent ankle jerks cannot be taken necessarily to indicate peripheral neuropathy. They suggested an alternative explanation. As the neuropathology of SMON has shown, distal degeneration (a central dying-back phenomenon) took place in the axons of the posterior and lateral columns of the spinal cord, they postulated that a similar degeneration must also be occurring in the short central process of the posterior root ganglia distributed to the anterior horn cells involved in the monosynaptic tendon reflex. This would explain the absent deep reflex without any peripheral neuropathy as such (i.e. degeneration of the peripheral processes of the posterior root ganglia). Shibasaki *et al.* (1982) have given recent support to this view by re-examining five long-standing cases of SMON in Japan. Studying short-latency somatosensory-evoked potentials on stimulating the median and posterior tibial nerve, they found abnormalities which suggested normal peripheral nerve conduction, but a marked attenuation of the cortical component and delayed central nerve conduction. They concluded that the pathophysiology of SMON was mainly 'a central distal axonopathy', as first demonstrated in clioquinol intoxication in dogs by Krinke *et al.* (1979). The Indian observation that there is very little neuropathy in SMON now seems substantiated.

PERIPHERAL NEUROPATHY (NEURONOPATHY) IN OLIVOPONTOCEREBELLAR DEGENERATION

Patients with heredo-familial spinocerebellar degeneration are seen regularly in our practice, and a variety of olivopontocerebellar degeneration distinguished by progressive cerebellar ataxia, slow saccadic eye movements and abnormal deep

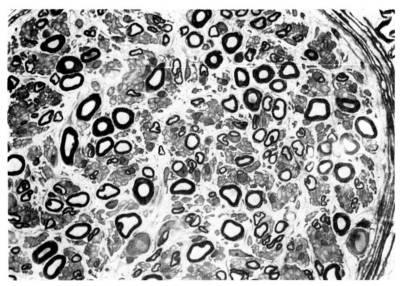

Figure 11.4 Semi-thin section through a sural nerve of a patient with olivopontocerebellar degeneration with slow saccades showing fall-out of myelinated fibres. 1% toluidine blue ×540

reflexes is even commoner than Friedreich's ataxia (Wadia and Swami, 1971). This disorder is uncommon outside India. In recent reviews (Wadia, 1983; Wadia, unpublished observations) of 23 families, attention is drawn to the fact that peripheral neuropathy was a constant feature of this degeneration. Electromyography showed denervation of muscles with normal motor conduction velocity in the related nerves, and abnormal or absent sensory action potentials. Sural nerve biopsy demonstrated a selective fall-out of large myelinated fibres in the early stages and of all fibres later (*Figure 11.4*), and autopsy revealed a variable degeneration of the anterior horn cells and of the posterior columns. It was postulated that in these patients a selective fall-out of the large sensory neurons in the posterior root ganglia occurred with a distal and central dying-back degeneration of axons, a neuronopathy. A study of these families illustrated that, when looked for, clinical or subclinical peripheral neuropathy may not be as rare an accompaniment of spinocerebellar degeneration as previously thought.

RABIES

Tangchai and Vejjajiva (1971) demonstrated inflammatory changes caused by the rabies virus in the peripheral nerves, spinal nerve roots and dorsal root ganglia of patients with classical rabies. They found leucocytic infiltration, proliferation and hypertrophy of Schwann cells, degeneration of nerve fibres and oedema in the peripheral nerves especially of the limb or face where the animal had bitten.

By contrast, Chopra *et al.* (1980) from India recently drew attention to peripheral nerve involvement in paralytic rabies without hydrophobia which clinically simulated Landry's paralysis but for the history of animal bite. The peripheral nerves showed segmental demyelination and remyelination, Wallerian degeneration, and myelinated fibre and axon loss. Segmental demyelination was the primary lesion in the majority, whilst both Wallerian degeneration and segmental demyelination were seen in some others. In no case was Wallerian degeneration seen alone. They postulated that these changes were not due to infection by the virus, but due to the protein component of the virus which produced primary demyelination by a cross-antigenic action on the myelin protein.

GENERAL OBSERVATIONS

In 25 years of urban neurological practice I have seen peripheral neuropathy as a common neurological disease, caused by most of the already well-known aetiological agents, with diabetes leading the field. Yet some differences, as mentioned earlier, have been evident. Drug toxicity and industrial poisoning have not appeared frequently as a cause in my experience. Sarcoidosis, although not a common cause of peripheral neuropathy in the West, is even rarer in India. I have seen it only once here. Similarly, 'nutritional' ataxic tropical peripheral neuropathy, so frequently reported from the West Indies (Montgomery *et al.*, 1964) and Africa (Money, 1961; Osuntokun, 1968), has not been reported. I have seen only one patient with severe sensory ataxia, optic atrophy and nerve deafness and he was an Arab ex-prisoner in whom severe malnourishment had occurred during his confinement. As anywhere else in the world it has not been possible to find an aetiological agent in nearly 30% of our hospital patients.

References

Antia, N. H. (1974) The significance of nerve involvement in leprosy. *Plastic and Reconstructive Surgery*, **54**, 55–63

Baumgartner, G., Gawel, M. J., Kaeser, H. E. *et al.* (1979) Neurotoxicity of halogenated hydroxyquinolines: clinical analysis of cases reported outside Japan. *Journal of Neurology, Neurosurgery and Psychiatry*, **42**, 1073–1083

Chopra, J. S., Banerjee, J. M., Murthy, J. M. K. and Pal, S. R. (1980) Paralytic rabies – a clinicopathological study. *Brain*, **103**, 789–802

Chuttani, P. N., Chawla, L. S. and Sharma, T. D. (1967) Arsenical neuropathy. *Neurology (Minneapolis)*, **17**, 269–274

Chuttani, P. N. and Chopra, J. S. (1979) Arsenic poisoning. In *Handbook of Clinical Neurology*, edited by P. J. Vinken and G. W. Bruyn, vol. 36, pp. 199–216. Amsterdam: North Holland Publishing Company

Dastur, D. K. (1976) Leprosy (an infectious and immunological disorder of the nervous system). In *Handbook of Clinical Neurology*, edited by P. J. Vinken and G. W. Bruyn, vol. 33, pp. 421–468 Amsterdam: North Holland Publishing Company

Dastur, D. K., Dewan, A., Manghani, D. K. and Udani, P. M. (1977a) Quantitative histology of nerve in protein-calorie malnutrition and well-nourished children. *Neuropathology and Applied Neurobiology*, **3**, 405–422

Dastur, D. K., Dewan, A., Santhadevi, N., Manghani, D. K. and Razzak, Z. A. (1977b) Malnutrition – alcoholism: histopathology of peripheral nerves and B vitamins in nerves, blood and CSF. In *Neurotoxicology*, edited by L. Roizin, H. Shiraki and N. Grecevic, pp. 529–547. New York: Raven Press

Dastur, D. K., Santhadevi, N., Quadros, E. V. *et al.* (1976) The B-vitamins in malnutrition with alcoholism. A model of intervitamin relationships. *British Journal of Nutrition*, **36**, 143–159

Dastur, D. K., Wadia, N. H., Bharucha, E. P. *et al.* (1972) Interim Report. *Studies on Nutritional Disorders of the Nervous System*, pp. 13–17. Bombay: Tata Press

Fite, G. L. (1943) Leprosy from the histologic point of view. *Archives of Pathology*, **35**, 611–644

Gopalan, C. (1969) Possible role for dietary leucine in pathogenesis of pellagra. *Lancet*, **1**, 197–199

Iyer, G. V., Taori, G. M., Kapadia, C. R., Mathan, V. I. and Baker, S. J. (1973) Neurological manifestations in tropical sprue: a clinical and electrodiagnostic study. *Neurology (Minneapolis)*, **23**, 959–966

Jeejeebhoy, K. N., Wadia, N. H. and Desai, H. G. (1967) Role of vitamin B_{12} deficiency in tropical 'nutritional' neuromyelopathy. *Journal of Neurology, Neurosurgery and Psychiatry*, **30**, 7–12

Jopling, W. H. (1978) The disease. In *Handbook of Leprosy*, 2nd ed, pp. 7–43. London: William Heinemann Medical Books

Kaur, U., Chopra, J. S., Prabhakar, S. and Radhakrishnan, K. (1982) Clinical spectrum of peripheral neuropathies. *Indian Journal of Medical Research*, **76**, 728–735

Krinke, G., Schaumberg, H. H., Spencer, P. S., Thomann, P. and Hess, R. (1979) Clioquinol and 2,5-hexanedione induce different types of distal axonopathy in the dog. *Acta Neuropathologica (Berlin)*, **47**, 213–221

Lancet (1977) Chemotherapy of leprosy. **2**, 77–78

Le Quesne, P. M. (1975) Neuropathy due to drugs. In *Peripheral Neuropathy*, edited by P. J. Dyck, P. K. Thomas and E. H. Lambert, vol. II, pp. 1264–1266. Philadelphia: W. B. Saunders

Miyakawa, T., Sumiyoshi, S., Murayama, E., Ishikawa, H., Miyakawa, K. and Tatesu, S. (1970) Ultrastructural study of a nerve and muscle biopsy from a case of 'subacute myelo-opticoneuropathy'. *Acta Neuropathologica*, **16**, 17–24

Money, G. L. (1961) Etiology of funicular myelopathies in tropical Africa. *World Neurology*, **2**, 526–535

Montgomery, R. D., Cruickshank, E. K., Robertson, W. B. and McMenemey, W. H. (1964). Clinical and pathological observations on Jamaican neuropathy. *Brain*, **87**, 425–462

Morehead, C. (ed.) (1860) *Clinical Researches on Diseases in India*, pp. 695–698. London: Longman, Green, Longman and Roberts

Noordeen, S. K. (1980) Epidemiology. In *A Manual of Leprosy*, edited by R. H. Thangaraj, pp. 3–9. New Delhi: Printaid

Osuntokun, B. O. (1968) An ataxic neuropathy in Nigeria – a clinical, biochemical and electrophysiological study. *Brain*, **91**, 215–248

Pallis, C. A. and Lewis, P. D. (1974a) Other vitamin deficiencies. In *The Neurology of Gastrointestinal Disease*, pp. 98–123. London: W. B. Saunders

Pallis, C. A. and Lewis, P. D. (1974b) Neurological complications of infective diarrhoeas. In *The Neurology of Gastrointestinal Disease*, pp. 175–188. London: W. B. Saunders

Pearson, J. M. H. (1981) The problem of dapsone-resistant leprosy. *International Journal of Leprosy*, **49**, 417–420

Rao, P. N., Chopra, J. S., Mehta, S. K. and Sawhney, B. B. (1981) Peripheral neuropathy in tropical sprue – a clinical electrodiagnostic and histopathological study. *Indian Journal of Medical Research*, **74**, 915–925

Sachdev, K. K., Taori, G. M. and Pereira, S. M. (1971) Neuromuscular status in protein-calorie malnutrition: clinical, nerve conduction and electromyographic studies. *Neurology (Minneapolis)*, **21**, 801–804

Schaumburg, H. H. and Spencer, P. S. (1980) Clioquinol. In *Experimental and Clinical Neurotoxicology*, edited by P. S. Spencer and H. H. Schaumburg, pp. 395–406. Baltimore; Williams and Wilkins

Shah, D. R. and Singh, S. V. (1967) Pellagra in Udaipur district. *Journal of Association of Physicians of India*, **15**, 1–7

Shah, D. R., Singh, S. V. and Jain, I. L. (1971) Neurological manifestations in pellagra. *Journal of Association of Physicians of India*, **19**, 443–446

Shetty, V. P., Mehta, L. N., Antia, N. H. and Irani, P. F. (1977) Teased fibre study of early nerve lesions in leprosy and in contacts, with electrophysiological correlates. *Journal of Neurology, Neurosurgery and Pshychiatry*, **40**, 708–711

Shibasaki, H., Kakigi, R., Ohnishi, A. and Kuroiwa, Y. (1982) Peripheral and central nerve conduction in subacute myelo-opticoneuropathy. *Neurology (New York)*, **32**, 1186–1189

Sobue, I., Ando, K., Iida, M., Takayanagi, T., Yamamura, Y. and Matsuoka, Y. (1971) Myeloneuropathy with abdominal disorders in Japan. *Neurology (Minneapolis)*, **21**, 168–173

Stefanini, M. (1948) Clinical features and pathogenesis of tropical sprue. Observations on series of cases among Italian prisoners of war in India. *Medicine (Baltimore)*, **27**, 379–427

Tangchai, P. and Vejjajiva, A. (1971) Pathology of the peripheral nervous system in human rabies – a study of nine autopsy cases. *Brain*, **94**, 299–306

Tsubaki, T., Honma, Y. and Hoshi, M. (1971) Neurological syndrome associated with clioquinol. *Lancet*, **1**, 696–697

Wadia, N. H. (1973) Is there SMON in India? *Neurology India*, **21**, 95–103

Wadia, N. H. (1977) Some observations on SMON from Bombay. *Journal of Neurology, Neurosurgery and Psychiatry*, **40**, 268–275

Wadia, N. H. (1979) Nutritional disorders of the nervous system. In *Progress in Clinical Medicine*, edited by M. M. S. Ahuja, pp. 487–510. New Delhi: Arnold – Heinemann

Wadia, N. H. (1983) A variety of olivopontocerebellar degeneration distinguished by slow eye movements and peripheral neuropathy. In *Olivopontocerebellar Atrophies*, edited by R. C. Duvoisin and A. Plaitakis. New York: Raven Press (in press)

Wadia, N. H. and Swami, R. K. (1970) Pattern of nutritional deficiency disorders of the nervous system in Bombay. *Neurology India*, **18**, 203–218

Wadia, N. H. and Swami, R. K. (1971) A new form of heredo-familial spinocerebellar degeneration with slow eye movements (nine families). *Brain*, **94**, 359–374

WHO (1976) Expert committee of leprosy. Fifth Report. *WHO Technical Report Series*, No. 607

WHO Study Group (1982) Chemotherapy of leprosy for control programmes. *WHO Technical Report Series*, No. 675

12
Geographical patterns of neuropathy: Japan

Akio Ohnishi

INTRODUCTION

The association of polyneuropathy with 'dysglobulinemia' (dysproteinemia and paraproteinemia) is well known (Silverstein and Doniger, 1963; Driedger and Pruzanski, 1980; Kelly *et al.*, 1981a, b). Since 1969 over 80 patients with the symptom complex – skin hyperpigmentation, edema and polyneuropathy associated with plasma cell dyscrasia – were found amongst the Japanese (Fukase *et al.*, 1969; Iwashita, 1976; Nishitani *et al.*, 1976; Iwashita *et al.*, 1977; Nakanishi, Ozaki and Muramoto, 1982). Similar cases have been reported in non-Japanese (Scheinker, 1938; Crow, 1956; Morley and Schweiger, 1967; Waldenström *et al.*, 1978; Trillet *et al.*, 1980; Ohnishi and Dyck 1981). The symptom complex seems to be a specific form of 'dysglobulinemic' neuropathy.

Clinical, immunological, neurophysiological and histopathological features of the symptom complex, especially of polyneuropathy, are reviewed herein and the possible pathogenic mechanisms are briefly discussed in the light of recent advances in immunochemical and immunohistochemical procedures (Propp *et al.*, 1975; Swash, Perrin and Schwartz, 1979; Asbury and Lisak, 1980; Latov *et al.*, 1981a, b; Abrams *et al.*, 1982).

A CASE REPORT

Clinical findings

A 61-year-old Japanese man presented in August 1973 with a 1-year history of progressive bilateral weakness and tingling sensation in the lower limbs and edema in the feet. He was diagnosed as having a polyneuropathy of unknown etiology. In January 1974 he noticed that his face, upper limbs and back had become increasingly pigmented, and he began to have tingling and weakness in his hands. Weakness in the lower limbs was progressively worse, so that he could not walk at the time of his admission in September 1974.

On admission, his skin showed dark-brownish pigmentation over his whole body (*Figure 12.1*); the breasts were slightly swollen with induration (gynecomastia). The skin of his fingers and forearms was thickened, and his fingernails and toenails were white. There was marked pitting edema, especially in distal areas of the upper and lower limbs (*Figure 12.2*). The facial skin was somewhat reddish and

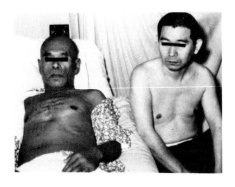

Figure 12.1 The patient (*left*) with diffuse skin hyperpigmentation, compared with the control patient (*right*). (From Iwashita *et al.*, 1977, courtesy of the Editor and Publishers, *Neurology (Minneapolis)*)

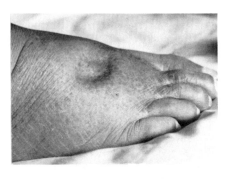

Figure 12.2 Marked pitting edema on the dorsum of the foot. (From Iwashita *et al.*, 1977, courtesy of the Editor and Publishers, *Neurology (Minneapolis)*)

thickened. Hyperhidrosis was present on the face, neck and back. There was an unusual hypertrichosis (rough hair) on the upper portion of the legs and knees (*Figure 12.3*) which had not been present a few years previously. The abdomen was swollen and the liver was palpable four fingerbreadths below the costal margin. The spleen and lymph nodes were not palpable or swollen. There were a few dark reddish verrucous eruptions of millet to pea-size over the chest, abdomen and back. Neurologically, he was alert and well oriented. Slight venous engorgement and arteriosclerosis were found in the retina. Papilledema was absent but developed later. The pupils were miotic and not responsive to light, but reacted well to accommodation (Argyll-Robertson pupil). Muscle weakness of a moderate to severe degree was present in the hands and below the knees, especially in the anterior tibial and peroneal muscles. The weak muscles were slightly to moderately atrophic. He could not pick up small objects with his fingers. Deep tendon reflexes in the four limbs were absent with no pathologic reflexes. Standing was difficult, and he could not walk even with canes. Moderate to severe degrees of impairment of touch and temperature sensations as well as dysalgesia and delayed pain were found in the hands and below the knees in a glove-stocking fashion. Vibration

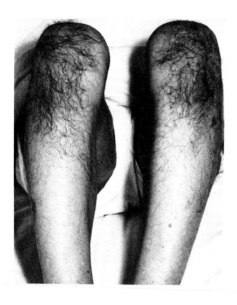

Figure 12.3 Hypertrichosis on the anterior surface of the upper parts of legs and knees. (From Iwashita *et al.*, 1977, courtesy of the Editor and Publishers, *Neurology* (*Minneapolis*))

sensation was totally absent below the neck and so was position sensation in the fingers and toes. There was no abnormality in coordination and sphincter function was normal.

On laboratory examination, erythrocyte sedimentation was 11 mm in 1 hour, 33 mm in 2 hours. When trace amounts of protein were present, no Bence Jones protein (boiling method with buffer) was found. However, an immunoelectrophoretic analysis of 100-fold concentrated urine showed lambda type Bence Jones protein with a clear M-bow formation. There was no glucosuria. Serum total protein was 6.0 g/100 ml (normal range 6.5–8.5) and its cellulose-acete electrophoresis showed an albumin level of 53.3% (54.0–62.0); α_1-globulin 4.2% (3.0–6.0); α_2-globulin 10.2% (8.0–12.0); β-globulin 8.5% (8.0–12.0) and γ-globulin 23.3% (14.0–21.0). Immunoglobulin quantitation was IgG 2120 mg/100 ml (1.160–2.080); IgA 304 mg/100 ml (140–350), and IgM 250 mg/100 ml (60–380). There was no monoclonal pattern in the γ-globulin region, but a slight polyclonal increase of IgG was seen. Immunoelectrophoresis of serum protein revealed an M-bow-forming precipitating line of Bence Jones protein of lambda type. There was no M-bow-formation in IgG, IgA or IgM precipitating lines. Bone marrow puncture of the sternum showed 2.4% plasma cells (less than 1.9) without other abnormalities. Serum estrogen (estradiol) was 12.5, 17.5 and 50.0 pg/ml (17–41) on three occasions. Roentgenologic examinations of the whole skeleton revealed osteosclerotic lesions of the eleventh and twelfth vertebral bodies, as shown in *Figure 12.4*. A biopsy specimen from the eleventh vertebral body contained a nest of immature plasma cells. On cerebrospinal fluid examination, protein content was 167.5 mg/100 ml (10–40). Electrophoresis of CSF protein showed pre-albumin 2.1% (2.8–6.0); albumin 57.5% (55.9–65.3); α-globulin 5.3% (3.5–8.3); α_2-globulin 5.9% (4.3–6.3); β-globulin 10.6% (12.1–15.1) and γ-globulin 18.6% (7.6–9.8). CSF IgG was 29.6 mg/100 ml (0.4–4.2); IgA 2.8 mg/100 ml (0.5–1.0) and IgM 1.0 mg/100 ml (0–0.5).

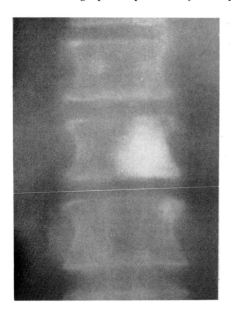

Figure 12.4 Tomogram of the spine shows localized osteosclerotic lesions in the eleventh and twelfth thoracic vertebral bodies. (From Iwashita *et al.*, 1977, courtesy of the Editor and Publishers, *Neurology* (*Minneapolis*))

On needle electromyography, denervation of clinically involved muscles was apparent. Conduction velocity of motor fibers of the left ulnar nerve was 18.0 m/sec. Measurement of conduction velocity of the left tibial and sural nerves was not possible because an electrical response was not obtained from these nerves. Fascicular biopsy of the right and left sural nerves was performed at ankle level, on August 17, 1973 (first biopsy) and April 14, 1975 (second biopsy). Quantitative histological data for both nerves are shown in *Table 12.1*. In both biopsies the densities (numbers/mm^2 of fascicular area) of both large and small myelinated fibers were moderately and markedly decreased, respectively, although the density of unmyelinated fibers was within normal limits on two occasions. No onion-bulb formation was noted. Teased fiber analysis was not performed at the first biopsy. At the second, the myelinated fibers in the specimen were not well enough osmicated to be classified by the criteria described by Dyck (1975).

Table 12.1 Number* of nerve fibers in sural nerves

	Total	Myelinated fibers		Unmyelinated fibers
		Large	Small	
Control†				
Mean ± SE	9452 ± 931	3827 ± 465	5624 ± 585	31 825 ± 7078
Range	7393–13 247	2675–507	4379–8213	23 052–45 833
This case				
First biopsy	3733	1680	2053	22 045
Second biopsy	614	37	577	38 939

* Number/mm^2 of fascicular area
† Six controls for myelinated fibers and three controls for unmyelinated fibers

The diagnosis of osteosclerotic myeloma associated with polyneuropathy, skin hyperpigmentation, hypertrichosis and edema was made. After establishment of the diagnosis, prednisolone 60 mg was administered orally every other day for 2 weeks without noticeable decrease of edema or skin hyperpigmentation. There was also no change in muscle weakness of the upper and lower limbs. After irradiation (total dosage 3000 rad of cobalt) to the eleventh thoracic vertebral area (area of myeloma) for 17 days with continued prednisolone therapy, his grasping power increased and he could pick up small objects with his fingers and walk with canes. The thickened skin, white nails, gynecomastia and cutaneous hyperpigmentation were noticeably improved. Liver swelling decreased, and the hair on the legs and knees became softer. Edema was also decreased. Foot drop, however, remained unimproved. The prednisolone dosage was gradually reduced to 25 mg every other day. The roentgenologic findings in the eleventh and twelfth thoracic vertebral bodies remained unchanged. Bence Jones protein of the lambda type was still immunoelectrophoretically present in the urine.

He was seen in the outpatient clinic once a month and was kept on prednisolone 20–25 mg every other day. He continued to show the medical and neurologic improvement described until May 1976, when he noted an aggravation of the muscle weakness of the upper and lower limbs and generalized edema with easy fatigability and loss of appetite. By the third admission in May 1976, he had became almost bedridden with emaciation, mainly due to severe muscle weakness of the upper and lower limbs. The roentgenologic examination revealed additional osteosclerotic lesions of the twelfth vertebral body, the left fifth, sixth, seventh and eighth ribs and the left scapula. In December 1976 acute circulatory failure occurred and he died on the same day. The total clinical course was about 4 years' duration.

Autopsy findings

The presence of osteosclerotic lesions was confirmed on roentgenologic examination of the vertebral bodies and ribs. Nests of mature plasma cells with new bone formation in the surrounding area were demonstrated in the vertebral bodies.

Morphometric analysis (Ohnishi, Ikeda and Tateishi, 1979) was made on myelinated fibers on the fifth lumbar (L5) spinal roots, of Goll's tract and on nerve cells of L3 dorsal root ganglion.

L5 DORSAL AND VENTRAL ROOTS

In the teased fibers, the frequency of myelinated fibers showing segmental demyelination and remyelination (condition C, D, *Figure 12.5* and F) was greater than in the controls (*Table 12.2*) in both dorsal and ventral roots. There were no myelinated fibers showing linear rows of myelin ovoids. In the dorsal root, numbers of both large and small myelinated fibers per root were decreased compared with the control. In the ventral root, the number of large myelinated fibers per root was decreased, and that of small myelinated fibers was increased compared with controls (*Table 12.2*).

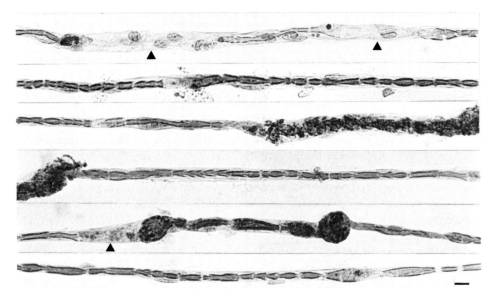

Figure 12.5 Consecutive portions of myelinated fibers of dorsal root. Demyelinated (solid triangles) and thinly myelinated portions are seen along a single myelinated fiber (condition D fiber). Bar represents 10 μm. (From Shibasaki *et al.*, 1982, *Annals of Neurology*, **12**, 355–360, courtesy of the Editor and Publishers)

Table 12.2 Number[a] of myelinated fibers and frequency (%) of fiber conditions in teased fibers in L5 spinal roots

		Dorsal root						
Myelinated fibers			*Fiber conditions*					
Large[b]	Small[c]	Total	A + B	C	D	E	F	G
This case								
1165	14 166	15 331	0	14	84	0	2	0
Control[d]								
Mean 14 332	27 694	42 026	95.9	0	0	0.1	3.0	1.0
SE[g] 923	1743	2066	1.0	0	0	0.1	0.8	0.6

		Ventral root						
Myelinated fibers			*Fiber conditions*					
Large[e]	Small[f]	Total	A + B	C	D	E	F	G
This case								
106	6518	6624	0	34	66	0	0	0
Control[d]								
Mean 6155	2024	8179	95.0	0	0	0.2	4.1	0.4
SE[g] 346	199	446	1.6	0	0	0.1	1.5	0.2

a: Number per root; b: diameter >5.62 μm; c: diameter ≤5.62 μm; d: 15 controls (ages 8–83 years) for number of myelinated fibers and nine controls (ages 23–71 years) for teased fibers; e: diameter >7.83 μm; f: diameter ≤7.83 μm; g: standard error.
Fiber conditions A–G as described by Dyck (1975)

FASCICULUS GRACILIS

The densities of total myelinated fibers at the fifth thoracic and the third cervical segment of fasciculus gracilis were 25 296 and 26 338/mm^2 of fascicular area, respectively, and were within normal limits. The size frequency distributions of myelinated fiber diameters were similar to those in the controls.

L3 DORSAL ROOT GANGLION

The total number of nerve cell bodies and their diameter size freqency distributions suggested a slight decrease of cell bodies over 60 μm diameter. Nageotte's residual nodules were rarely found.

ANTERIOR HORN OF LUMBAR SPINAL CORD

A significant number of large anterior horn cells showed central chromatolysis. A decrease in the number of anterior horn cells and astrogliosis in the anterior horn was not evident.

Infiltration of plasmacytoma cells or inflammatory cells in the peripheral and central nervous systems was nil and amyloid deposits were never detected.

OTHER AUTOPSY FINDINGS

An abscess (14 cm diameter) in the right upper pulmonary lobe, bilateral bronchopneumonia and membranoproliferative glomerulonephritis were observed. The cause of death was considered to be bilateral bronchopneumonia with right pulmonary abscess.

Comment

In this case the actual diagnosis should be chronic polyneuropathy associated with osteosclerotic myeloma. Such cases have been reported previously (Crow, 1956; Morley and Schweiger, 1967; Iwashita *et al.*, 1977; Waldenström *et al.*, 1978; Driedger and Pruzanski, 1980). There was a generalized skin hyperpigmentation, hypertrichosis and edema, in addition to polyneuropathy with osteosclerotic myeloma. Such a case is rare in the literature (Crow, 1956; Iwashita *et al.*, 1977; Waldenström *et al.*, 1978; Driedger and Pruzanski, 1980). Since 1969, special attention has been given to such cases in Japan, because they may constitute a syndrome in which an etiological factor unique to Japan may be revealed. The case presented herein is typical, and is termed the 'symptom complex' – skin hyperpigmentation, edema and polyneuropathy associated with plasma cell dyscrasia. The first case of this complex was described by Fukase *et al.* (1969).

Clinical features

The main clinical findings are summarized in *Table 12.3.*

Polyneuropathy is one of the main findings. The course is chronic, progressive and the onset is insidious. Almost all the cases presented with sensorimotor

Table 12.3 Clinical findings of the symptom complex in Japan

Cases	The first case in Japan	The case presented	Nine cases in Kyushu Univeristy	Eighty-three cases in Japan
Age (Mean age)	36	63	27–64 (51)	27–72 (46)
Sex (Numbers)	F	M	M (6), F (3)	M (57), F (26)
Physical findings				
Polyneuropathy	+	+	+,9/9	+,83/83
Skin hyperpigmentation	+	+	+,9/9	+,77/83
Pedal edema	+	+	+,8/9	+,73/81
Hypertrichosis	+	+	+,8/9	+,61/77
Papilledema	+	+	+,8/9	+,47/77
Hepatomegaly	+	+	+,6/9	+,62/80
Ascites	–	+	+,4/9	+,40/66
Lymphadenopathy	+	–	+,6/9	+,53/79
Gynecomastia		+	+,3/6	+,35/53
Laboratory findings				
Radiological skeletal findings	S	S	S,6/6 L,0/6	S,27/44 L, 5/44 S and L,12/44
Bone marrow plasmacytosis	+	+	+,4/7	+,24/75
Serum M-component	+ IgG,λ	+ BJ,λ	+,5/9	+,61/82
Increase of CSF protein (≥50 mg/100 ml)	+	+	+,7/8	+,75/77
Decrease of MCV (≥35 m/s)	+	+	+,8/8	+,55/61
Decrease of SCV (≥35 m/s)		+	+,6/6	+,27/31

MCV: Motor nerve conduction velocity; SCV: sensory nerve conduction velocity; S: sclerotic; L: lytic; BJ: Bence Jones protein

polyneuropathy. Protein in the cerebrospinal fluid was increased in almost all cases. Marked decrease of motor and sensory nerve conduction velocities occurred in the majority.

Monoclonal protein in the serum was found in 61 out of 82 cases. The numbers with IgG (λ type), IgA (λ type), IgG (κ type) and IgA (κ type) with monoclonal protein in the serum were 32, 24, 1 and 1, respectively. The light chain of the immunoglobulin was λ type in 56 out of 58 cases.

HISTOLOGICAL FINDINGS OF SURAL NERVE ON BIOPSY

Nine subjects were studied.

In teased fiber analysis (Dyck, 1975; Ohnishi *et al.*, 1979), myelinated fibers showing linear rows of myelin ovoids (axonal degeneration) and those with demyelinated and/or remyelinated segments were evident to varying degrees (*Figure 12.6*).

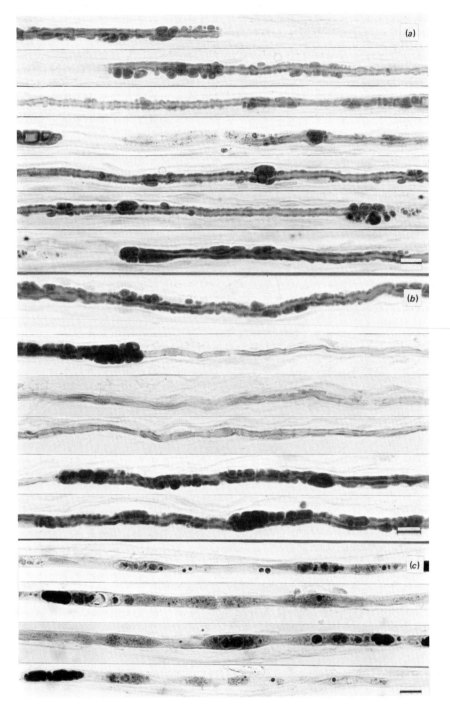

Figure 12.6 Consecutive portions of myelinated fibers of the sural nerve. Note the presence of three demyelinated portions with or without small myelin ovoids and thinly myelinated portions along a single myelinated fiber showing marked irregularities of myelin sheath (*a*), condition D fiber and the presence of internodes with thin myelin sheath along a single myelinated fiber showing marked irregularities of myelin sheath (*b*), condition F fiber. Note the presence of linear rows of various sizes of myelin ovoids (*c*), condition E fiber. Bar represents 10 μm

In epon-embedded sections, a decrease in the densities (numbers/mm^2 of fascicular area) of both large and small myelinated fibers was found in the majority of cases. The density of unmyelinated fibers remained within normal limits.

On electron microscopy, uncompacted lamellae in the myelin sheath of myelinated fibers were found in over half the cases studied. Of 50–100 myelinated fibers in transverse sections in each case, uncompacted lamellar structures were observed at frequencies of 3–8%. At the transitional border between compacted and uncompacted myelin, the major dense lines of compacted myelin sheaths opened up to form layers of stacked flat islands of Schwann cell cytoplasm (uncompacted lamellar structure; *Figures 12.7* and *12.8*). The uncompacted

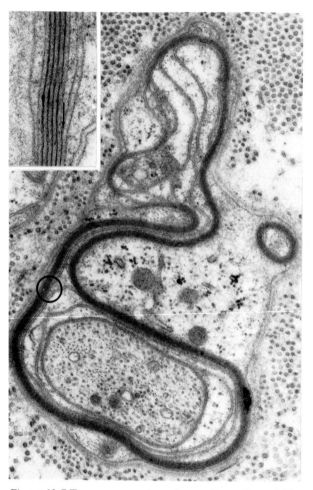

Figure 12.7 Transverse section of a small myelinated fiber rich in Schwann-cell cytoplasm with an abnormal myelin sheath (×20 000). An uncompacted portion of the lamellar structure continuous to the major dense line is shown at high magnification in the insert (arrow, ×62 000). (From Ohnishi and Hirano, 1981, courtesy of the Editor and Publishers, *Journal of the Neurological Sciences*)

lamellar structure was commonly seen in inner and middle layers of the myelin sheath, but was also seen in the outer layer. The intraperiod line could not usually be identified in between the uncompacted lamellae, although the partial formation of intraperiod line was observed on some fibers. The uncompacted lamellar structure was usually continuous with abnormal Schmidt-Lantermann incisures or paranode-like structures. Dense bodies and/or membranous structures were occasionally found in some of the islands of Schwann cell cytoplasm of the uncompacted portions of myelin sheaths and the paranodal area (*Figure 12.8*).

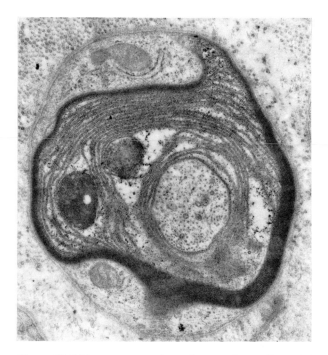

Figure 12.8 Transverse section of a small myelinated fiber with uncompacted lamellar structure. Two dense bodies are seen in islands of Schwann-cell cytoplasm (×13 000) (From Ohnishi and Hirano, 1981, courtesy of the Editor and Publishers, *Journal of the Neurological Sciences*)

Myelin sheath showing extra leaflets of the intraperiod line (Raine and Bornstein, 1979) and myelin sheath with a widened space between major dense lines (Sluga, 1974; Propp *et al.*, 1975; Julien *et al.*, 1978) were absent. Although macrophages containing myelin debris were occasionally seen in the endoneurium, there were no invading macrophages which penetrated the basal lamina of the Schwann cell or separated the groups of myelin lamellae from the main sheath. In fibers with an uncompacted lamellar structure, the transverse axonal area seemed to be small relative to the number of myelin lamellae. Definite abnormalities of axoplasmic organelles were not usual in axons of such myelinated fibers. The ongoing degeneration of unmyelinated axons was rare.

The presence of the debris of myelin breakdown was occasionally seen. Various abnormalities of axons of myelinated fibers, such as granular disintegration of axoplasmic organelles, axonal shrinkage and focal increase of myelin figures, vacuoles and dense bodies were sometimes noted.

The uncompacted lamellae of the myelin sheath are well explained by the irregular distribution of adaxonal, incisural and paranodal cytoplasm of the Schwann cell and may be understood by modifications of the configuration of the myelinating cell (Hirano and Dembitzer, 1967). The uncompacted lamellae of the myelin sheath seem to be due to the effect of dysglobulinemia on the Schwann cell (Ohnishi and Hirano, 1981).

STUDIES OF SOMATOSENSORY EVOKED POTENTIALS (SEPs) TO LOCALIZE DEGENERATION

Five patients were studied (Shibasaki, Ohnishi and Kuroiwa, 1982). Electromyograph (EMG) of affected muscles revealed fibrillation potentials and positive sharp waves at rest. During maximal contraction, the recruitment pattern was markedly reduced with long duration of the motor unit potentials. Motor nerve conduction velocity (CV) of the median nerve was reduced to 23–43 m/sec. Electrical stimulation of either peroneal or tibial nerve evoked no recognizable muscle action potential in most cases.

Sensory CV of the sural nerve could not be measured due to the absence of any recognizable response to electrical stimulation. To record SEP, the median nerve was electrically stimulated by a pair of cup electrodes placed on the wrist. The short latency SEPs were markedly abnormal in all cases. As shown in *Figure 12.9*, the

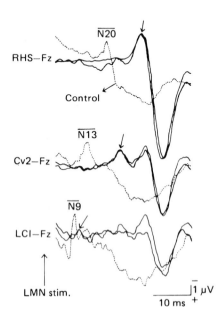

Figure 12.9 SEPs with left median nerve (LMN) stimulation in a patient with the symptom complex. SEPs in control are shown in dotted lines. RHS, right hand sensory area; Cv2, the second cervical spine; LC1, left clavicle; Fz, frontal midline. See text for explanation. (From Shibasaki, *et al.*, 1982, *Annals of Neurology*, **12**, 355–360, courtesy of the Editor and Publishers)

typical abnormality consisted of a markedly depressed amplitude and moderately delayed peak latency of the $\overline{N9}$ component (action potential through the brachial plexus), and significantly delayed peak latency of the components $\overline{N13}$ (action potential generated in the cervical cord of cuneate nucleus of the medulla oblongata) and $\overline{N20}$ (action potential generated in the postcentral gyrus). With respect to the amplitude of each component, $\overline{N9}$ was reduced in the majority of cases, but $\overline{N13}$ and $\overline{N20}$ were normal in all cases, although the amplitude of the component $\overline{N13}$ was close to the low normal range. With regard to the latency, the component $\overline{N9}$ showed a mild but significant delay in five out of six hands tested. In three hands, the latency measurement was impossible because of the polyphasic appearance of the $\overline{N9}$ component. The interpeak latency $\overline{N9}$ to $\overline{N13}$ was significantly prolonged, except in two hands (one case). The interpeak latency from $\overline{N13}$ to $\overline{N20}$ was normal in all cases.

The marked reduction in amplitude and moderately delayed peak latency of the $\overline{N9}$ component may indicate the presence of axonal degeneration and segmental demyelination in the peripheral nerves. These findings are in conformity with the pathological findings of the sural nerve described above. A prolongation of the interpeak latency from $\overline{N9}$ to $\overline{N13}$ suggests a marked conduction delay in the dorsal root. This finding is in good conformity with the pathological change found in the dorsal root, i.e. extensive segmental demyelination and remyelination. The normal interpeak latency from $\overline{N13}$ to $\overline{N20}$ is interpreted to reflect a normal central conduction, substantiated by normal neuropathological findings in the posterior columns. Therefore, the results in the studies of somatosensory evoked potentials are in good conformity with the pathological abnormalities revealed at autopsy.

AUTOPSY FINDINGS OF OTHER CASES

In two cases, the histopathological findings of the sural nerve, the fifth spinal lumbar (L5) roots, Goll's tract and the third lumbar (L3) dorsal root ganglion were similar to those of the case described above. In teased fibers, the frequencies of myelinated fibers showing segmental demyelination and remyelination were markedly greater in L5 dorsal and ventral roots as compared with the controls. The decrease of myelinated fibers was obvious in the sural nerve and L5 dorsal root. On the other hand, it was not obvious in the L5 ventral root and Goll's tract. A definite decrease was not found in the total numbers of cell bodies in the L3 dorsal root ganglion.

The histopathological changes at different levels of the peripheral nervous system in our studies led to the conclusion that the major findings are the segmental demyelination and remyelination in both dorsal and ventral roots and sural nerve, and the decrease of both large and small myelinated fibers of sural nerves (peripheral axons of primary sensory neuron) with preservation of myelinated fibers in fasciculus gracilis (central axons of primary sensory neuron) (Sato *et al.*, 1980).

Immunohistochemical findings

The histopathological studies suggest the possible primary involvement of the myelin sheath and/or Schwann cell in this symptom complex. In order to clarify whether the paraprotein is preferentially found in myelin sheath and/or endoneurium, we studied the distribution of IgG, IgM, IgA, light chain λ and light chain κ in spinal dorsal roots, kidney and cerebrum in four patients with this syndrome, four with multiple myeloma without polyneuropathy and five neurological controls (one case each of cerebral thrombosis, striatonigral degneration, tuberculous meningitis, cerebral contusion and senile dementia), by applying the peroxidase-antiperoxidase technique on paraffin sections (Sternberger et al., 1970; Doi et al., 1982). Serial sections of two spinal dorsal roots were alternately stained for the immunoglobulin in relation to the myelin sheath.

Strong immunostaining for immunoglobulins, especially of the same type of immunoglobulin as was elevated in the serum in each case, was observed in the spinal dorsal roots from all with the symptom complex and from two out of four with multiple myeloma without polyneuropathy. The immunostaining was found in the endoneurial tissue and some axons, but not in the myelin sheath. However, the reaction to the immunoglobulins was weak in spinal dorsal roots in the controls. Immunostaining was successfully blocked by the absorption studies, indicating specificity. As expected, the strong reaction to the immunoglobulins was observed equally in the renal tissue in all cases. On the other hand, only a weak reaction to immunoglobulin was found in the cerebral tissue, except the area directly involved by cerebral thrombosis or cerebral contusion.

Thus the deposition of immunoglobulins, especially the paraprotein which was elevated in the serum in each patient, was found in the endoneurial tissue and not in the myelin sheath in this symptom complex as well as in some cases of multiple myeloma without polyneuropathy. Therefore, the deposition of immunoglobulins alone does not seem to be responsible for the nerve fiber degeneration (Doi et al., 1982).

TREATMENT AND PROGNOSIS

Surgical removal of the myeloma, radiation to the area of the myeloma, chemotherapy (steroids, melphalan and cyclophosphamide) or their combination have been prescribed. Improvement of the clinical signs and symptoms and decrease in the serum monoclonal protein have followed this treatment (Iwashita et al., 1977; Bosch et al., 1982; Nakanishi, Ozaki and Muramoto, 1982).

Among 73 patients in Japan, 23 (32%) were rehabilitated and 33 (45%) died. The mean duration of the symptom complex from onset to death was 2.9 years (Nakanishi, Ozaki and Muramoto, 1982).

PATHOGENESIS

In this symptom complex, the causal relationship of plasma cell dyscrasia or dysglobulinemia to skin hyperpigmentation, edema and polyneuropathy has not been elucidated (Swash, Perrin and Schwartz, 1979; Asbury and Lisak, 1980; Latov *et al.*, 1981a; Bosch *et al.*, 1982; Doi *et al.*, 1982). The recent immunochemical and immunohistochemical studies strongly suggest that the monoclonal immunoglobulins with λ type, which were most frequently found among the patients with this symptom complex, may be antibodies which specifically react with human peripheral nerve myelin and/or axon and subsequently may initiate the segmental demyelination and/or axonal degeneration (Besinger *et al.*, 1981; Latov *et al.*, 1981a, b; Abrams *et al.*, 1982).

Although the occurrence of the symptom complex seems to be more frequent in Japan than in any other country, similar or almost identical cases have been recorded in the literature from various countries (Crow, 1956; Morley and Schweiger, 1967; Waldenström *et al.*, 1978; Trillet *et al.*, 1980; Ohnishi and Dyck, 1981).

The biochemical and immunological nature of monoclonal immunoglobulins produced in plasma cell dyscrasia may be variable among different races and various genetic backgrounds. Therefore, a certain monoclonal immunoglobulin, which is unique to the Japanese, may be related to the development of this symptom complex.

Acknowledgements

We thank Professors Y. Kuroiwa and J. Tateishi for continuous encouragement and M. Ohara for reading the manuscript.

References

Abrams, G. M., Latov, N., Hays, A. P., Sherman, W. and Zimmerman, E. A. (1982) Immunocytochemical studies of human peripheral nerve with serum from patients with polyneuropathy and paraproteinemia. *Neurology (New York)*, **32**, 821–826

Asbury, A. K. and Lisak, R. P. (1980) Demyelinating neuropathy and myelin antibodies. *New England Journal of Medicine*, **303**, 638–639

Besinger, U. A., Toyka, K. V., Anzil, A. P. *et al.* (1981) Myeloma neuropathy: passive transfer from man to mouse. *Science*, **213**, 1027–1030

Bosch, E. P., Ansbacher, L. E., Goeken, J. A. and Cancilla, P. A. (1982) Peripheral neuropathy associated with monoclonal gammopathy. Studies of intraneural injections of monoclonal immunoglobulin sera. *Journal of Neuropathology and Experimental Neurology*, **41**, 446–459

Crow, R. S. (1956) Peripheral neuritis in myelomatosis. *British Medical Journal*, **2**, 802–804

Doi, H., Itoyama, Y., Yoshinaga, T., Sato, Y. and Ohnishi, A. (1982) Endoneurial deposition of immunoglobulins in cases of plasma cell dyscrasia associated with polyneuropathy, edema and pigmentation. *Clinical Neurology (Tokyo)*, **22**, 237–243

Driedger, H. and Pruzanski, W. (1980) Plasma cell neoplasia with peripheral neuropathy. A study of five cases and review of the literature. *Medicine (Baltimore)*, **59**, 301–310

Dyck, P. J. (1975) Pathologic alterations of the peripheral nervous system of man. In *Peripheral Neuropathy*, edited by P. J. Dyck, P. K. Thomas and E. H. Lambert, pp. 296–336. Philadelphia: W. B. Saunders

Fukase, M., Tsunematsu, T., Nishitani, H., Imura, H., Matsuoka, T. and Fukumashi, H. (1969) Report of a case of solitary plasmacytoma in the abdomen presenting polyneuropathy and endocrinological disorders (abstract). *Clinical Neurology (Tokyo)*, **9**, 657

Hirano, A. and Dembitzer, H. M. (1967) A structural analysis of the myelin sheath in the central nervous system. *Journal of Cell Biology*, **34**, 555–567

Iwashita, H. (1974) Polyneuropathy associated with dermatoendocrinological changes and dysglobulinemia. *Advances in Neurological Sciences (Tokyo)*, **20**, 709–726

Iwashita, H., Ohnishi, A., Asada, M., Kanazawa, Y. and Kuroiwa, Y. (1977) Polyneuropathy, skin hyperpigmentation, edema, and hypertrichosis in localized osteosclerotic myeloma. *Neurology (Minneapolis)*, **27**, 675–681

Julien, J., Vital, C., Vallat, J.-M., Lagueny, A., Deminiere, C. and Darriet, D. (1978) Polyneuropathy in Waldenström's macroglobulinemia. *Archives of Neurology (Chicago)*, **35**, 423–425

Kelly, J. J. Jr, Kyle, R. A., Miles, J. M., O'Brien, P. C. and Dyck, P. J. (1981a) The spectrum of peripheral neuropathy in myeloma. *Neurology (New York)*, **31**, 24–31

Kelly, J. J. Jr, Kyle, R. A., O'Brien, P. C. and Dyck, P. J. (1981b) Prevalence of monoclonal protein in peripheral neuropathy. *Neurology (New York)*, **31**, 1480–1483

Latov, N., Braun, P. E., Gross, R. B., Sherman, W. H., Penn, A. S. and Chess, L. (1981a) Plasma cell dyscrasia and peripheral neuropathy: identification of the myelin antigens that react with human paraproteins. *Proceedings of National Academy of Sciences USA*, **78**, 7139–7142

Latov, N., Gross, R. B., Kastelman, J. *et al.* (1981b) Complement-fixing antiperipheral nerve myelin antibodies in patients with inflammatory polyneuritis and with polyneuropathy and paraproteinemia. *Neurology (New York)*, **31**, 1530–1534

Morley, J. B. and Schweiger, A. C. (1967) The relation between chronic polyneuropathy and osteosclerotic myeloma. *Journal of Neurology, Neurosurgery and Psychiatry*, **30**, 432–442

Nakanishi, T., Ozaki, Y. and Muramoto, O. (1982) Chronic polyneuropathy with skin hyperpigmentation, hypertrichosis, edema and abnormal immunoglobulins. Summary of 83 reported cases. *The Proceedings of the Annual Meeting of Peripheral Neuropathy Research Group*, 121–148

Nishitani, H., Konishi, T., Noguchi, S., Suzuki, M. and Kijima, S. (1976) Clinicopathological study upon 8 cases of myelomatous polyneuropathy associated with skin pigmentation. *Advances in Neurological Sciences (Tokyo)*, **20**, 727–733

Ohnishi, A. and Dyck, P. J. (1981) Two cases of solitary myeloma with polyneuropathy, skin hyperpigmentation, hypertrichosis and edema in USA. *Neurological Medicine (Tokyo)*, **14**, 582–584

Ohnishi, A. and Hirano, A. (1981) Uncompacted myelin lamellae in dysglobulinemic neuropathy. *Journal of the Neurological Sciences*, **51**, 131–140

Ohnishi, A., Ikeda, M. and Tateishi, J. (1979) Morphometry of myelinated fibers of sural nerve, L5 spinal roots and fasciculus gracilis and of cytons of L5 spinal ganglion of man. *Neurological Medicine (Tokyo)*, **11**, 160–168

Ohnishi, A., Yamashita, Y., Goto, I., Kuroiwa, Y., Murakami, S. and Ikeda, M. (1979) De- and remyelination and onion bulb in cerebrotendinous xanthomatosis. *Acta Neuropathologica (Berlin)*, **45**, 43–45

Propp, R. P., Means, E., Deibel, R., Sherer, G. and Barron, K. (1975) Waldenström's macroglobulinemia and neuropathy – deposition of M-components on myelin sheaths. *Neurology (Minneapolis)*, **25**, 980–988

Raine, C. S. and Bornstein, M. B. (1979) Experimental allergic neuritis – ultrastructure of serum-induced myelin aberrations in peripheral nervous system cultures. *Laboratory Investigation*, **40**, 423–432

Sato, Y., Ohnishi, A., Tateishi, J., Iwashita, H. and Shii, H. (1980) The pathology of the peripheral nervous system in two autopsy cases of osteosclerotic myeloma associated with polyneuropathy, skin hyperpigmentation, hypertrichosis and edema. *Clinical Neurology (Tokyo)*, **20**, 742–749

Scheinker, I. (1939) Myelom und Nervensystem – über eine bisher nicht beschriebene, mit eigentümlichen Hautveränderungen einhergehende Polyneuritis bei einem plasmazellulären Myelom des Sternums. *Deutsche Zeitschrift für Nervenheilkunde*, **147**, 247–273

Shibasaki, H., Ohnishi, A. and Kuroiwa, Y. (1982) The use of somatosensory evoked potentials to localize degeneration in a rare polyneuropathy. Studies on polyneuropathy associated with pigmentation, hypertrichosis, edema and plasma cell dyscrasia. *Annals of Neurology*, **12**, 355–360

Silverstein, A. and Doniger, D. E. (1963) Neurologic complications of myelomatosis. *Archives of Neurology (Chicago)*, **9**, 534–544

Sluga, E. (1974) *Polyneuropathien – Typen und Differenzierung, Ergebnisse bioptischer Untersuchungen*. Berlin: Springer-Verlag

Sternberger, L. A., Hardy, P. H. Jr, Cuculis, J. J. and Meyer, H. G. (1970) The unlabeled antibody-enzyme method of immunocytochemistry. Preparation and properties of soluble antigen-antibody complex (horseradish peroxidase-antihorseradish peroxidase) and its use in identification of spirochetes. *Journal of Histochemistry and Cytochemistry*, **18**, 315–333

Swash, M., Perrin, J. and Schwartz, M. S. (1979) Significance of immunoglobulin deposition in peripheral nerve in neuropathies associated with paraproteinemia. *Journal of Neurology, Neurosurgery and Psychiatry*, **42**, 179–183

Trillet, M., Fischer, C., Charhon, S., Bady, B., Kopp, N. and Schott, B. (1980) Polyradiculonévrite chronique avec signes cutanés et endocriniens révélatrice d'une dyscrasie plasmocytaire à IgA. *Revue Neurologique (Paris)*, **136**, 247–258

Waldenström, J. G., Adner, A., Gydell, K. and Zettervall, O. (1978) Osteosclerotic 'plasmocytoma' with polyneuropathy, hypertrichosis and diabetes. *Acta Medica Scandinavica*, **203**, 297–303

13
Geographical patterns of neuropathy: Africa

B. O. Osuntokun

INTRODUCTION

In Africa, a continent of approximately 400 million people, there are a number of distinct races. The main ones are the Arabs, found mainly in the northern parts, and the Negroes – the West African type in West and Central Africa and the Bantus in East and South Africa. Socio-economic differences are rampant. Some of the least developed countries in the world are found in the continent. Malnutrition is widespread. The standards and availability of modern health care are variable, being poor in many countries, and hence reliable data on patterns of disease are not available for many areas. Often the information on the spectrum of diseases is based on hospital populations which are unrepresentative of the communities. In Nigeria, for example, a country with a current estimated population of 100 million, 80% of the population, regardless of social status, consult the native doctor first and may not be seen in the hospital at all. As would be expected there is no uniformity in the pattern of diseases for all parts of Africa: this is certainly the case for peripheral nerve disorders (PND).

FREQUENCY OF PERIPHERAL NERVE DISORDERS

There are very few community-based studies of neurological diseases reported from Africa (Osuntokun, 1971; Osuntokun et al., 1982). However, experience in hospital populations suggests that PND are common. In a population study, the prevalence rate of symmetrical polyneuropathy (PN) was 7 per 1000 (Osuntokun et al., 1982). Peripheral nerve disorders constituted 8% of 4519 neurological admissions in Senegal, 4.7% cent among the Bantus in Natal, South Africa and 0.3% of the hospital population at Ibadan, Nigeria. Peripheral neuropathy, especially the Guillain-Barré syndrome (GBS), is said to be common in Ghana and Uganda where the overall frequency of peripheral neuropathy is thought to be less than in Caucasians (Spillane, 1973).

Age and sex distribution

In many African countries life expectancy is still low – about 45 years – and half the population is less than 20 years of age. Yet PND are very rare in children in the first decade. The peak prevalence of PND in published series occurs in the fourth and fifth decades. Peripheral nerve disorders are more commonly seen in males than females. Male predimonance occurs in hospital populations in most parts of Africa, because males, as bread winners, readily seek medical care in hospitals. Hence male predominance has been reported in nearly all neurological diseases (except migraine and polymyositis) documented in hospital populations.

AETIOLOGICAL FACTORS

Leprosy

As a nosological entity, leprosy is the commonest cause of PND in Africa. It is estimated that 12 million people throughout the world suffer from leprosy, a chronic bacillary (*Mycobacterium leprae*) disease, and over 1 million of these are in the African continent. It is little recognized that leprosy is primarily a disease of peripheral nerves, since in *all* cases the peripheral nerves are involved. For example, in a series of 11 000 patients, 4.3% had involvement of the peripheral nerves without any cutaneous manifestations (Dongre, Ganapati and Cholawala, 1976). Primary neuritic leprosy is not uncommon. However, most patients in Africa who suffer from leprosy are treated in special centres (Leprosaria) and are rarely seen by neurologists except when they present as primary neuritic leprosy. Therefore, in most series of PND reported by neurologists, the importance of leprosy as the commonest cause of PND is not likely to be obvious.

Table 13.1 shows the frequencies of aetiological factors reported in one series of 358 patients with PND (Bademosi and Osuntokun, 1981)

Table 13.1 Frequencies of aetiological factors in 358 patients with PND

Aetiology	Frequency (%)
Undetermined	26.5
Guillain-Barré syndrome	15.6
Diabetes mellitus	10.9
Nutritional deficiencies	10.1
Malignancy	6.7
Leprosy	6.2
Pressure and trauma	4.5
Drugs	3.6
Alcohol	3.4
Infections (post-meningitis, herpes zoster, typhoid)	2.5
Vascular	2.5
Endocrine disturbance	1.4
Porphyria	1.1
Amyloidosis	0.8
Miscellaneous (renal and hepatic failure, lead poisoning, hereditary neuropathies, etc.)	4.2

Leprosy is usually associated with diminished sensation in localized hypopigmented skin lesions, palpable enlargement of peripheral nerves in the absence of any history of injury and the presence of acid-fast bacilli in skin smears obtained by the standard slit and scrape technique and stained by the Ziehl-Neelson method.

In tuberculoid leprosy in which the cutaneous infiltrates contain well-organized epithelioid and giant cell granulomas, and the predominant helper/inducer T-cell subset, bacilli or remnants of them are scanty; on the other hand, in lepromatous leprosy the cutaneous infiltrates consist of macrophages heavily parasitized with bacilli, the suppressor/cytotoxic T-cell subset (Van Voorhis *et al.*, 1982) is predominant and bacilli are numerous. The indeterminate and borderline types of leprosy are variations between the 'immune-competent' tuberculoid leprosy and the immune-deficient lepromatous leprosy. Electron microscopy demonstrates bacilli in Schwann cells and nerve terminals. In leprosy, sensorimotor or sensory neuropathy and mononeuritis simplex or multiplex are the usual presentations or manifestations. Motor neuropathy without sensory disturbance is rare. The nerves which are commonly palpably enlarged and felt are the dorsal cutaneous branch of the radial as it runs over the lateral side of the lower end of the radius, the ulnar nerve just behind and proximal to the medial epicondyle of the humerus, the common peroneal nerve behind the head of the fibula and the great auricular nerve over the sternomastoid muscle at the anterior border of the posterior triangle of the neck.

Recent advances in the chemotherapy of leprosy, using once-monthly rifampicin and clofazimine, and daily dapsone with or without ethionamide and protionamide and other drug regimens have considerably improved the cure rate and have been reviewed in detail elsewhere (*Lancet*, 1982; WHO, 1982). A vaccine effective against leprosy is likely to be available in the near future. Immunization with BCG vaccine offers some protection, at least in Ugandans.

Nutritional neuropathies

In nutritional neuropathies there is usually evidence of predisposing factors such as poverty, lack of care and food, diarrhoea, malabsorption, excessive vomiting from pregnancy or disease states, mental illness, anorexia, and compounding factors such as periodic drought, famine, wars (one-third of the 130 wars since the end of World War II in 1945 have been fought in Africa) and ignorance. Precipitating conditions include pregnancy, lactation, febrile illnesses and alcoholism. Clinical evidence of malnutrition usually includes mucocutaneous lesions such as glossitis, cheilosis, angular stomatitis, follicular hyperkeratosis, changes in colour and texture of hair, pigmented and seborrhoeic dermatosis, and pitting oedema; weight loss, anaemia and circulatory disturbances may be present. Sensorimotor neuropathy is the usual presentation; the lower limbs are affected earlier than the upper limbs and the distal parts more severely than the proximal. Sensory manifestations usually precede motor disorders and patients frequently complain of paraesthesiae (numbness, tight bands), dysaesthesiae (pins and needles, burning sensation), loss of or altered sensation (inability of the bare-footed to 'feel' the ground, or the ground feels like cotton wool, or the sensation of some ointment smeared on the soles of the feet). Paraesthesiae or dysaesthesiae alone are difficult to evaluate and are common in many anxious, neurotic and depressed patients in Africa. They may suggest in some patients that sensory nerve function could be disturbed. However, paraesthesiae or dysaesthesiae alone without sensory loss, tendon areflexia, muscle weakness and wasting or demonstrable clinical neurophysiological findings of abnormal nerve function cannot be accepted as evidence of neuropathy.

Autonomic dysfunction or neuropathy is rare in nutritional neuropathy. A chronic state of malnutrition may affect the central as well as the peripheral nervous system and there may be associated lesions of the spinal cord, optic and auditory nerves and the cerebellum. In the experience of most physicians in Africa, central nervous manifestations such as the Wernicke-Korsakoff syndrome are not usually associated with nutritional symmetrical polyneuropathy. Symptoms and signs of heart disease, such as those in beriberi, are rarely associated with nutritional neuropathies in Africa.

Investigations of nutritional peripheral neuropathy (PN) are very difficult for several reasons (WHO, 1980). The disease process (both onset and recovery) is very slow, being measured in terms of weeks or months. The underlying biochemical lesion or metabolic insult usually antedates the onset of clinical symptoms and signs, the abnormal physiological findings and the pathological changes. By the time a patient is seen, the underlying biochemical defect may already have been corrected or masked by previous treatment, either self-administered or given by non-medical personnel. For example, a single dose of thiamine will correct the abnormal transketolase activity of red blood cell haemolysate in thiamine deficiency. Therefore, measurement of vitamin levels or vitamin-dependent variables such as enzymes (transketolase, transaminases, etc.) may be misleading, but whenever such data indicate abnormalities, the nutritional deficiency is further confirmed.

It is now generally agreed that deficiencies of thiamine, pyridoxine, pantothenic acid, biotin, vitamin B_{12} and possibly folate are associated with PND. It is rare for deficiency of a single vitamin (with the exception of vitamin B_{12}) to be the sole cause of PN, since nutritional deficiencies are usually multiple. The commonest demonstrable vitamin deficiencies in nutritional neuropathies in Africans are thiamine and drug-induced (isoniazid) pyridoxine deficiency. Addisonian vitamin B_{12} deficiency is extremely rare in black Africans although it has been reported from Kenya and Zambia; folate deficiency is not rare, but is an uncertain cause of PN since it is very common in pregnancy states without PN. It is doubtful whether isolated deficiency of riboflavin, folate, biotin or protein-energy malnutrition cause PN, although protein-energy malnutrition may cause reversible peripheral nerve dysfunction (Dastur *et al.*, 1982).

In nutritional neuropathies, cerebrospinal fluid examination is usually normal. Clinical neurophysiological studies may provide some clues as to whether the underlying pathological process involves the axon or the myelin sheath. Nerve biopsies contribute to knowledge of the neuropathic process but often yield no aetiological clues.

Tropical neuropathy

Symmetrical peripheral sensorimotor neuropathy is a variable component of the tropical neuropathy syndrome first described in Jamaica, at the end of the nineteenth century, in which bilateral optic atrophy, perceptive deafness, myelopathy, and mucocutaneous evidence of malnutrition are also present. The tropical neuropathy has been described from virtually all African countries south of the Sahara and north of the Zambezi river, and usually in poor communities. Aetiological factors though variable from country to country have malnutrition as a common factor and include chronic cyanide intoxication derived mainly from the cassava diet in Nigeria, Tanzania and Mozambique (in which a large epidemic was reported following a drought in 1981) and multiple vitamin deficiences in Senegal (Osuntokun, 1981). Occasionally cases of pellagra with dementia, dermatitis, and diarrhoea as the main symptoms are seen, especially among maize-eaters. They may show either a spinal spastic ataxia or a symmetrical polyneuropathy; it is uncertain whether polyneuropathy is due solely to a basic deficiency of nicotinic acid in such cases.

Alcoholism

Alcoholism is becoming increasingly common in Africa. Peripheral neuropathy in alcoholism is probably due to a deficiency of thiamine caused by abnormal vitamin metabolism and inadequate vitamin intake in the presence of a high calorie diet (derived from alcohol). Deficiencies of other vitamin B components such as pyridoxine, folate and pantothenic acid may also play a role. There is substantial evidence that alcohol *per se* is directly neurotoxic and that individual susceptibility to the neurotoxicity of alcohol may be genetically determined (Blass and Gibson, 1977).

Guillain Barré syndrome

The Guillain Barré syndrome (GBS) or acute infective polyneuropathy appears to be as common in Africans as in Caucasians. The precipitating factors, clinical manifestations and prognosis are similar to those reported in Caucasians. It is the commonest identifiable form of PND in Uganda (Spillane, 1973) and in Nigeria (Bademosi and Osuntokun, 1981).

Diabetes mellitus

In diabetes mellitus PND are common complications in Africans and were found in 48% of 832 Nigerian diabetics. Peripheral neuropathy was the initial presentation of glucose intolerance in 25 of these patients (Osuntokun *et al.*, 1971). Diabetes mellitus was the second commonest identifiable cause of PN in Nigerians (Bademosi and Osuntokun, 1981). Vascular disease, including microangiopathy, is rare in African diabetics with or without PN.

Drugs

Drugs commonly incriminated as causing PN in Africans are isoniazid, nitrofurantoin, anticancer drugs such as vincristine, and chloramphenicol. Isoniazid is widely used in the treatment of tuberculosis which still has a high prevalence in Africans. Peripheral neuropathy due to isoniazid which induces pyridoxine deficiency is relatively uncommon since most Africans are fast acetylators of the drug (Salako and Aderounmu, 1978). Chloramphenicol (commonly used for the treatment of typhoid fever, a highly prevalent infection in tropical Africa) is known to induce vitamin B_{12} deficiency but is an uncommon cause of PN in Africans. Nitrofurantoin which inhibits thiamine pyrophosphate is popular for the treatment of urinary infections; it causes PN, especially in the elderly, in those with impaired renal function and as a result of prolonged therapy. Phenytoin is widely prescribed for the treatment of epilepsy, the incidence of which in Africans is several times that in Caucasians, but PN as a complication is rare in Africans. Chloroquine is widely used as an antimalarial drug, but neuropathy is rare because prolonged therapy is hardly ever indicated. Drugs containing clioquinol (a halogenated hydroxyquinoline and incriminated as a cause of subacute myelo-opticoneuropathy (SMON) in the Japanese and some other races) are still frequently used by Africans for the treatment of diarrhoeal diseases. However, prolonged therapy is rare and neurotoxicity leading to PN is virtually unknown.

Industrial toxins

With the exception of lead, most of the industrial neurotoxins and environmental factors recognized in the developed countries as causally related to PND are not important in the aetiology of PN in Africans. The industries in Africa that involve the manufacture or use of polymers, plasticizers, pigment, rayon, organic solvents, rubber, or electronics are few, although such industries are bound to grow in number and size. Physicians in Africa should be aware of these occupational hazards. Farmers in African countries increasingly use herbicides, insecticides, rodenticides (which are usually derivatives of organophosphates, hexachlorophene, pyrethrum, thallium, and arsenic). There are no systematic studies and hence no reliable data on the extent of the hazards and neurotoxicity (including polyneuropathy) associated with these substances.

Porphyria

Acute intermittent porphyria described in West and East Africa and symptomatic porphyria cutanea tarda linked with liver disease and alcoholism in the South African Bantus are occasionally causes of PN.

Miscellaneous causes

Other relatively uncommon causes of PN include renal and hepatic failure, collagen disease and amyloidosis. Peripheral neuropathy as a complication of malignant diseases occurs as frequently in Africans as in Caucasians, usually associated with neoplasms of the gastrointestinal tract, breast, or in myelomatosis, lymphomas and leukaemias. Carcinoma of the lung is relatively rare in Africans although it has increased in frequency in the last decade. Burkitt's lymphoma, the commonest malignancy of childhood in many parts of West, East and Central Africa, may present initially as cranial neuropathy with symmetrical sensorimotor or motor PN, with cyto-albuminologic dissociation in the CSF, mimicking the Guillain-Barré syndrome. In such cases malignant pleocytosis is usually present.

Peripheral neuropathy may complicate acute infections such as typhoid fever. Peripheral nerve disorders are rare in parasitic infections but have been described in association with malarial infections; the causal relationship is, however, tenuous and doubtful. Unlike South American trypanosomiasis (Chagas' disease) in which autonomic neuropathy is common, PN is not a feature of African trypanosomiasis. None of the other parasitic diseases (leishmaniasis, filariasis, taeniasis, nematode infestations, schistosomiasis, etc.) highly prevalent in Africa, have been incriminated in the aetiology of peripheral nerve disorders in Africans.

Hereditary neuropathies

Reports of PND in Africans show a low incidence of the hereditary neuropathies, genetically-determined metabolic aberrations and diseases due to enzymic defects in which peripheral neuropathy is either the sole or predominant feature, or a significant concomitant component of their pathological manifestations. There are a few case reports of peroneal muscular atrophy (Charcot-Marie-Tooth disease) from Senegal, Uganda, Rhodesia and Nigeria, and of ataxia telangiectasia from Nigeria. However, peroneal muscular atrophy and variants are common in Tunisian Arabs. Many diseases such as hereditary sensory neuropathies, Roussy-Levy syndrome, Refsum's disease, giant axonal neuropathy, adreno-leucodystrophy, metachromatic leucodystrophy, Fabry's disease, Tangier disease, Bassen-Kornzweig disease, and familial dysautonomia have been virtually unrecognized in all parts of Africa. This may be related to scarcity of trained personnel, tolerance of the disease by Africans who are often 'non-complaining', or inadequate facilities for investigations.

Isolated diseases of cranial nerves

The commonest causes of isolated diseases of cranial nerves are malignancies affecting the paranasal sinuses, Burkitt's lymphoma, haemoglobinopathies (especially HbSS and HbS-C disease), infective and carcinomatous meningitides, neurosarcoidosis, medial sphenoidal ridge meningiomas, pituitary tumours, aneurysms of the internal carotid and posterior communicating arteries, and diabetes mellitus. Transient cranial nerve palsies are often encountered in African patients with migraine and are common in those who have the sickle-cell trait (HbAs), and the painful ophthalmoplegic (Tolosa-Hunt) syndrome.

Isolated optic atrophy, a not uncommon finding in Africans, may be due to bilateral retrobulbar neuritis (probably a *forme fruste* of neuromyelitis optica), choroidoretinitis, onchocerciasis, trauma, methyl alcohol and unidentified toxins in home-made alcoholic brew. However, no identifiable causes are found in 20–50% (Spillane, 1973). Neurosyphilis may account for some. Multiple sclerosis is virtually unknown in black Africans although three autopsy-verified cases and a dozen clinical impressions have been reported from Senegal and Uganda, respectively.

Impaired vision with or without optic atrophy can occur in the absence of ocular causes, with or without painful dysaesthetic peripheral neuropathy and the mucocutaneous lesions of malnutrition. It has been labelled the tropical amblyopia syndrome and may represent a variant or *forme fruste* of the tropical neuropathies.

Sciatica

Sciatica due to ruptured intervertebral disc is rare in black Africans (Spillane, 1973). When seen it is usually found in the upper socio-economic classes and usually at the level of L4–5 instead of L5–S1 as commonly seen in Caucasians (spondylosis is only half as common in Africans as in Caucasians). The rarity of ruptured disc as a cause of sciatica has been attributed to unusually increased mobility of the lumbar spine in the black African compared with the Caucasian, to the conditioning effects of life-long strenuous manual work and physical exertion, and to the habit of peasants sleeping on mats spread on the bare ground. Pelvic malignant disease is a common cause of sciatica in African adult females.

Facial palsies

Idiopathic infranuclear facial (Bell's) palsy is common in Africans and has a good prognosis irrespective of treatment with corticosteroids. Other causes of infranuclear facial palsy in Africans are herpetic infection (Ramsay-Hunt syndrome) trauma, malignancies and occasionally severe hypertension and diabetes mellitus. Leprosy may cause a mononeuritis simplex affecting the facial nerve in which the upper part of the face is more severely affected than the lower part.

Entrapment syndromes

The frequencies and manifestations of the various entrapment syndromes are similar to those described in Caucasians.

Obstetric neurapraxia occurs commonly, following prolonged labour, in short primiparous women with cephalo-pelvic disproportion. It is usually unilateral but occasionally bilateral and as a rule the result of prolonged labour. The prognosis is good except when associated with genito-vesico-rectal fistulas – evidence of severely obstructed labour. Neurological, pelvimetric and clinical neurophysiological assessments as well as intravenous pyelographic investigation indicate that the pathogenesis is essentially a neurapraxia of the lumbosacral plexus, sometimes accompanied by transient hydroureter and transient palsy of the femoral and obturator nerves and ascending reversible ischaemic dysfunction of the lower lumbosacral segments of the spinal cord (Bademosi *et al.*, 1980).

References

Bademosi, O., Osuntokun, B. O., van der Werd, H. L. and Ojo, O. A. (1980) Obstetric neuropraxia: a study of 34 patients at Ibadan. *International Journal of Gynaecology and Obstetrics*, **17**, 611–614

Bademosi, O. and Osuntokun, B. O. (1981) Diseases of peripheral nerves as seen in the Nigerian Africans. *African Journal of Medical Sciences and Clinical Medicine*, **10**, 33–38

Blass, J. P. and Gibson, J. E. (1971) Deleterious aberrations of a thiamine-requiring enzyme in four patients with Wernicke-Korsakoff's syndrome. *New England Journal of Medicine*, **297**, 1367–1370

Dastur, D. K., Manghani, D. K., Osuntokun, B. O., Sourander, P. and Kondo, K. (1982) Neuromuscular changes in malnutrition: a review. *Journal of the Neurological Sciences*, **55**, 207–230

Dongre, V. Y., Ganapati, R. and Cholawala, R. G. (1976) A study of mononeuritic lesions in a leprosy clinic. *Leprosy in India*, **18**, 132–137

Lancet (1982) Chemotherapy of leprosy. **2**, 77

Osuntokun, B. O. (1971) Epidemiology of tropical nutritional neuropathy. *Transactions of the Royal Society of Tropical Medicine and Hygiene*, **65**, 454–479

Osuntokun, B. O. (1981) Cassava diet, chronic cyanide intoxication and neuropathy in the Nigerian Africans. *World Review of Nutrition and Dietetics*, **36**, 141–173

Osuntokun, B. O., Akinkugbe, F. M., Francis, T. I., Reddy, S., Osuntokun, O. and Taylor, G. O. L. (1971) Diabetes mellitus in Nigerians: a study of 832 patients. *West African Medical Journal*, **20**, 295–312

Osuntokun, B. O., Schoenberg, B. S., Nottidge, V. A. *et al.* (1982) Research protocol for measuring the prevalence of neurologic disorders in developing countries: results of a pilot study in Nigeria. *Neuroepidemiology*, **1**, 143–153

Salako, L. A. and Aderounmu, A. F. (1978) Determination of the isoniazid acetylator phenotype in a West African population. *Tubercle*, **58**, 109–112

Spillane, J. D. (Ed.) (1973) *Tropical Neurology*. London: Oxford University Press

Van Voorhis, W. C., Kaplan, A., Sarno, E. N. *et al.* (1982) The cutaneous infiltrates of leprosy: cellular characteristics and the predominant T-cell phenotypes. *New England Journal of Medicine*, **307**, 1593–1597

WHO (1980) Peripheral neuropathies. *WHO Technical Report Series*, No. 654. Geneva: WHO

WHO (1982) Chemotherapy of leprosy for control programmes, *WHO Technical Report Series*, No. 673. Geneva: WHO

Index